AF393364

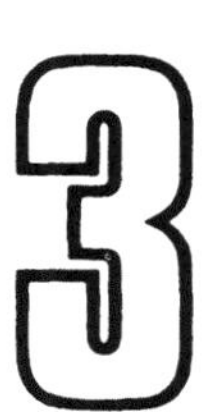

3 AIR INSTRUMENT SURGERY

FACIAL, ORAL AND RECONSTRUCTIVE SURGERY

Compiled and edited by Robert M. Hall
Santa Barbara, California

With contributors and 242 illustrations by
Ted Bloodhart, Medical Illustrator

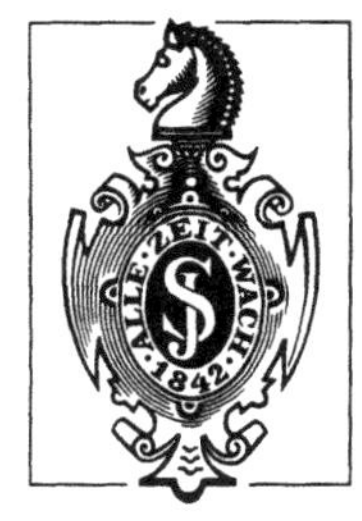

Springer-Verlag Berlin · Heidelberg · New York 1973

Additional information concerning these instruments and techniques is available from Hall International Inc., P.O.Box 4307, Santa Barbara, California 93103/USA, Telephone (805) 969-4777, Cable: HINTL.
Outside of the United States contact 3M Company in your country.

ISBN-13:978-3-642-65565-4   e-ISBN-13:978-3-642-65563-0
DOI: 10.1007/978-3-642-65563-0

Library of Congress Catalog Card Number 70-132149.

This Atlas is dedicated to JUDITH BÄHR, née Green, R. N., and
TED BLOODHART, medical illustrator.

During the last three years, they have devoted their outstanding talents
to the preparation of Air Instrument Surgery, Volumes I, II and III. Their
loyalty, hard work and friendship are deeply appreciated.

Foreword

The use of the compressed air-driven turbine for the activation of surgical burs and saws as developed by Dr. Robert M. Hall has been a boon for the plastic, maxillofacial, and oral surgeon. The development of air instrument surgery coincided with the opening of new vistas in surgery in the area of craniofacial surgery. Craniofacial osteotomies for orbital (ocular) hypertelorism, for the deformities of craniostenosis (Cronzon's disease, Apert's syndrome) and subcranial osteotomies at various levels of the facial skeleton have brought about dramatic improvements in the form of the facial substructure in patients with gross deformities. In many of these maxillofacial deformities the facial skeleton and dento-alveolar processes must be advanced, recessed or expanded in the lateral dimension. In such cases malocclusion of the teeth is usual; this is corrected by intermaxillary fixation of the mobilized bony structures which also reestablishes adequate relationships between the dento-alveolar processes of the upper and lower jaws.

This brings us to the subject of surgical orthodontics, a field that is just beginning to expand; its development should bring about closer collaboration between surgeon and orthodontist, resulting in rapid and efficient improvement of malocclusion.

The absence of vibration characteristic of the air-driven turbine, in contrast to the mechanically driven drill, allows the surgeon to carry out delicate and precise surgical procedures with less fatigue to himself.

The techniques made possible by air instrumentation are not restricted to bone surgery: the plastic surgeon is able to carve costal cartilage for the fabrication of a framework for a missing ear, or to activate the dermatome for cutting skin grafts. Again, the absence of vibration makes the air-driven instrument a more efficient tool in dermabrading areas such as the eyelids, nose and lips.

Dr. Hall has collected and illustrated in this volume the applications of air instrument surgery in a variety of surgical corrective procedures for deformity of the bony framework of the face and jaws.

John Marquis Converse, M. D.
Lawrence D. Bell Professor of Plastic Surgery and Director of the Institute of Reconstructive Plastic Surgery, New York University Medical Center.

Preface

We are living in an age of change. This change is evident in every aspect of modern living. It is almost beyond the realm of human comprehension to realize that ninety-five percent of all the scientists who ever lived are alive today. Their fertile minds are truly unlocking the secrets of the universe. It has been stated that we can expect more scientific and technological developments in the next twenty-five years than have occurred in the previous two thousand five hundred years.

Changes are particularly evident in the health sciences. It is estimated that medical and dental knowledge doubles every five years. It is evident that the modern dentist and physician must work diligently to keep abreast of the new developments in health sciences.

Without doubt, one of the greatest advances in oral and maxillofacial surgery has been the development of air instrumentation. The man who has contributed most to this field is Dr. Robert M. Hall. I vividly recall a visit in Pittsburgh several years ago where I saw Dr. Hall removing a torus palatinus with a bur activated by a conventional dental air rotor. This was undoubtedly one of the first oral surgical procedures utilizing air rotors. I was so impressed with the ease of the operation that I suggested to Dr. Hall that he produce a motion picture demonstrating the technique so others could benefit from his experience and become proficient in the use of air instruments. Fortunately Dr. Hall had the vision, motivation and ability to do this, and he was primarily responsible for the introduction of this instrument into oral surgery practice. His interest thus aroused, he did extensive research and development of various air-driven instruments which resulted in the development of the current range of Hall Air Instruments.

It is difficult to measure the contributions Dr. Hall has made to surgery. By utilization of his instruments many time-consuming laborious procedures have been simplified, and procedures that were once considered impractical or impossible are now performed with relative ease.

Since many of the procedures in oral and maxillofacial surgery involve the osseous structures, air instruments have received wide acceptance in these fields. This volume documents many of the practical uses of the instruments and provides guidelines for their efficient utilization.

Everyone who practices oral and maxillofacial surgery is deeply indebted to Dr. Hall. His innovative mind, his technical skill and his ability to transpose his ideas into efficient instruments and practical procedures represent a dramatic breakthrough in our search for perfection.

The introduction and utilization of the air instruments developed by Dr. Hall must be considered a major development in this important and rapidly expanding field of surgery.

Robert B. Shira, D.D.S.
Dean, Tufts University
School of Dental Medicine
Boston, Massachusetts

Contents

Contents

SECTION III. TEMPORAL BONE SURGERY

SECTION IV. HAND RECONSTRUCTIVE SURGERY

SECTION V. SOFT TISSUE SURGERY

SECTION VI. EQUIPMENT GUIDE

SECTION VII. POWER SYSTEMS

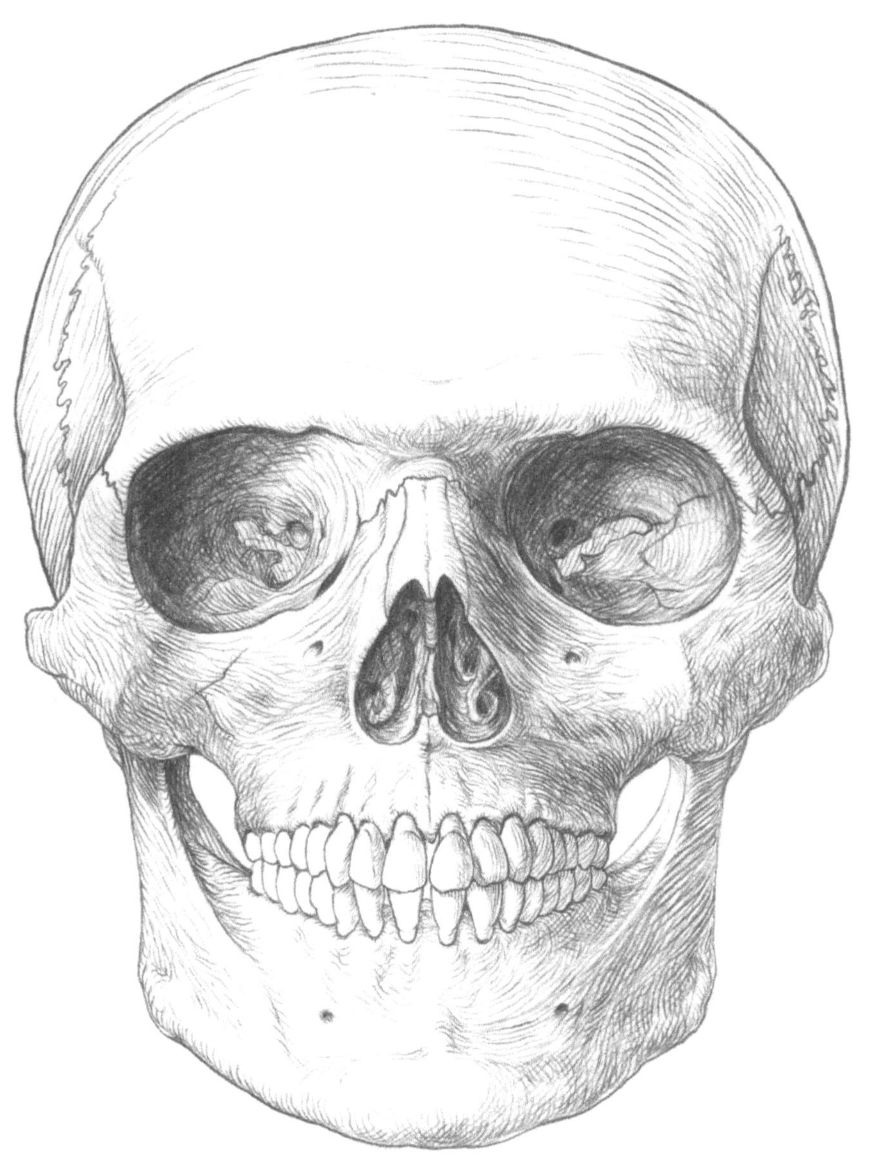

Contents

Fixation of a Fractured Zygoma and Orbital Floor

Assemble the air drill, 90° angle, and 26 wire-pass bur*.

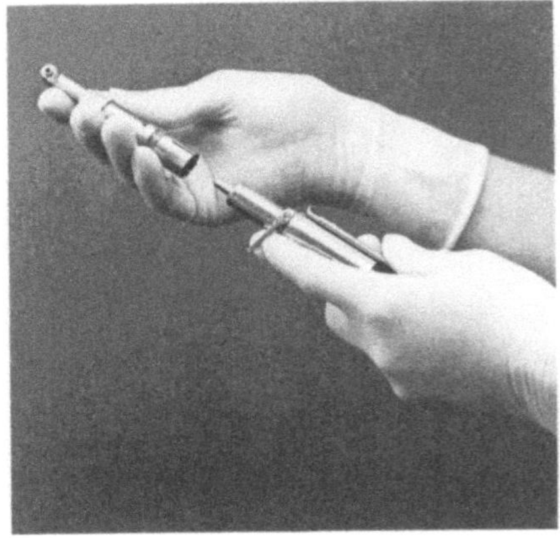

1. Push bur release lever forward 90° to assemble attachment. Completely seat.

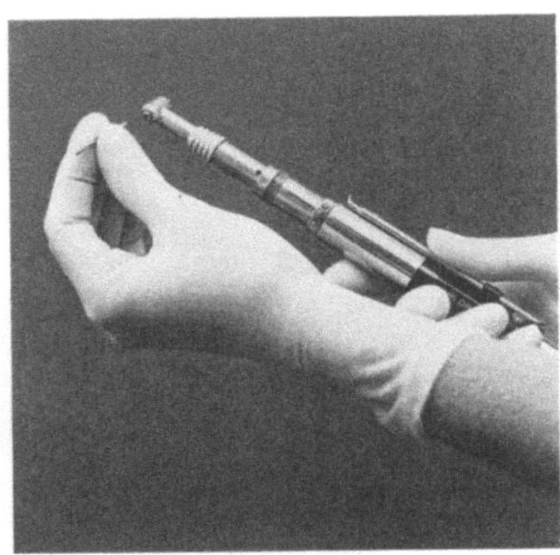

3. Place wire pass bur into collet.

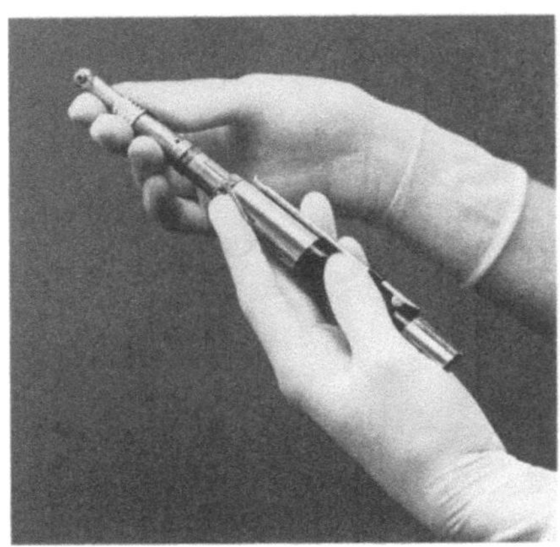

2. Return lever flush against drill to lock attachment.

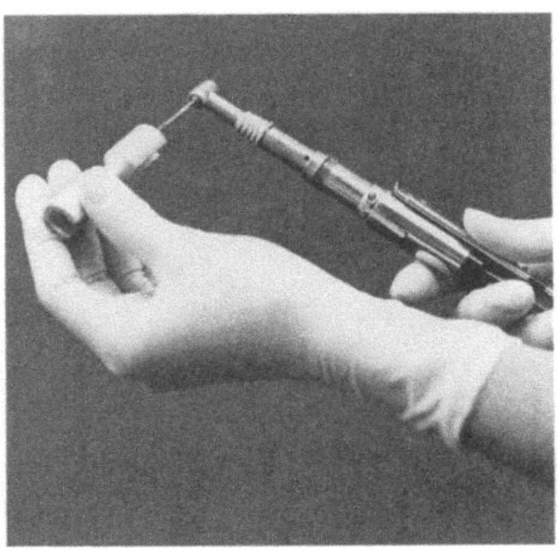

4. Slide hollow side of bur changer over bur. Press the bur firmly into place.

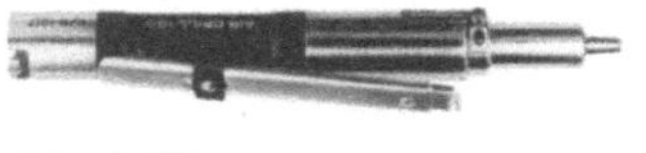

Air drill

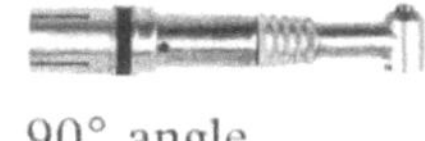

90° angle

26 short wire pass bur

Symposium: Malunited Fractures of the Zygoma; Repair of Deformity. R. O. Dingman, AB, DDS, MS, MD. **Tr Am Acad Ophth,** 57: 889-896, 1953.

* Throughout this book, the word "bur" is used to denote the small cutting tool, while "burr" refers to the act of cutting or sculpting bone.

5. A deformity due to malunion fracture with dislocation of the left zygomatic bone and orbital floor. Line of incisions is indicated.

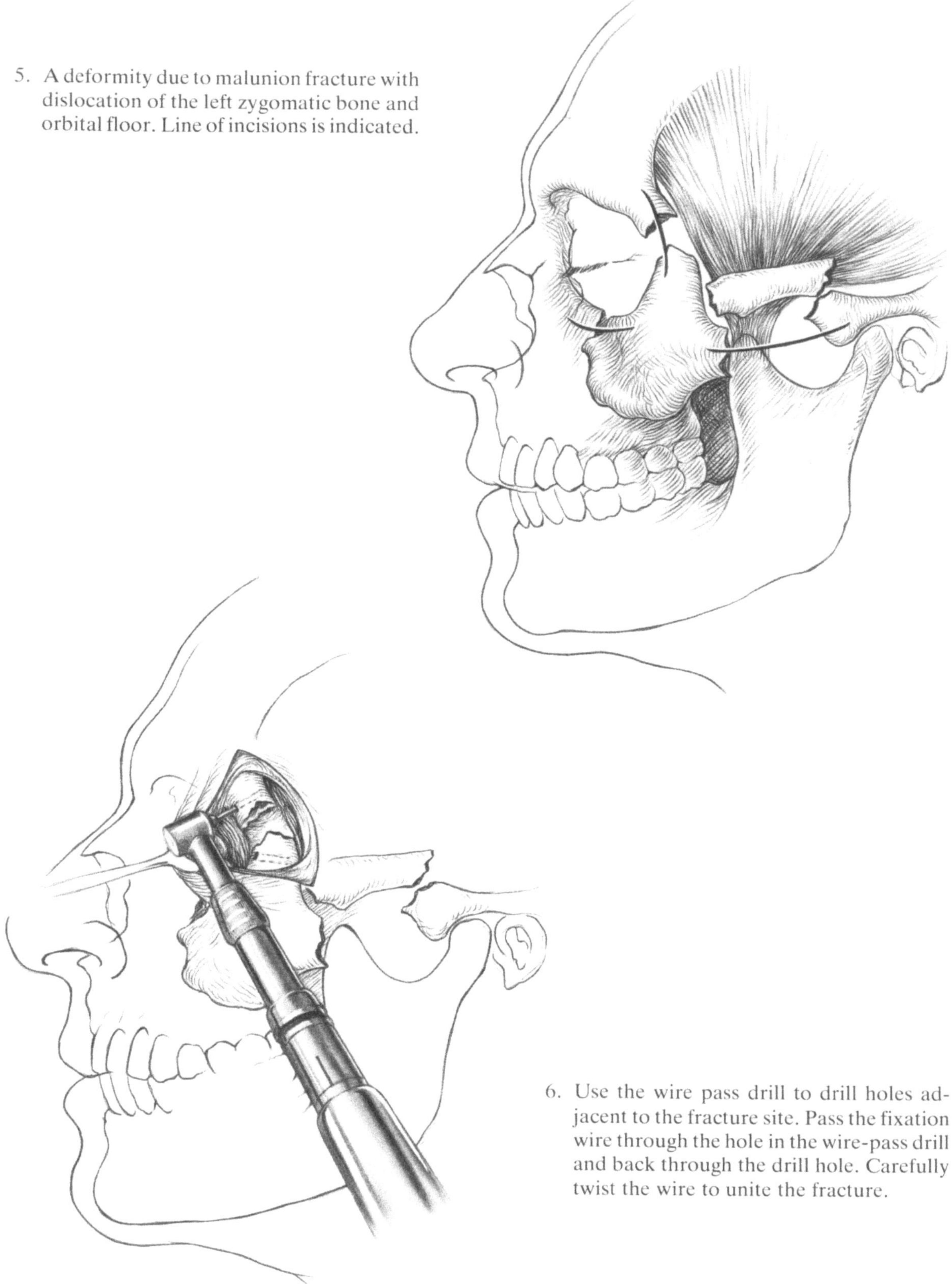

6. Use the wire pass drill to drill holes adjacent to the fracture site. Pass the fixation wire through the hole in the wire-pass drill and back through the drill hole. Carefully twist the wire to unite the fracture.

Fixation of a Fractured Zygoma and Orbital Floor *(continued)*

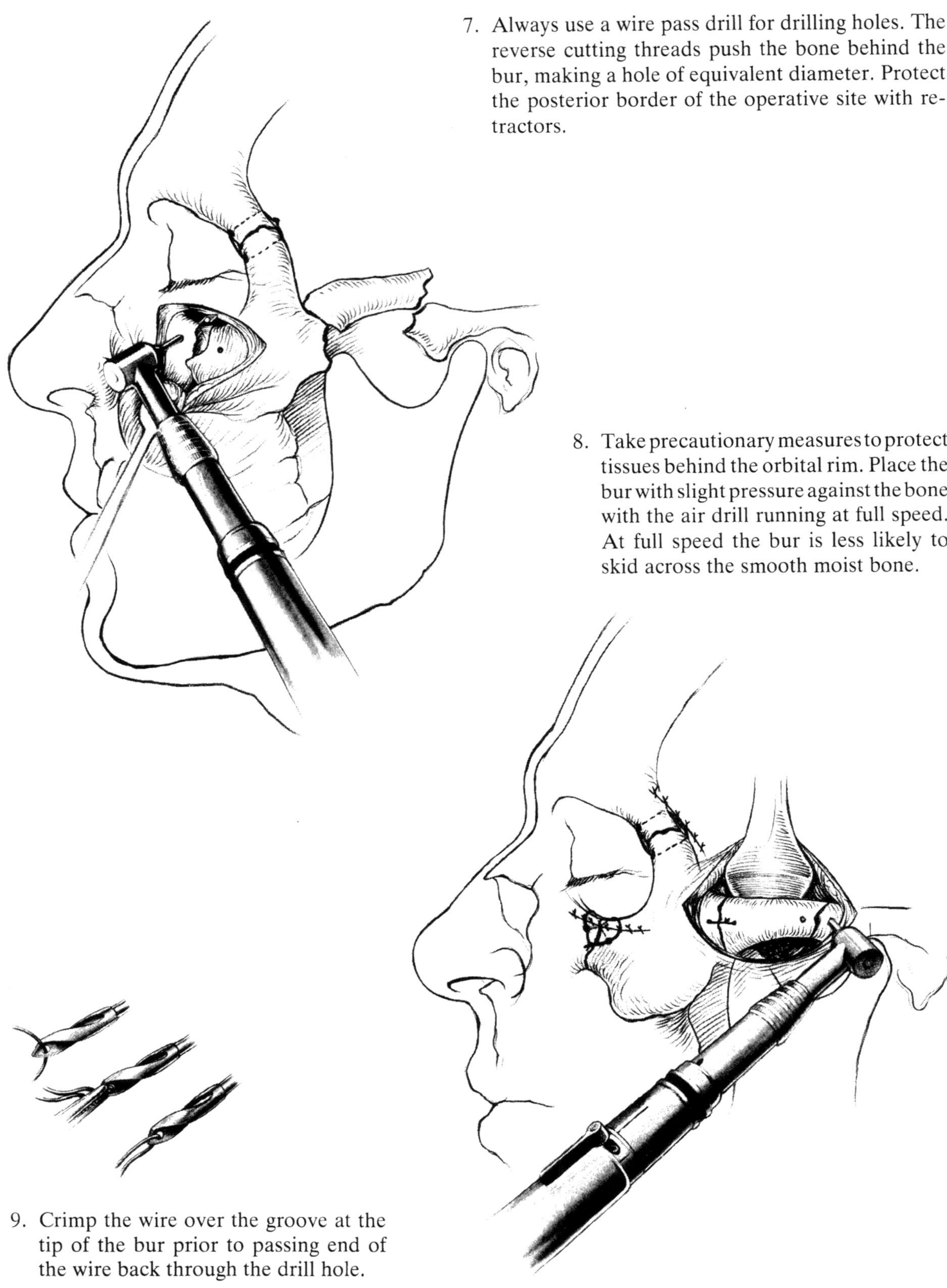

7. Always use a wire pass drill for drilling holes. The reverse cutting threads push the bone behind the bur, making a hole of equivalent diameter. Protect the posterior border of the operative site with retractors.

8. Take precautionary measures to protect tissues behind the orbital rim. Place the bur with slight pressure against the bone with the air drill running at full speed. At full speed the bur is less likely to skid across the smooth moist bone.

9. Crimp the wire over the groove at the tip of the bur prior to passing end of the wire back through the drill hole.

Caldwell-Luc

1. Cut a maxillary window into the antrum with the air drill and 07 steel bur. Do not apply pressure to the bur; this will cause the bur to slow down, producing increased friction and heat.
   The combination of a delicate touch and the high speed cuts the bone with ease.

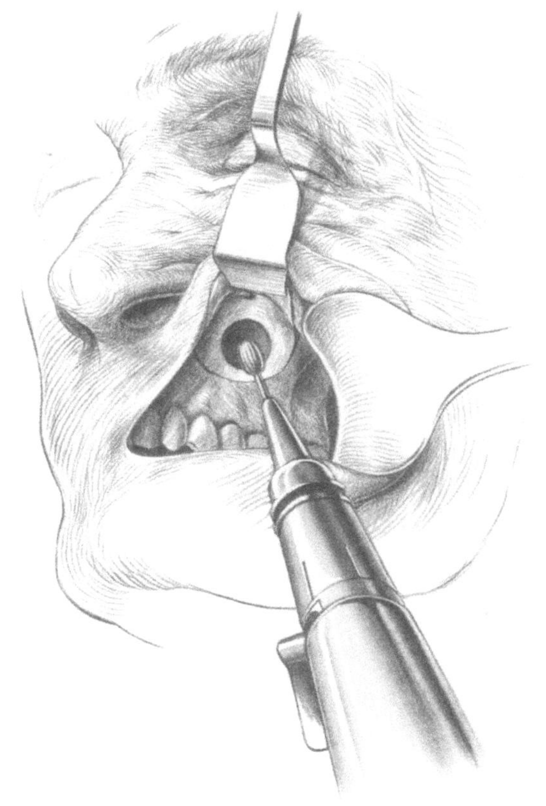

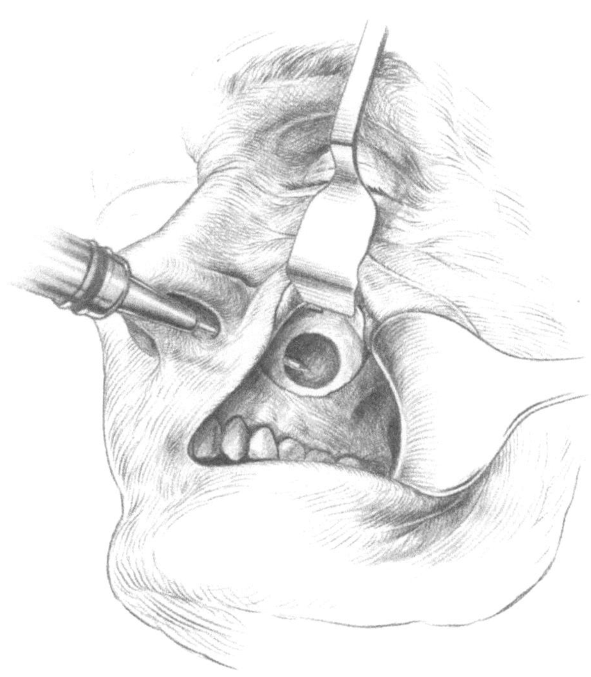

2. Make an intranasal antrostomy by moving the 28 wire pass bur downward beneath the inferior turbinate and through the surgical defect in the naso-antral wall. The passage may now be enlarged with a rasp.

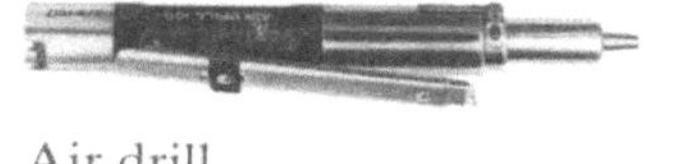

Air drill

Medium bur guard

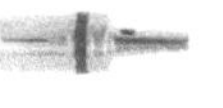

07 steel bur

28 wire-pass bur

Alloplastic Restoration of a Fractured Orbital Floor*

1. Through a Caldwell-Luc approach, support the fractured orbital floor with packing.

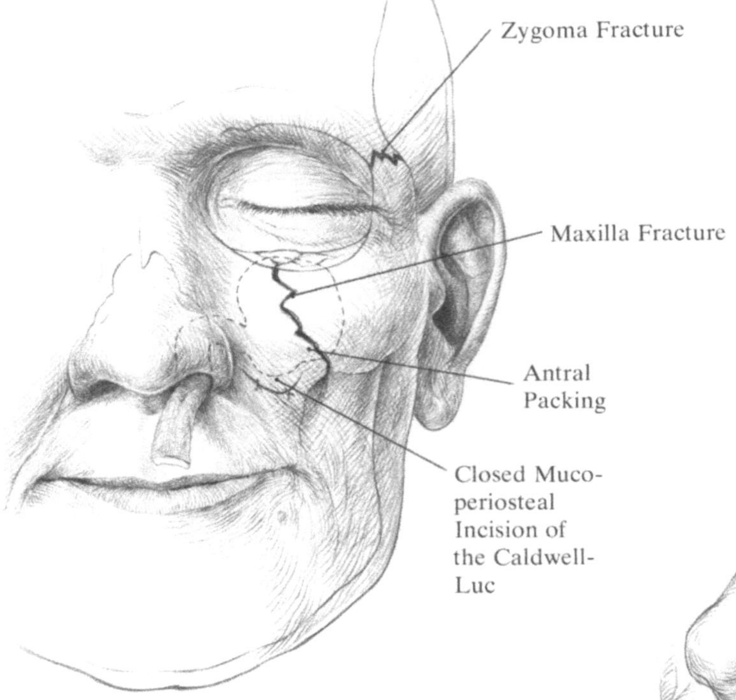
Zygoma Fracture
Maxilla Fracture
Antral
Packing
Closed Muco-
periosteal
Incision of
the Caldwell-
Luc

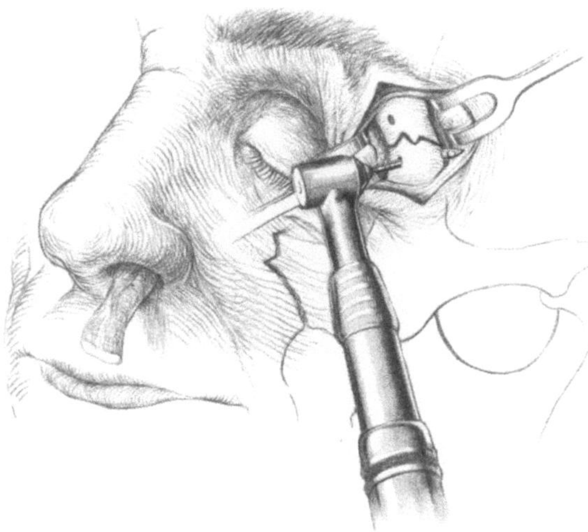

2. Drill two holes and pass the wire across the fractured zygoma.

Air drill

Long bur guard

90° angle

20 long diamond bur

28 short wire-pass bur

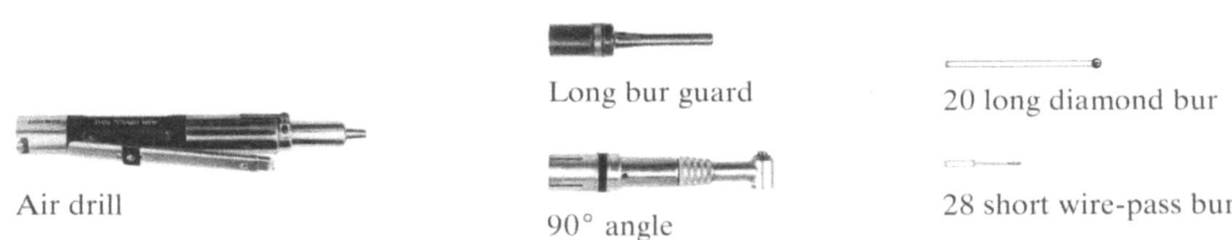

* Cdr. F. E. Jackson, MC, U.S.N.; Cdr. H. J. Sazima, D.C., U.S.N.; LCdr. M. L. Grafft, D.C., U.S.N.R.; and LCdr. James B. Back, M.C. U.S.N.R.: Management of Combined Intracranial Injuries and Extensive Orbital-Facial Fractures. **Military Med,** 134:7, July 1969.

3. With the 90° angle and wire-pass bur make holes for wiring maxilla and anchoring alloplastic material to the orbital floor.

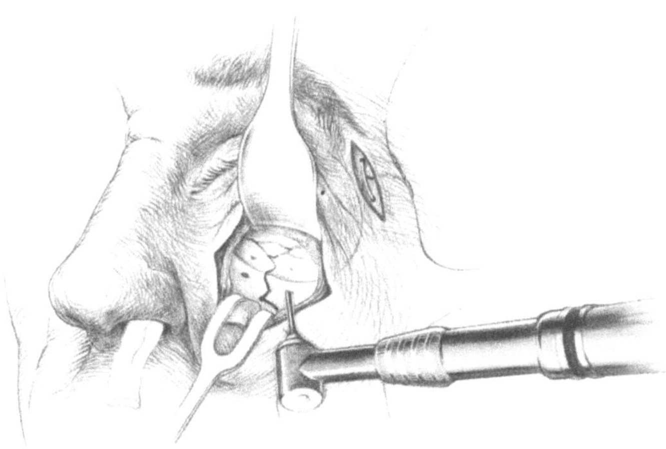

4. Always crimp the wire around the tip of the bur before drawing one end of the wire back through the drill hole.

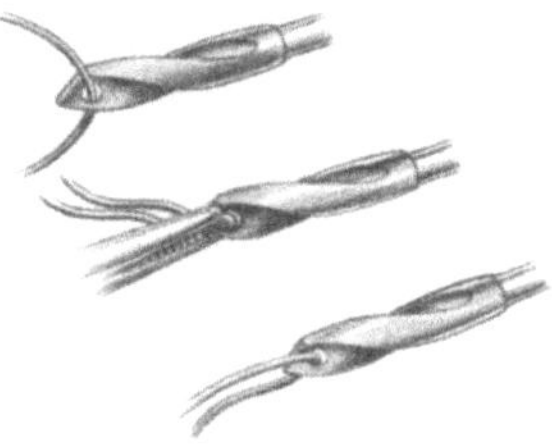

5. Grasp the implant with the protected tips of the forceps. Drill holes in the implant. Not too many as they will weaken the implant. When necessary the implant can be sculpted with a diamond bur to modify the shape. Secure the implant to the orbital floor with the fine 28 wire pass bur and fixation wire.

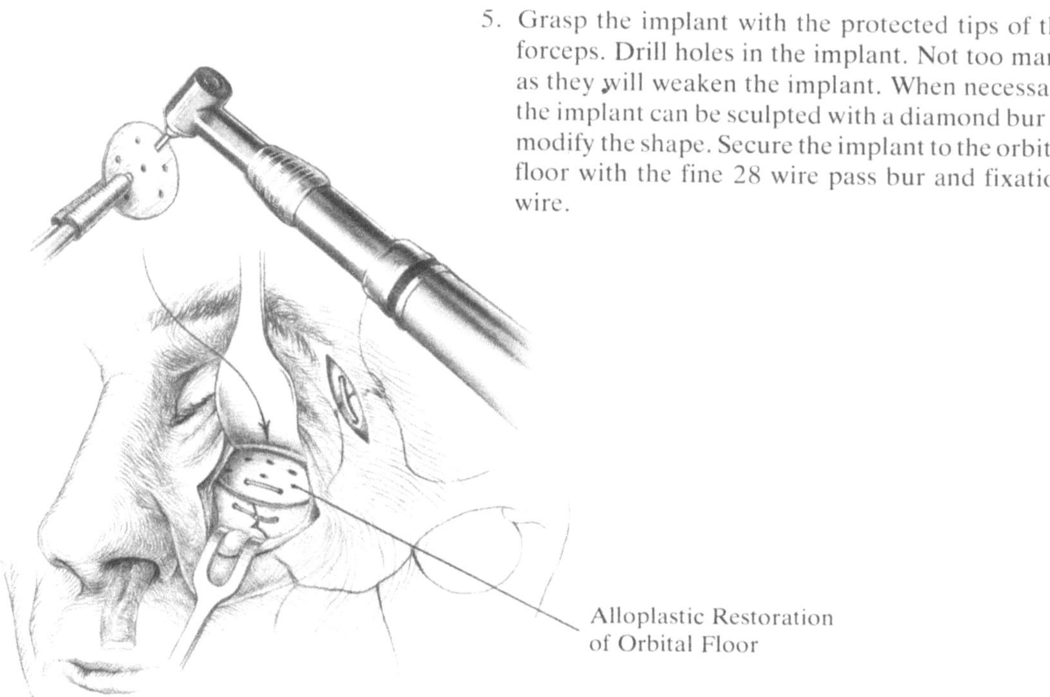

Alloplastic Restoration
of Orbital Floor

Segmental Mandibular Resection*

As an alternative to the air drill, specifically in the heavier bone resection and reconstruction procedures, the air driver with saw attachment can be used. Maneuverability may be limited compared with the lighter, smaller air drill. However, the angle variability of the blades and the high torque of the air driver often gives this instrumentation precedence.

Assemble the oscillating saw and blade:

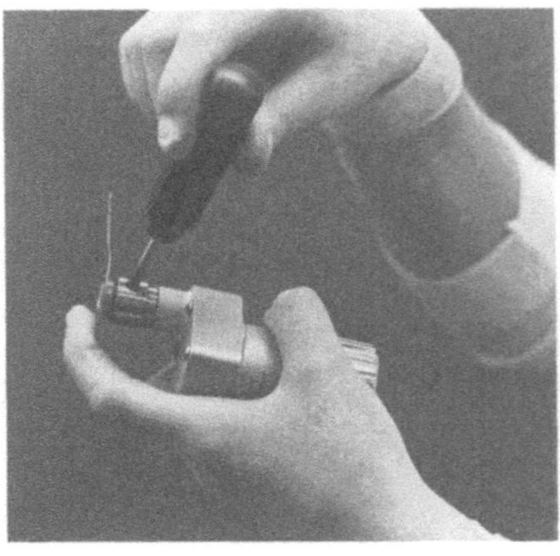

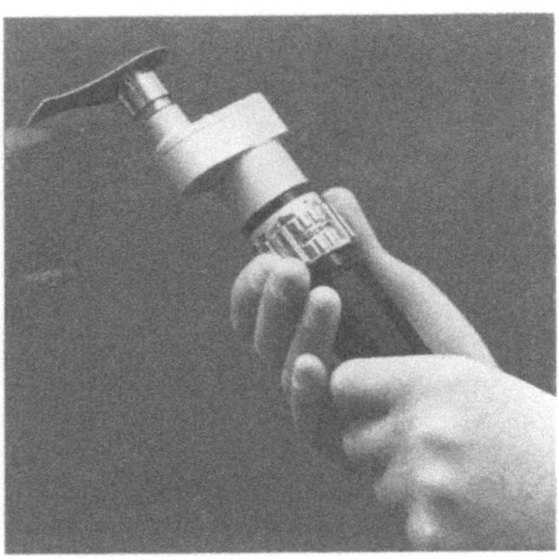

1. Set the blade at the correct angle and tighten securely with the hex wrench.

2. Seat attachment over air driver and lock. Run the motor at full speed.

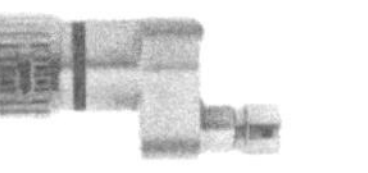

Oscillating saw attachment

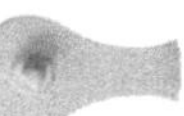

Wide deep oscillating blade

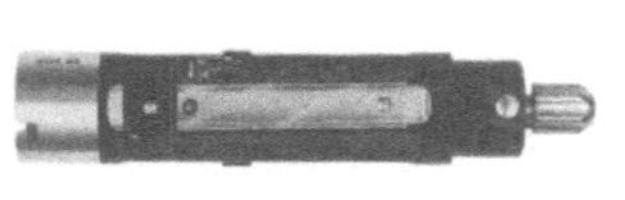

Air driver

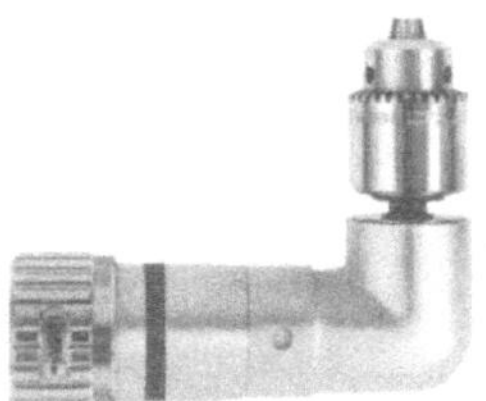

Wire and pin driver

Fixation pin

---

* Robin M. Rankow, DDS, MD. **An Atlas of Surgery of the Face, Mouth and Neck. W. B. Saunders Co.,** Philadelphia, Pa., USA, 1968.

3. Make a midline lip-splitting incision;
   then, with the air driver, oscillating saw
   and blade section the exposed mandible. Move the blade gently in motion
   with the oscillating action to keep the
   blade from stalling between the two
   raw bone surfaces. Irrigate intermittently with isotonic saline.

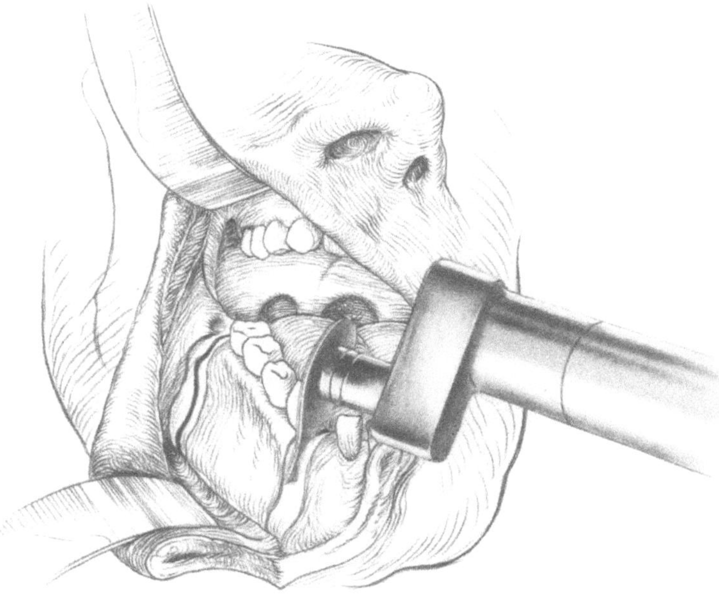

4. Change to the wire and pin driver attachment and with a Kirschner wire
   penetrate deep into the posterior mandibular fragment. Set the speed selector
   ring at half speed (.5) and control the
   speed at the throttle. Drill a hole in the
   anterior fragment.

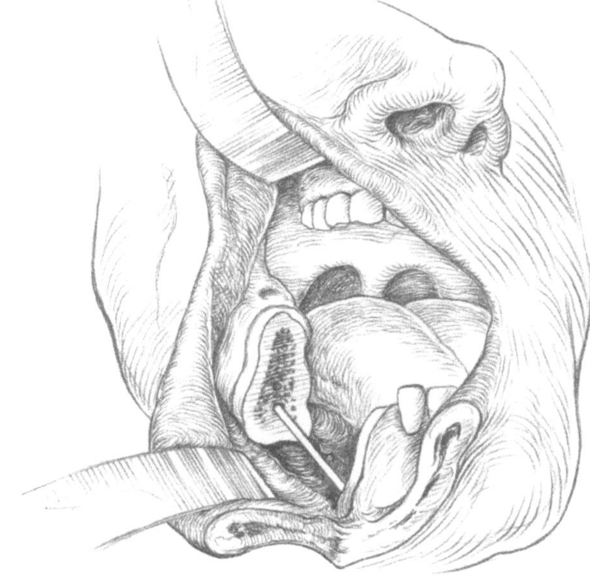

5. Bend the protruding wire to the contour of
   the mandible and insert it into the drill hole
   in the anterior segment. The exposed portion
   of the wire maintains mandibular contour
   and retains the space created by removal of
   the surgical specimen.

Retromaxillism*

Assemble the air drill and 12 long steel bur:

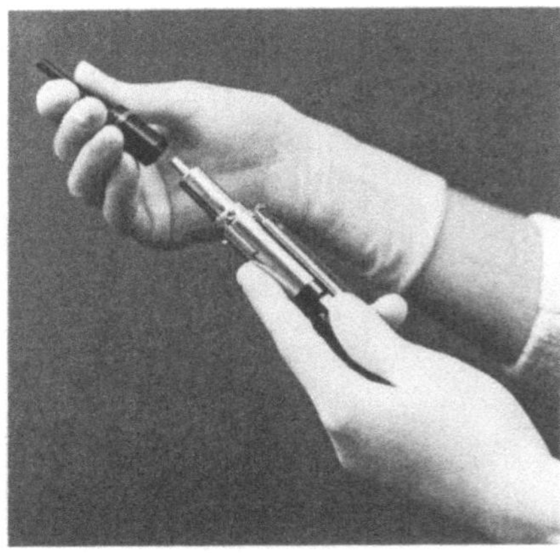

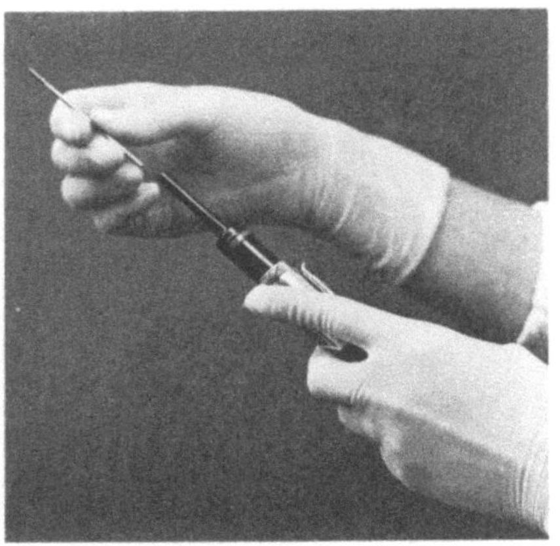

1. Place the long bur guard securely over the drill shoulder.

2. Push bur release lever forward 90° to insert bur. Return lever flush against the drill.

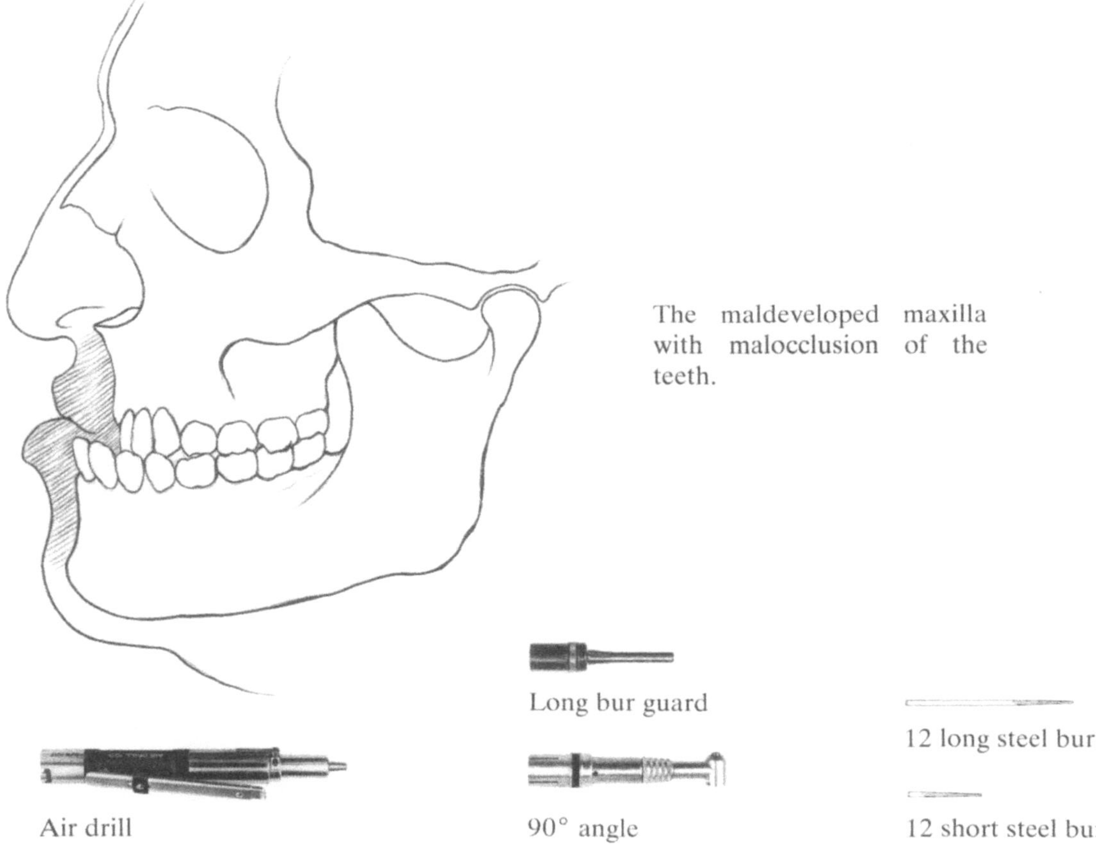

The maldeveloped maxilla with malocclusion of the teeth.

---

* H. L. Obwegeser, M.D., D.M.D.: Surgical Correction of Small or Retrodisplaced Maxillae. **Plastic** & **Recon Surg,** 43:351-365, April 1969.

3. With the 12 long steel bur define the line of osteotomy extending from the pyriform aperture to the maxillary tuberosity on the other side.

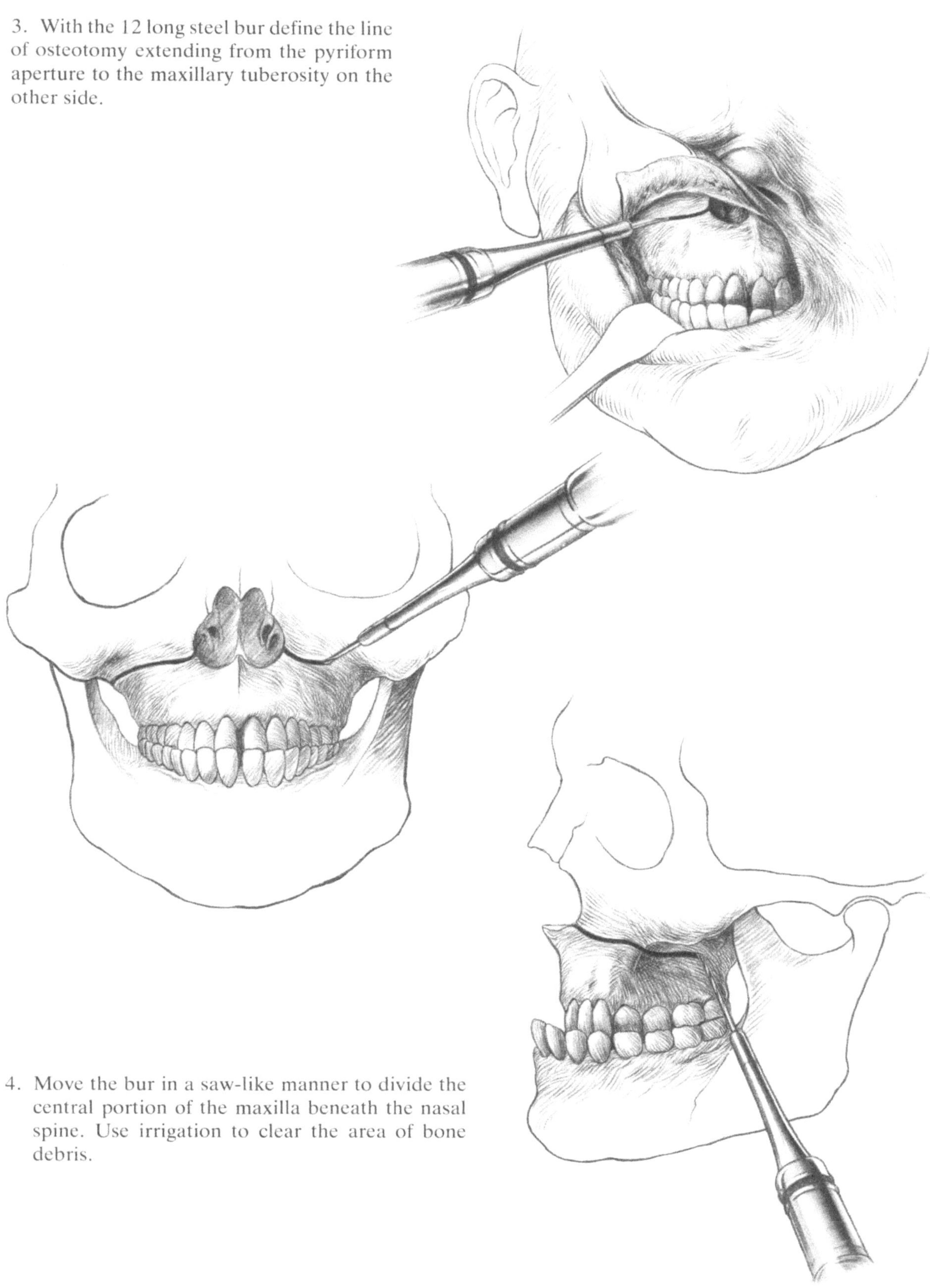

4. Move the bur in a saw-like manner to divide the central portion of the maxilla beneath the nasal spine. Use irrigation to clear the area of bone debris.

Retromaxillism *(continued)*

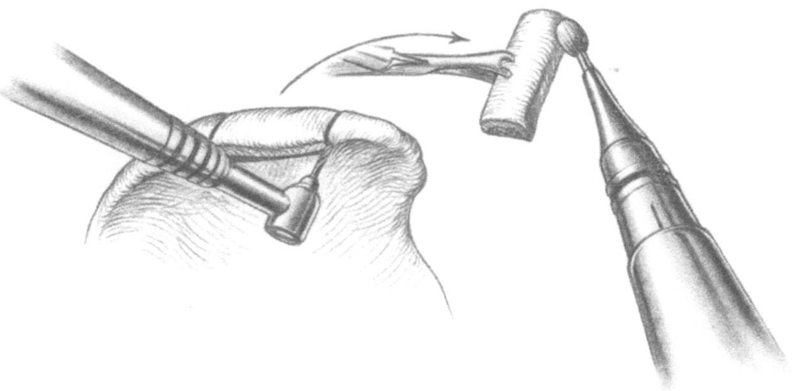

5. Excise a graft from the ilium with the 90° angle
   and 12 short steel bur. Shape the graft with the
   oval 07 steel bur.

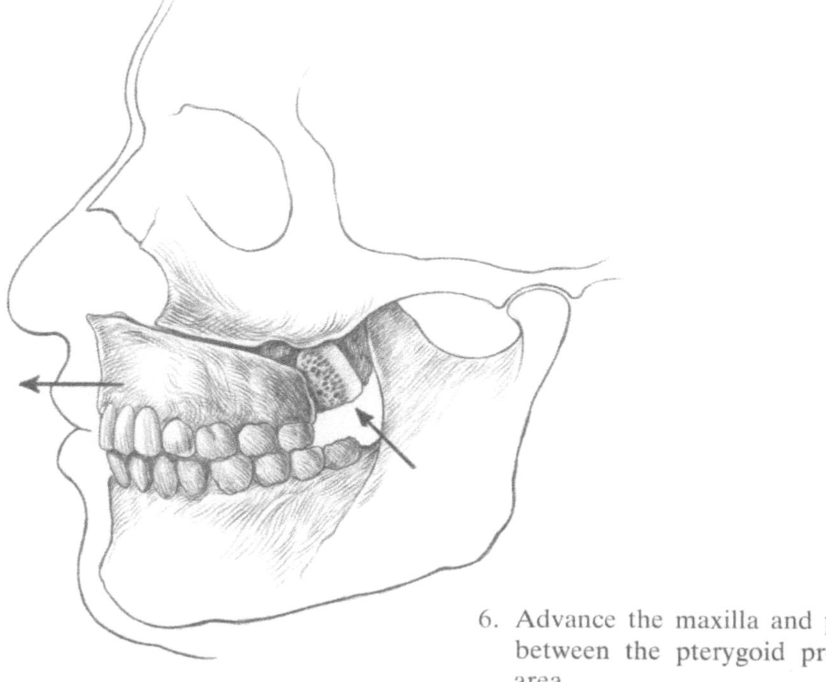

6. Advance the maxilla and place the bone block
   between the pterygoid process and tuberosity
   area.

Reconstruction of a "Dish Face" Deformity*

The defect loosely known as "dish face" is a developmental condition in which the central third of the face does not grow forward in the normal fashion.

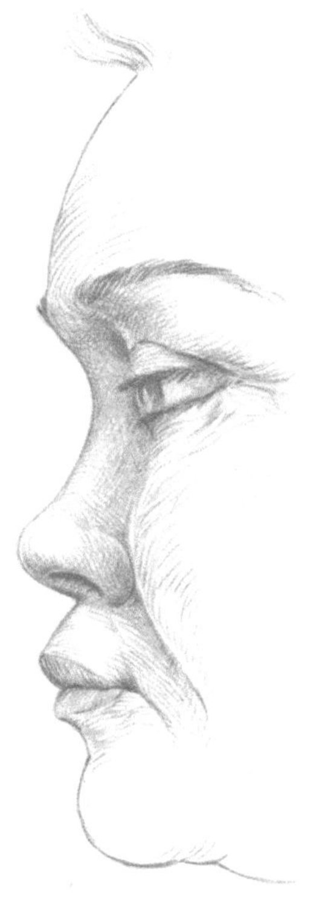

1. Take a large graft from the ilium with the air drill. Carve the graft with the 06 carbide-tip bur so that the single graft consists of two parts. Continue to shape the maxillary graft with the 07 steel bur; bow the graft by sculpture to fit the contour of the upper jaw.

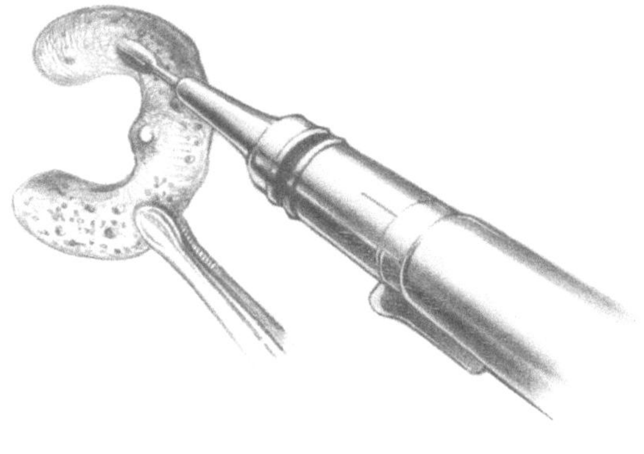

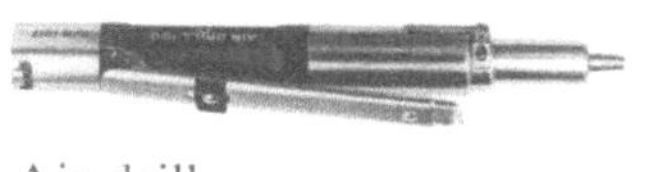

Air drill

Medium bur guard

06 carbide-tip bur

07 steel bur

26 wire-pass bur

---

* The late Herbert Conway, M.D. New York City, October 1964 (Personal Communication). K. L. Pickrell M.D.: Reconstructive Plastic Surgery of the Face. **Clin Symposia** 19:71-99, July - September 1967.

Reconstruction of a "Dish Face" Deformity *(continued)*

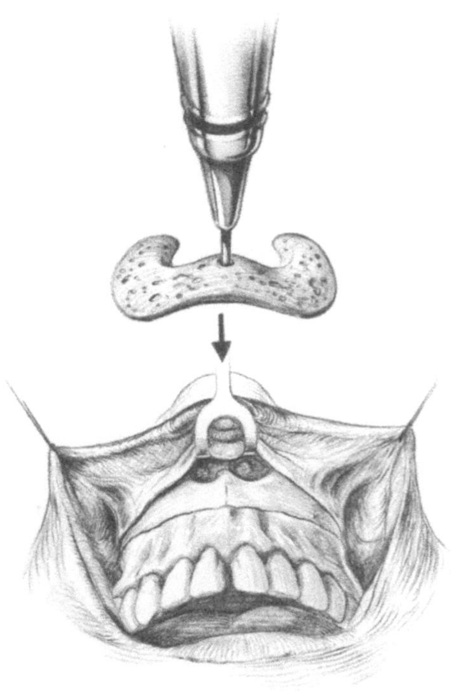

2. Drill an interlock hole in the implant with the wire-pass bur. The high speed of the drill prevents fracture of the graft. Through an intraoral incision just anterior to the gingivolabial sulcus, insert the implant.

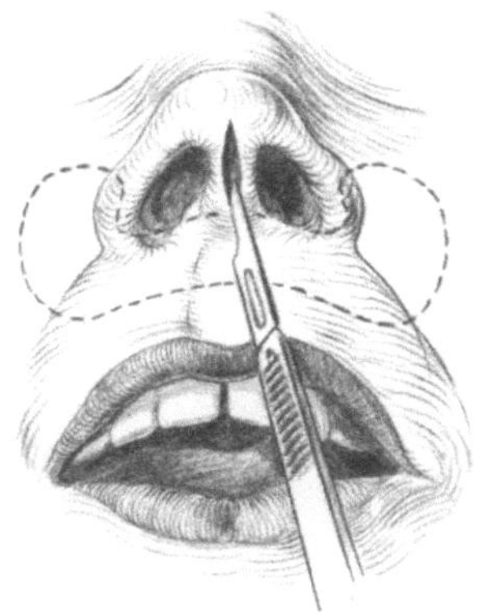

3. With the maxillary graft positioned, make an incision into the columella for insertion of the nasal strut.

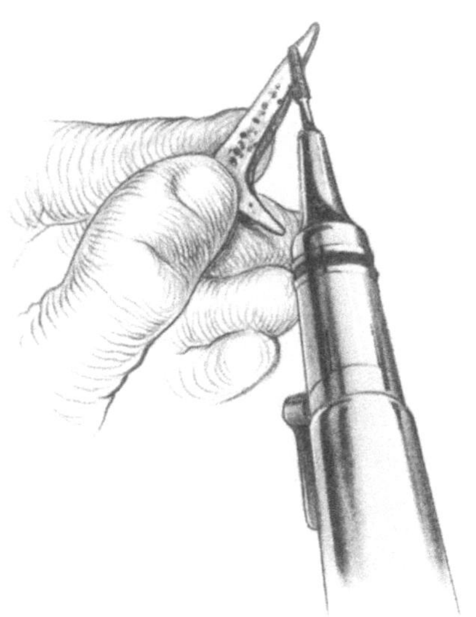

4. With additional bone from the ilium sculpt an L-shaped strut.

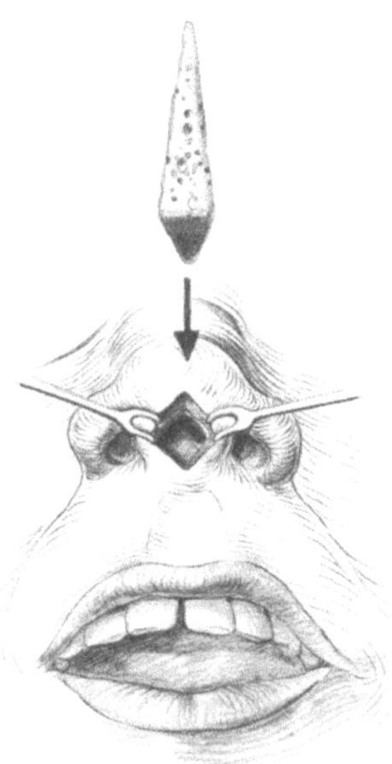

5. Insert the L-shaped graft into the dorsal area of the nose through the incision into the columella.

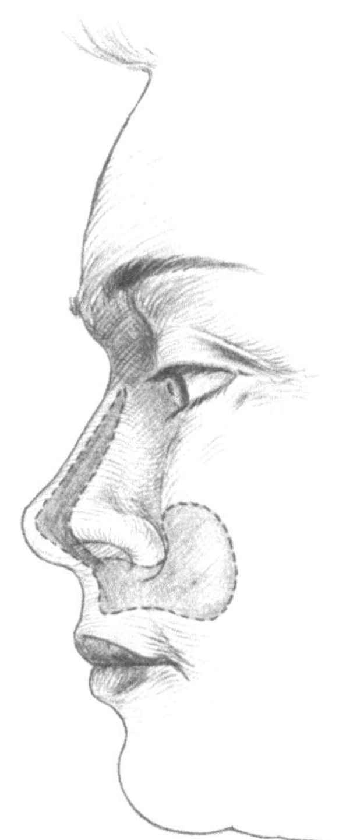

6. The strut brings the nose forward with its short arm so positioned that it rests in the small hole on the anterior surface of the maxillary graft.

Excision of a Tumor of the Ascending Ramus

Assemble the 20° angle and 06 carbide-tip bur:

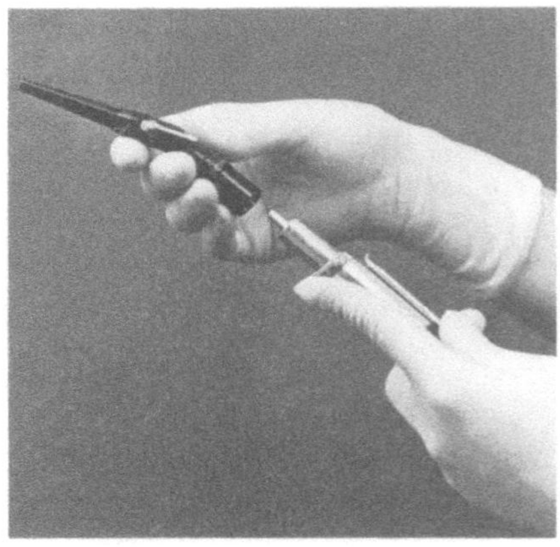

1. Slip the 20° angle snugly over the shoulder of the drill, while raising the release lever 90°.

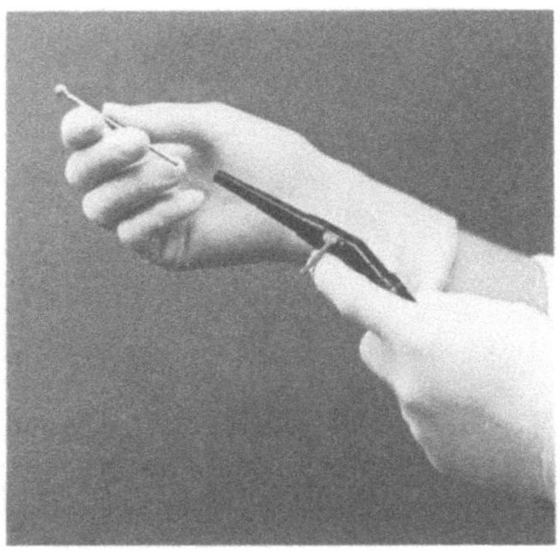

3. Insert the long bur with the release lever raised on the 20° angle.

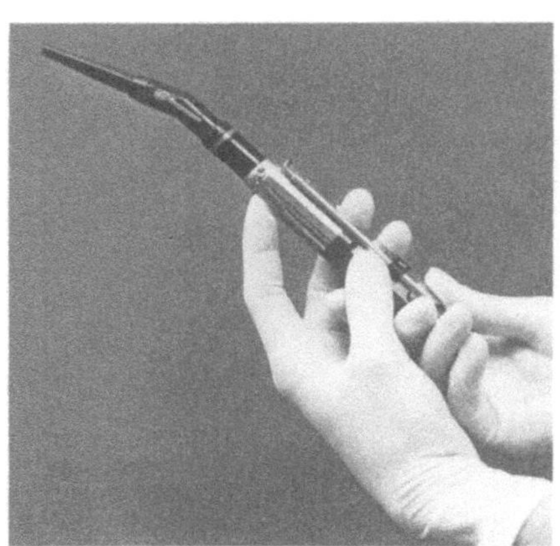

2. Return lever flush against drill to lock attachment.

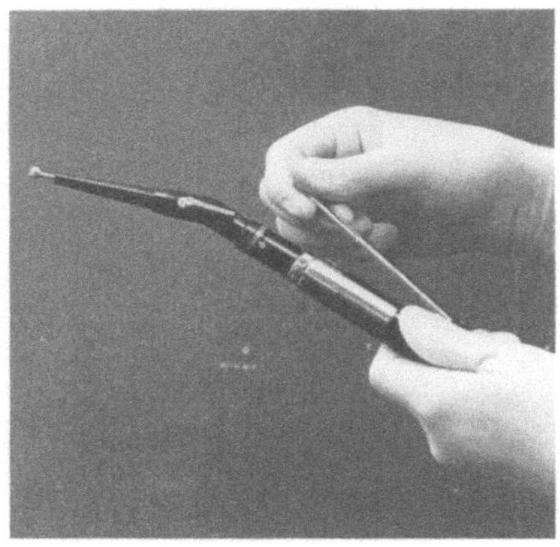

4. Use extension on the throttle for additional finger-tip control.

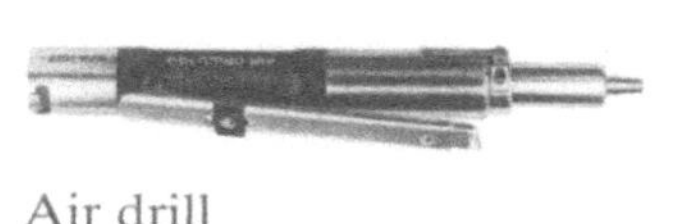

Air drill

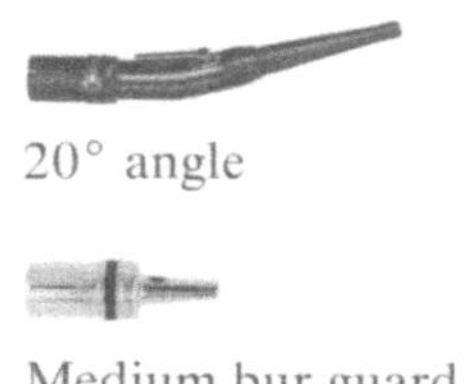

20° angle

Medium bur guard

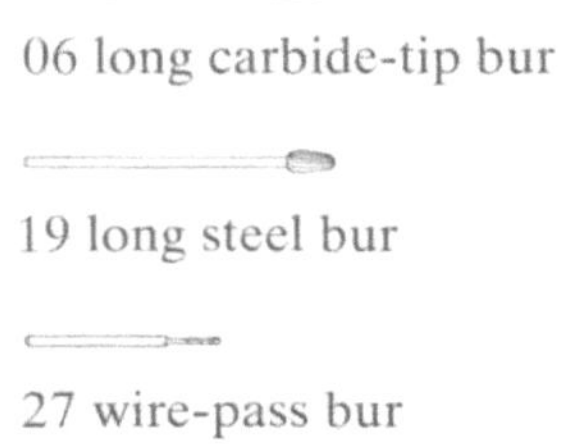

06 long carbide-tip bur

19 long steel bur

27 wire-pass bur

5. Gently, without pressure on the bur, cut through the neck of the condylar process with the 06 carbide-tip bur.

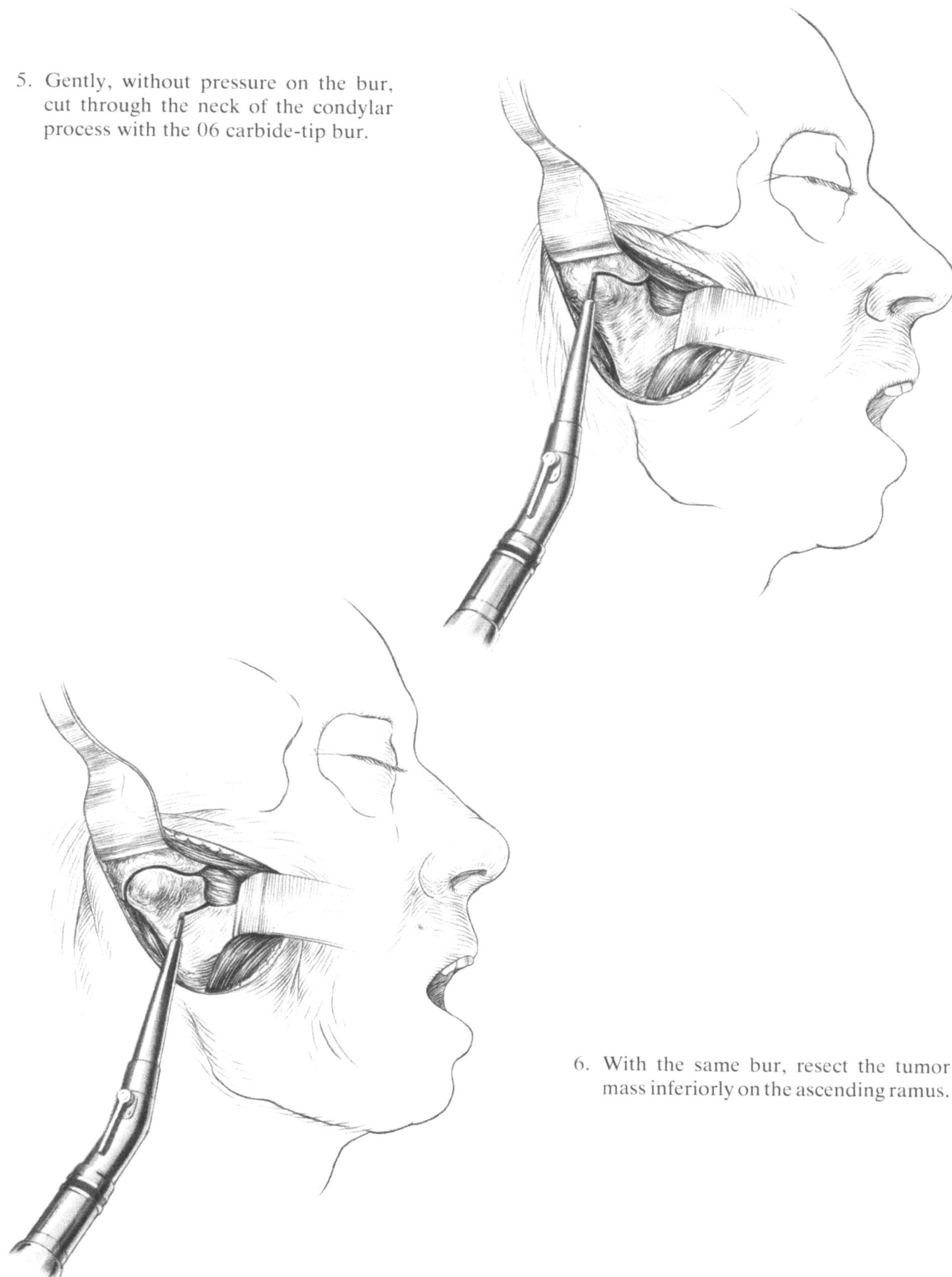

6. With the same bur, resect the tumor mass inferiorly on the ascending ramus.

Excision of a Tumor of the Ascending Ramus *(continued)*

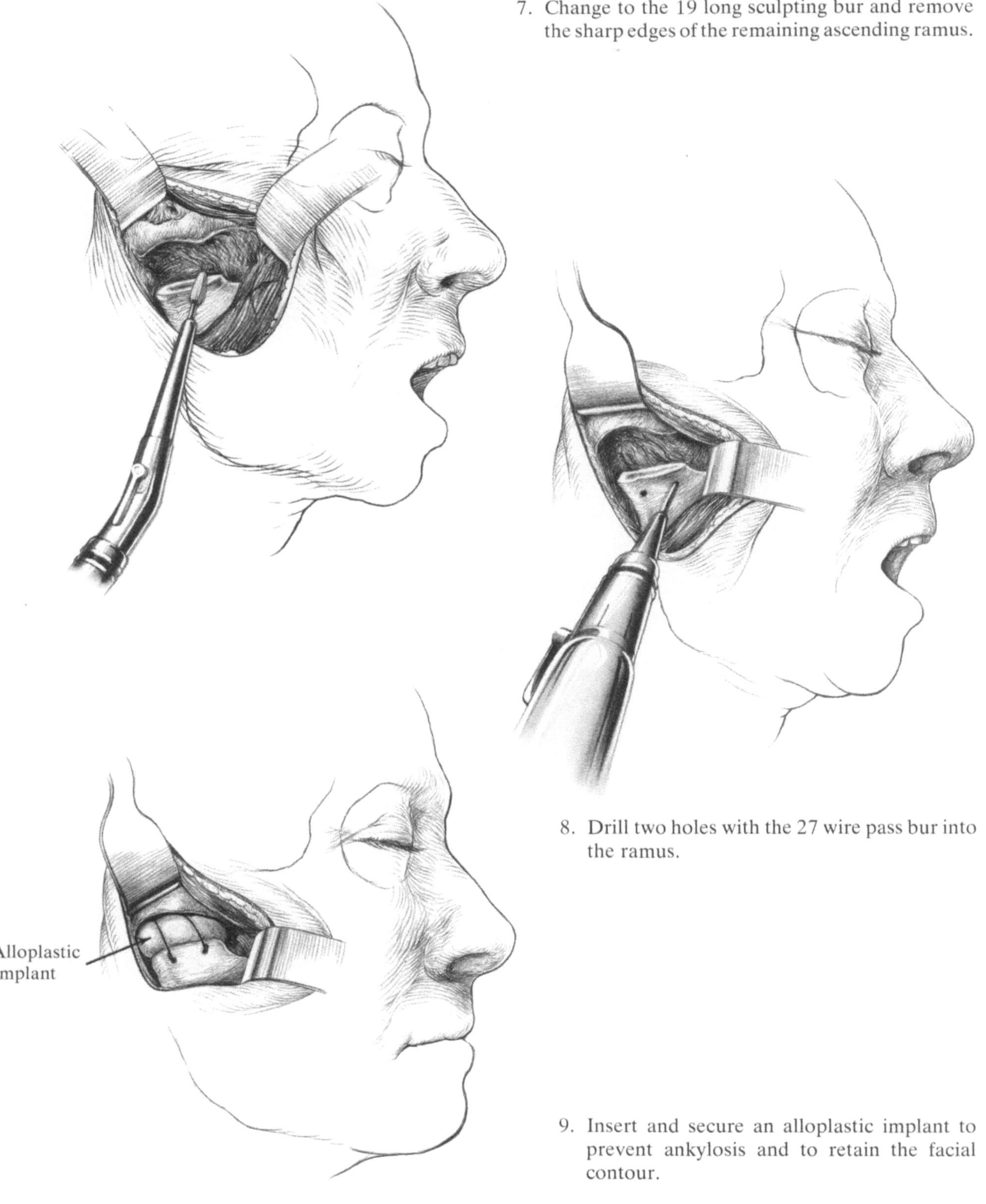

7. Change to the 19 long sculpting bur and remove the sharp edges of the remaining ascending ramus.

8. Drill two holes with the 27 wire pass bur into the ramus.

9. Insert and secure an alloplastic implant to prevent ankylosis and to retain the facial contour.

Advancing Mandibular Symphysis

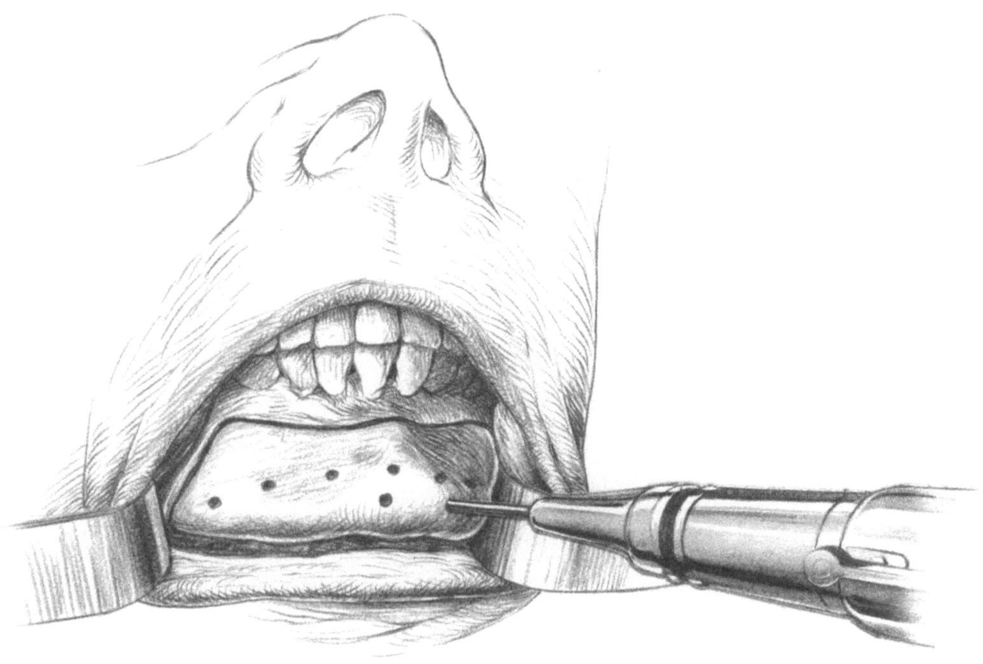

1. For advancement of the mandibular symphysis drill connecting holes across the area of mandibular resection with the wire pass drill. Before uniting the holes, drill two additional holes in the advancing bone section.

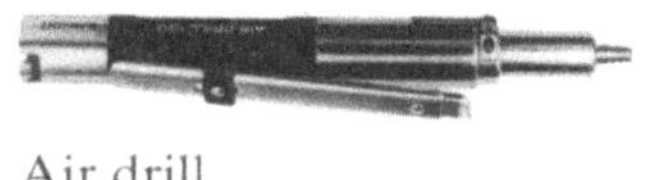

Air drill

Medium bur guard

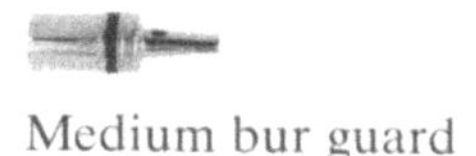

06 carbide-tip bur

27 wire-pass bur

Advancing Mandibular Symphysis *(continued)*

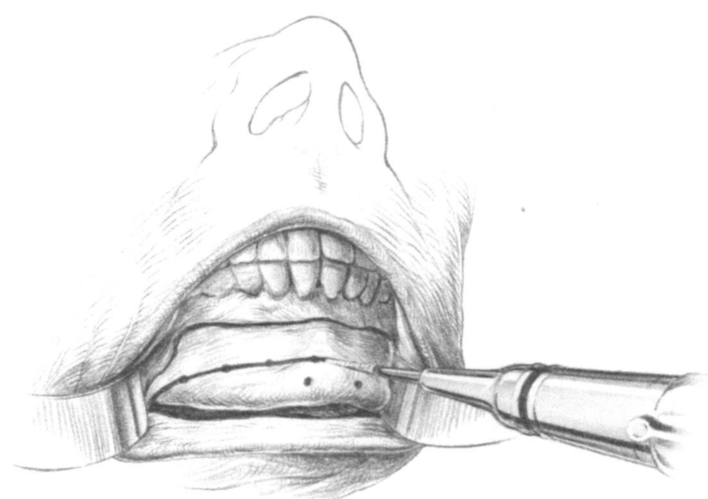

2. Connect the drill holes with the 06 carbide-tip bur. Do not exert too much lateral pressure on the bur; it will reduce the speed of the bur and increase the friction and heat at the bur tip. Allow the high speed and sharp bur to incise a path through the bone.

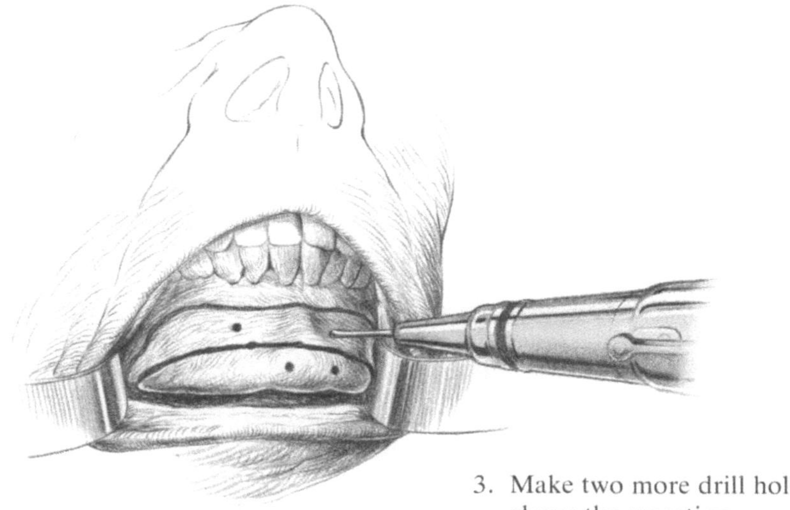

3. Make two more drill holes in the bone above the resection.

4. Divide the resected bone between the drill holes with the 06 bur.

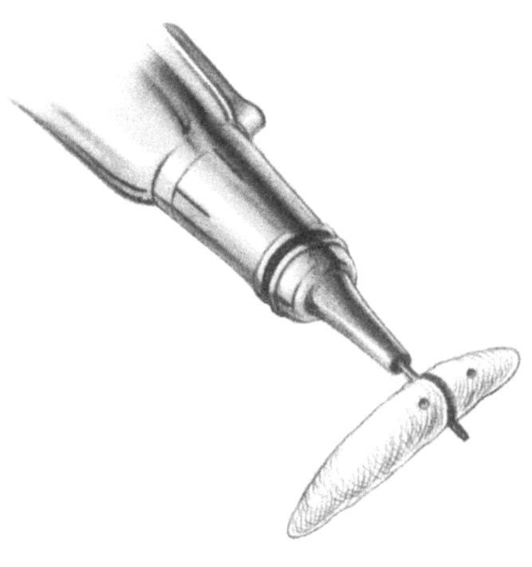

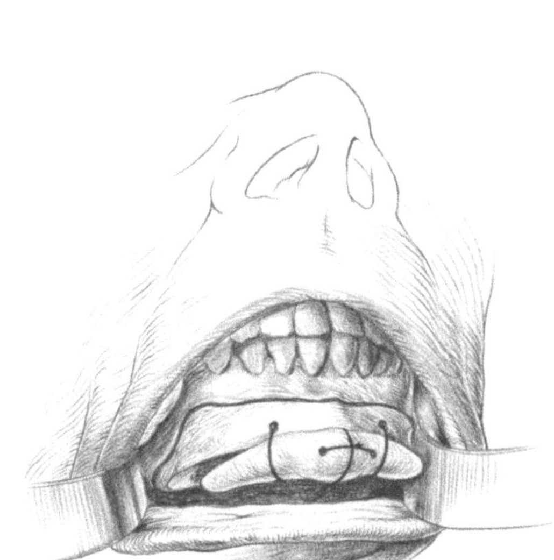

5. Pass a wire across the graft to realign it. Wire the graft into its new position against the mandible.

Total Maxillectomy

Extensive bone excision as in total maxillectomy can be performed with the air drill and osteotomy burs.

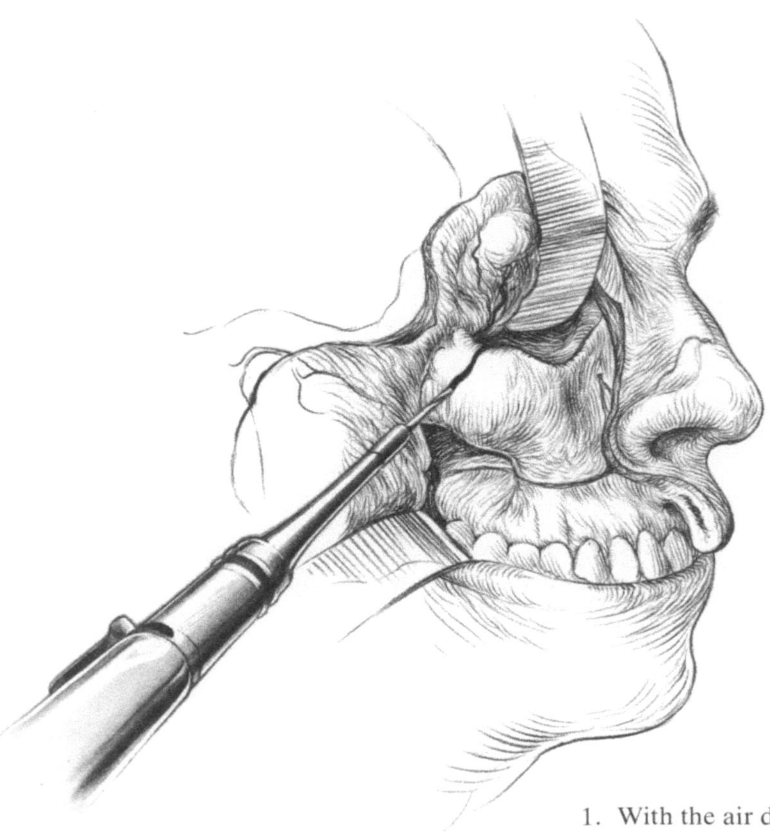

1. With the air drill and 12 long steel bur, section the zygoma vertically, extending the incision medially and obliquely to the inferior orbital fissure.

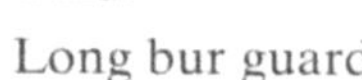

Air drill   Long bur guard   12 long steel bur

2. Using the same bur, section the nasofrontal process vertically from the maxilla onto the infraorbital surface.

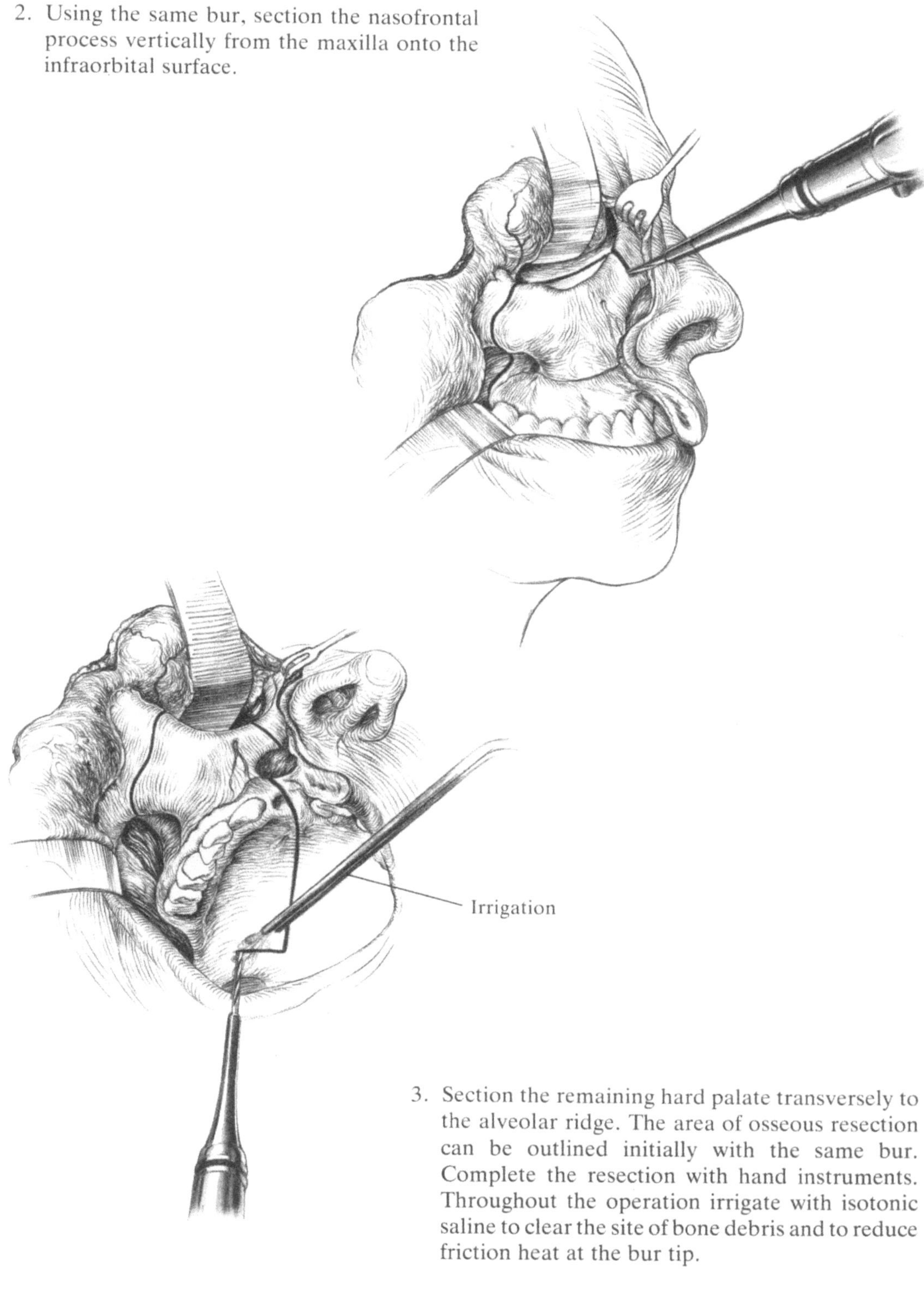

3. Section the remaining hard palate transversely to the alveolar ridge. The area of osseous resection can be outlined initially with the same bur. Complete the resection with hand instruments. Throughout the operation irrigate with isotonic saline to clear the site of bone debris and to reduce friction heat at the bur tip.

Ridge Onlay Graft for Microgenia

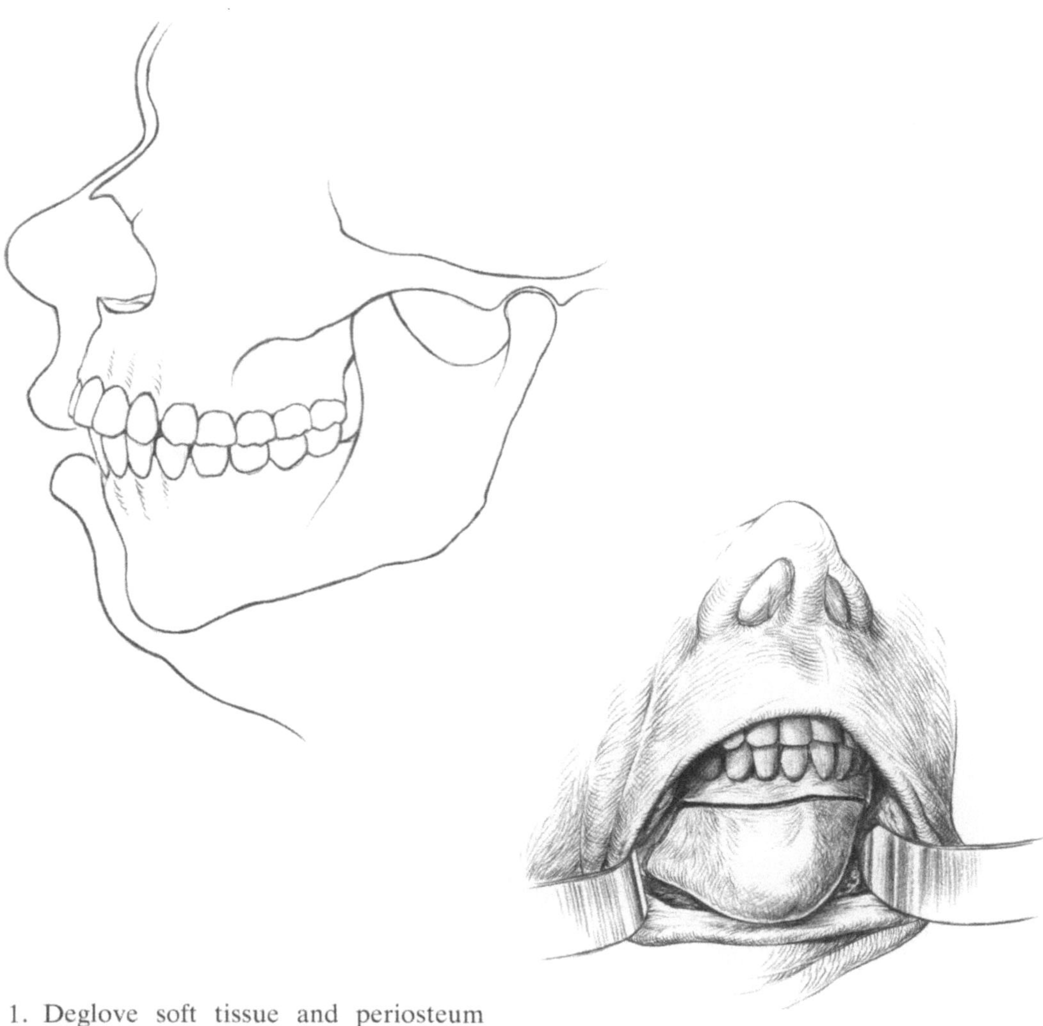

1. Deglove soft tissue and periosteum from the mandible.

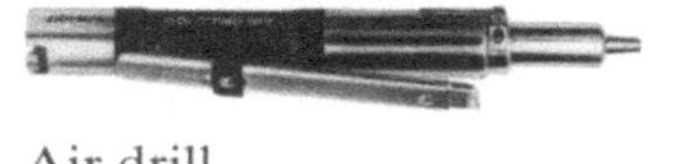

Air drill

Medium bur guard

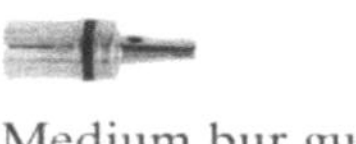

02 carbide-tip bur

27 wire-pass bur

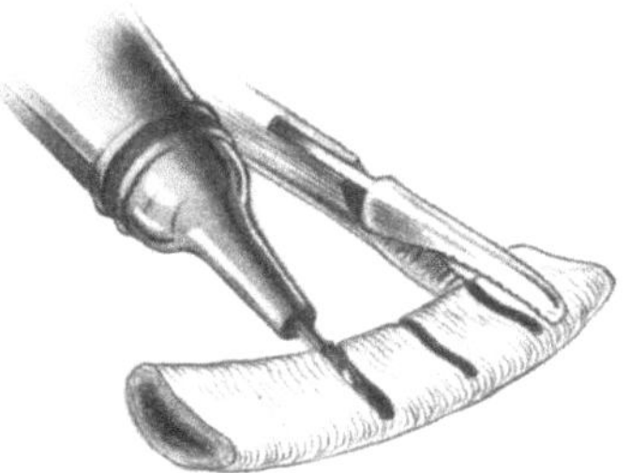

2. Take a bone graft from the rib and score the rib with the 02 carbide-tip bur. This will increase its flexibility and enhance the fusion of the graft to the mandible.

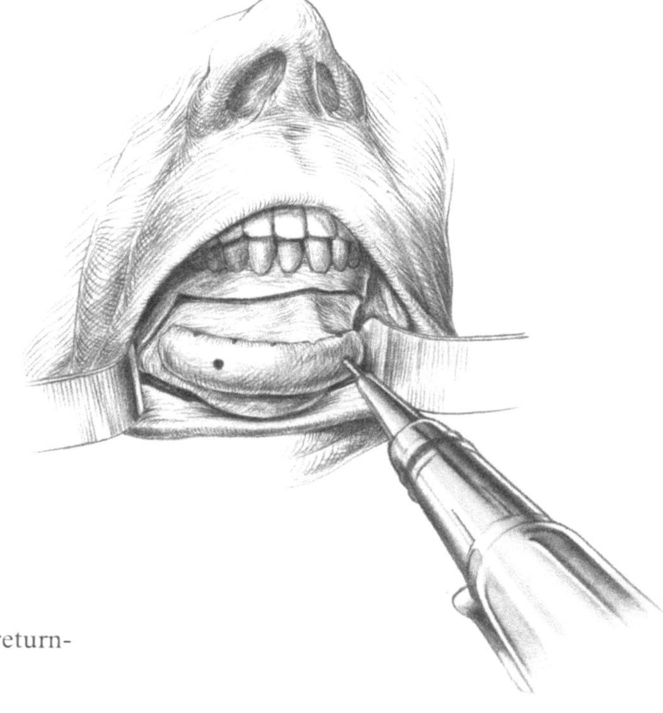

3. Drill holes with the wire-pass bur through the graft and the mandible.

4. Crimp the wire into the bur groove before returning the wire through the bone.

5. Make fine grooves on the anterior surface of the graft to seat the wires. Tighten and secure the fixation wires.

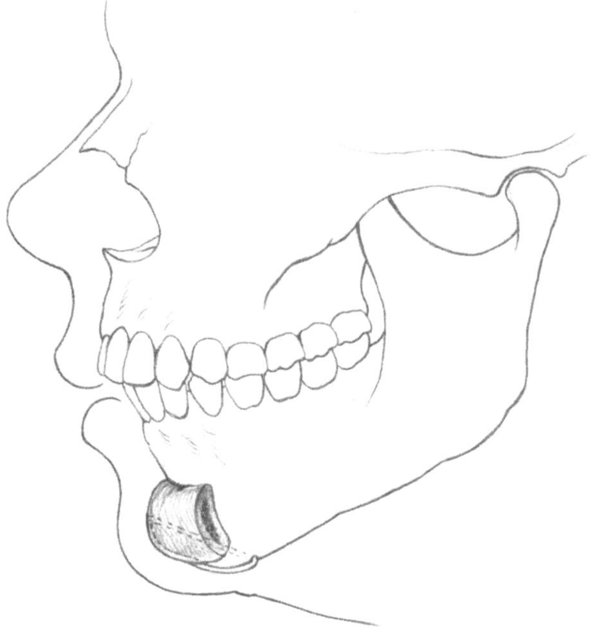

Nasal Reconstruction

In many nasal reconstructive techniques the overlying nasal mucosa and soft tissue remain intact. Attachments have been designed for the air drill to protect this soft tissue from the rotating bur. The tissue retractor guard accepts an oval steel sculpting bur for reconstruction of the nasal hump. For rhinoplasty the attachment is designed with a side-cutting diamond bur for lateral osteotomy of the nasal cartilage.

Assemble the tissue retractor guard and 19 long steel bur:

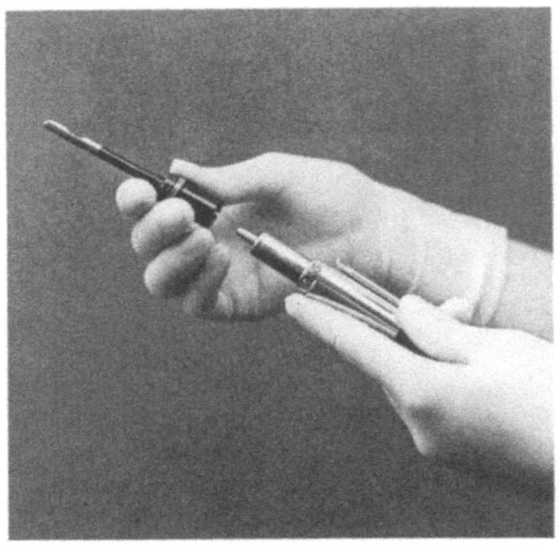

1. Seat the tissue retractor guard over the air drill shoulder.

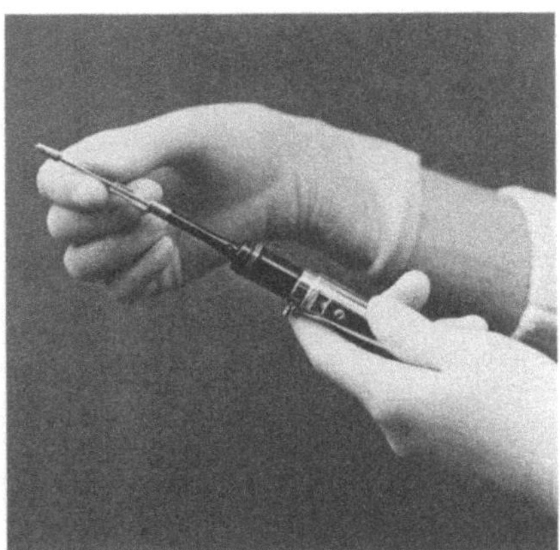

2. Insert the 19 long steel bur into the attachment and air drill collet with the bur release lever raised 90 degrees. Return lever flush against drill to lock bur.

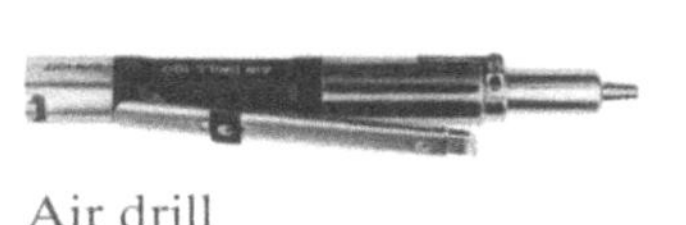

Air drill

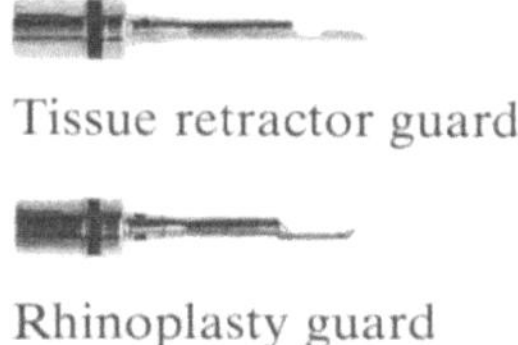

Tissue retractor guard

Rhinoplasty guard

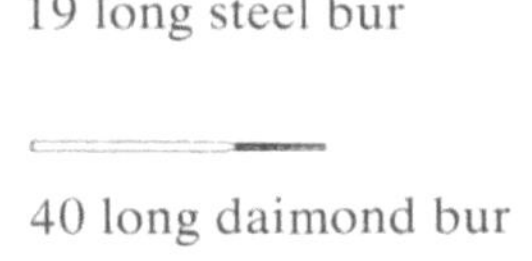

19 long steel bur

40 long daimond bur

Removal of a Nasal Hump

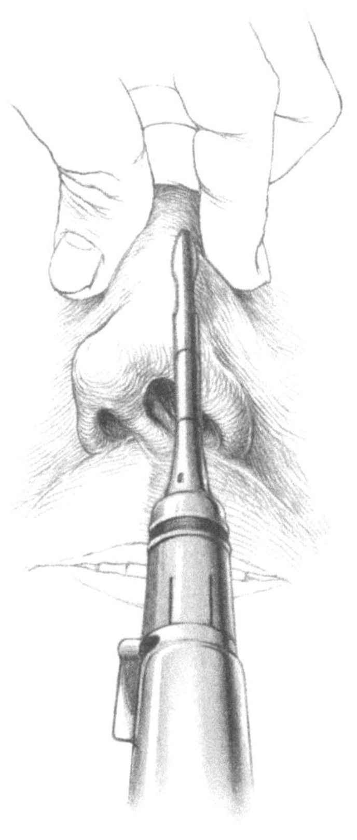

1. Elevate the soft tissue and periosteum from the nasal bone. Insert the tissue retractor guard and bur under the soft tissue. Sculpt away the excess bone.

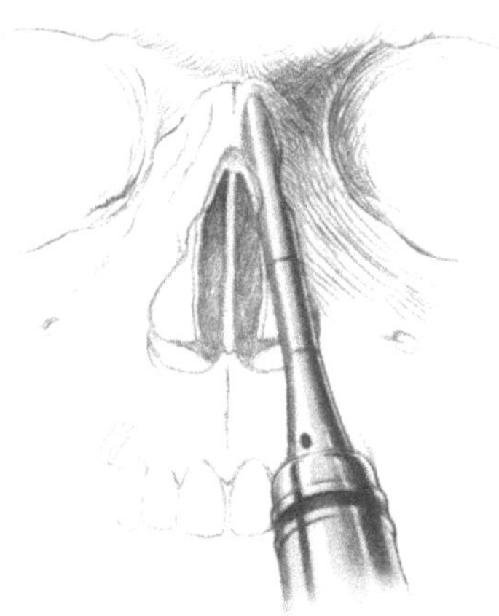

2. Move the bur gently over the nasal arch. Do not apply heavy pressure against the bur, as this will reduce speed and cutting efficiency.

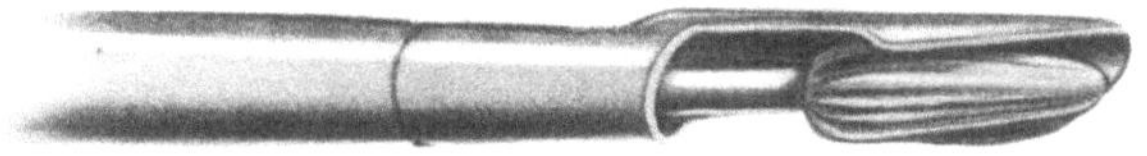

The tissue retractor guard acts as a tissue elevator and protector while the bur removes the bone.

Lateral Nasal Osteotomy (Rhinoplasty)

1. Assemble the air drill with the 40 long diamond bur and rhinoplasty guard.

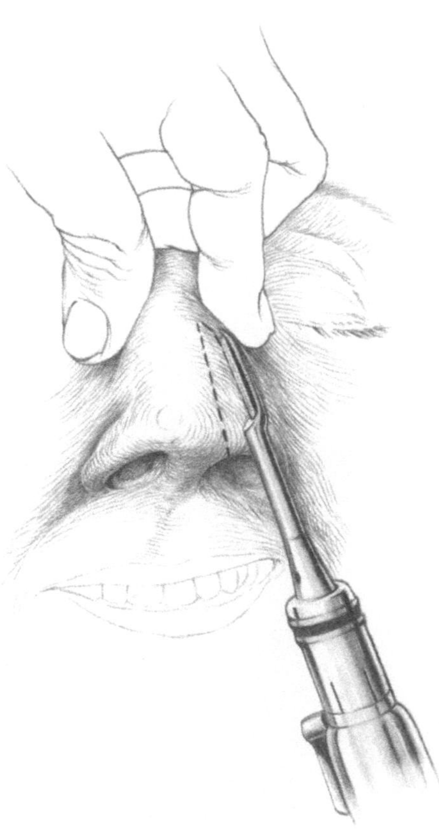

2. Manually elevate the nasal soft tissue and periosteum. Insert the rhinoplasty guard and bur laterally under the elevated tissue.

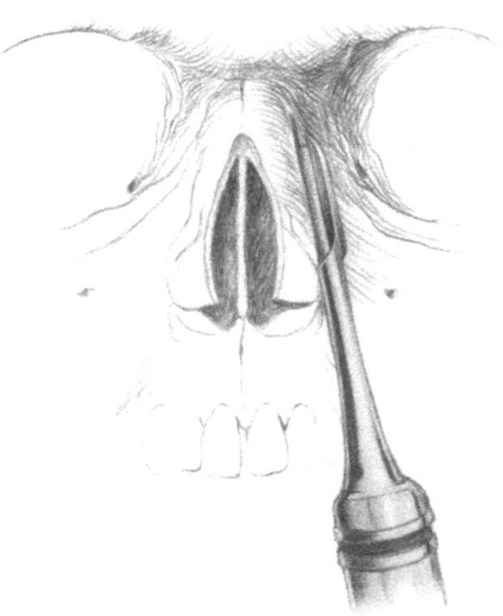

3. The bur will incise a groove in the nasal cartilage and osteotomy is completed with manual pressure of the fingers. Do not apply heavy manual side pressure against the bur, as this may cause the bur to bend and reduce its cutting efficiency.

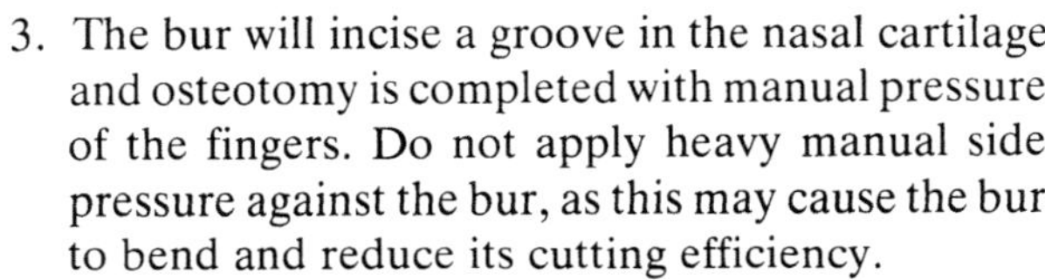

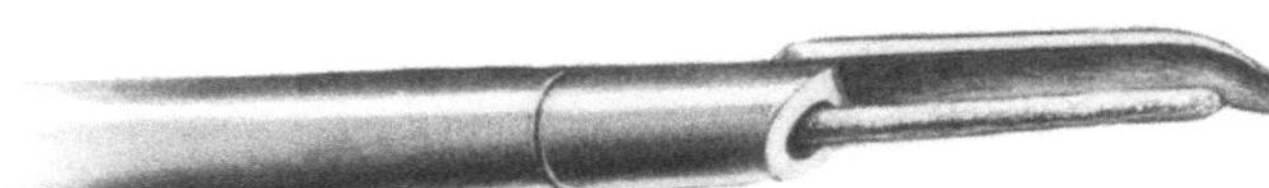

The rhinoplasty guard is designed to elevate the periosteum and soft tissue and protect these structures from the rotating bur.

Cartilage or Bone Grafting Following Subtotal Nasal Reconstruction

Assemble the air drill with the medium bur guard and 04 carbide-tip bur:

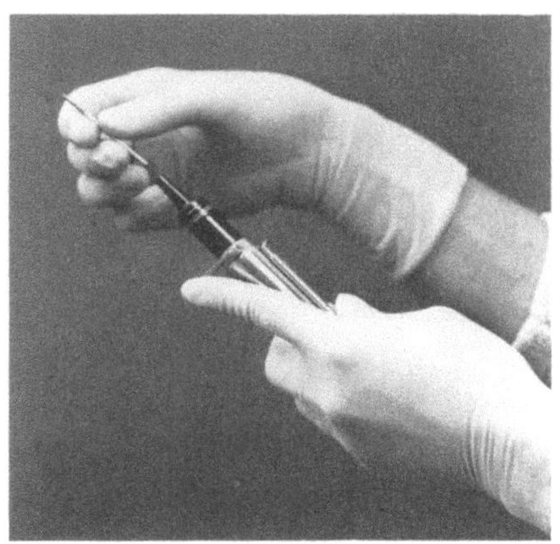

1. Seat the medium bur guard firmly over the air drill shoulder.

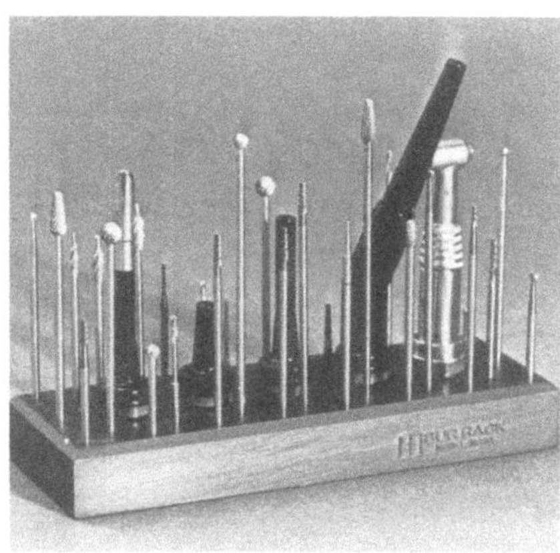

3. Use the throttle extension for close finger-tip control.

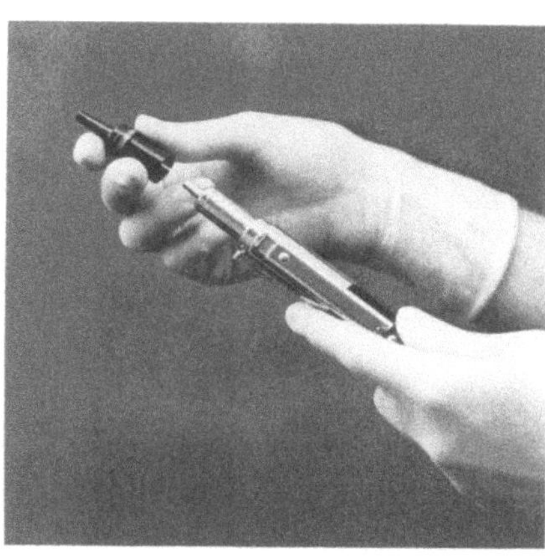

2. Push bur release lever forward 90 degrees to insert the bur. Return lever flush against drill to lock bur.

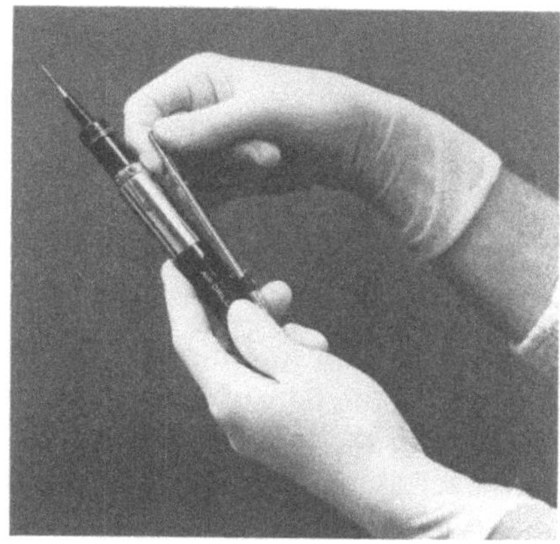

4. When not in use, the burs and attachments should be placed in the bur and attachment rack.

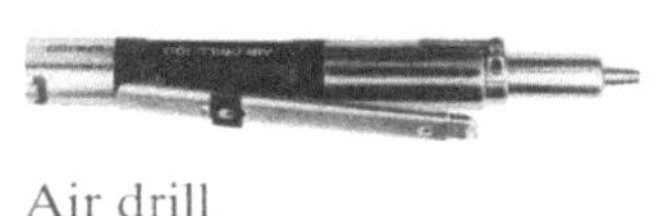

Air drill

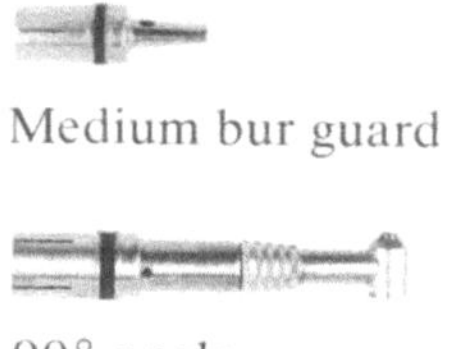

Medium bur guard

90° angle

04 carbide-tip bur

27 short wire-pass bur

Cartilage or Bone Grafting Following Subtotal Nasal Reconstruction *(continued)*

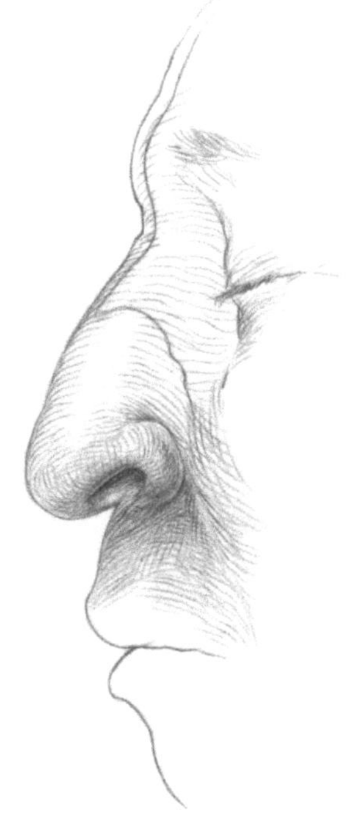

Preoperative appearance

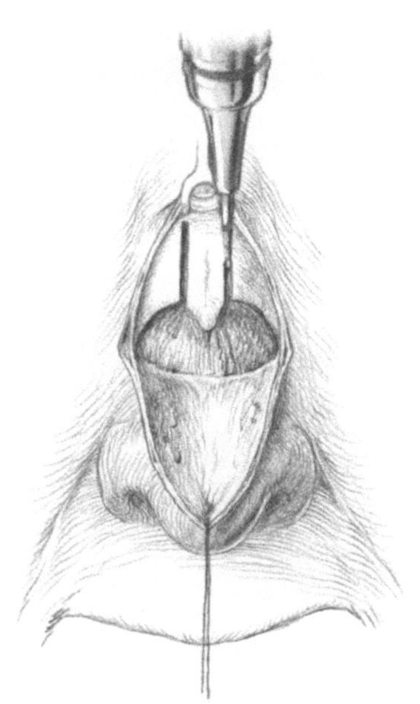

5. Make a skin flap exposing the full extent of the nasal bone. With the 04 carbide-tip bur excise a wedge of bone in the midline through the entire length of the nasal bones. Remove the bone without penetrating the lining of the mucous membrane.

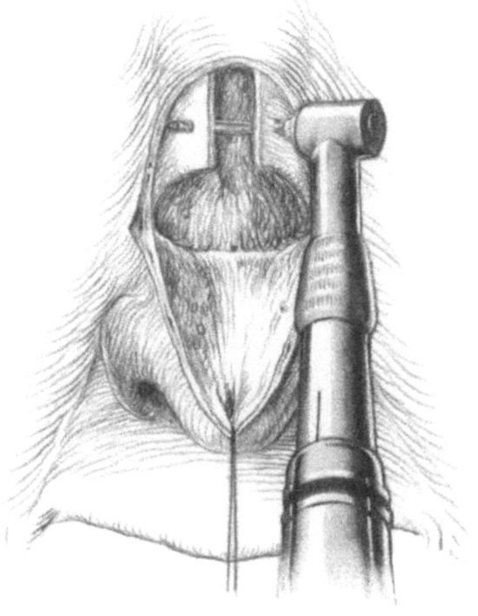

6. Change burs, and with the wire pass bur drill a hole across the resected bone.

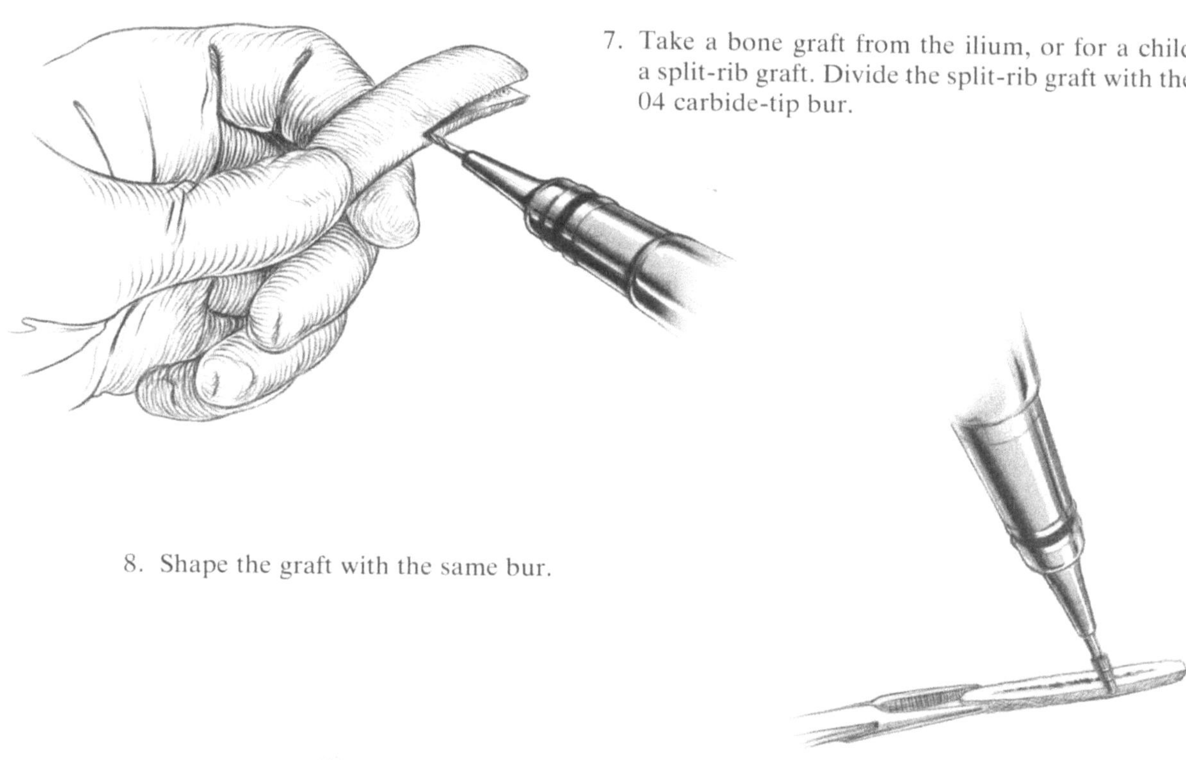

7. Take a bone graft from the ilium, or for a child a split-rib graft. Divide the split-rib graft with the 04 carbide-tip bur.

8. Shape the graft with the same bur.

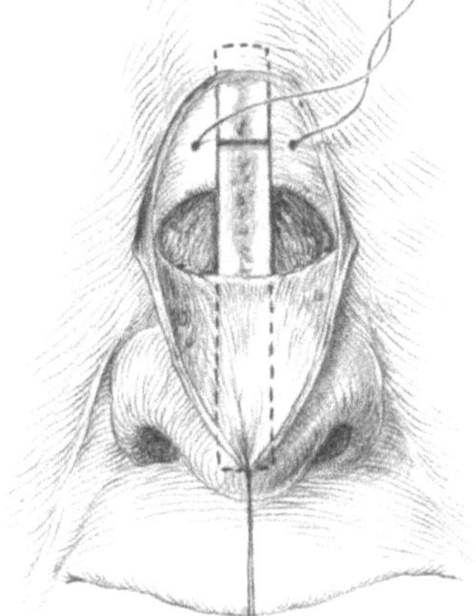

9. Cut a groove to support the fixation wire. Pass the wire through the drill holes.

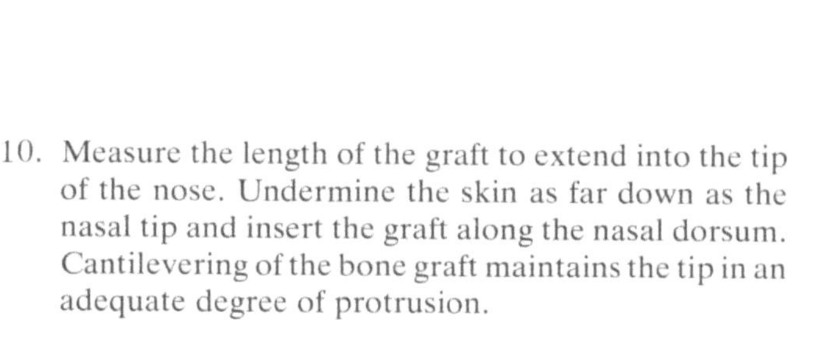

10. Measure the length of the graft to extend into the tip of the nose. Undermine the skin as far down as the nasal tip and insert the graft along the nasal dorsum. Cantilevering of the bone graft maintains the tip in an adequate degree of protrusion.

Krönlein Procedure

The incision

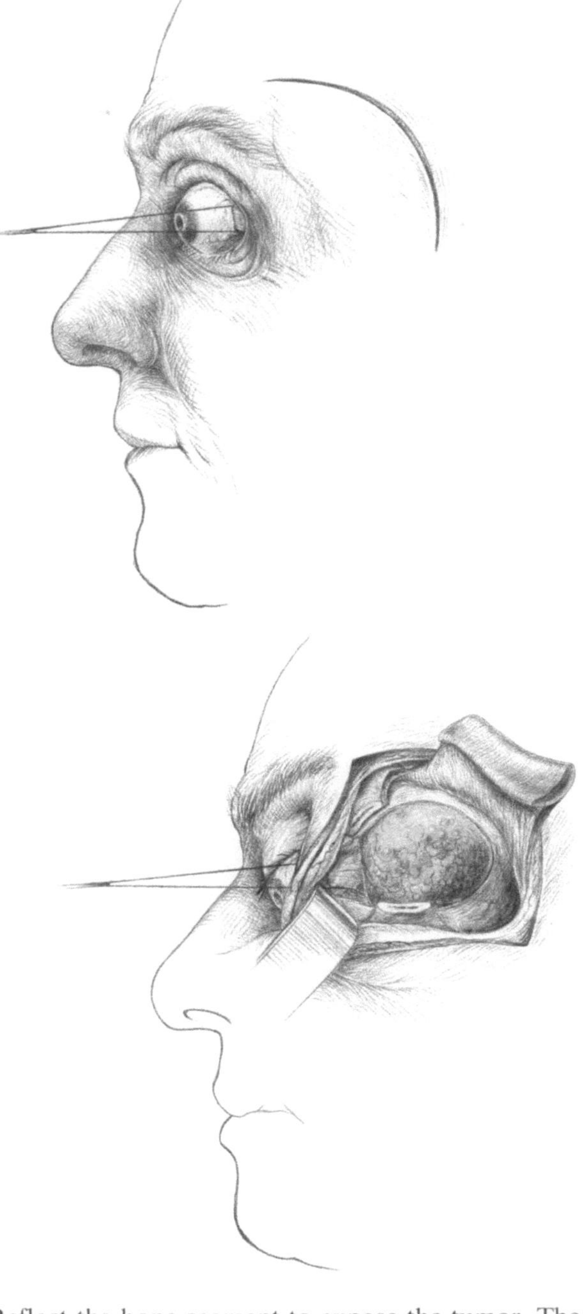

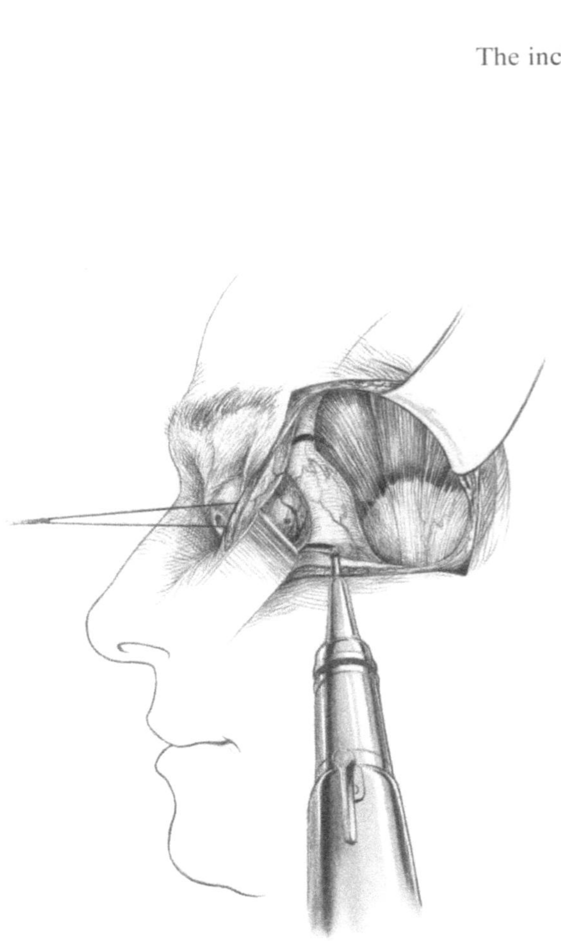

With a retractor reflecting the soft tissue, and a guard behind the orbital rim, take the 04 carbide-tip bur and incise the bone. It is possible to incise the bone for two-thirds of its depth; a gentle tap with a chisel will complete the separation.

Reflect the bone segment to expose the tumor. The amount of bone removed during excision is so minimal that accurate replacement of the bone is possible.

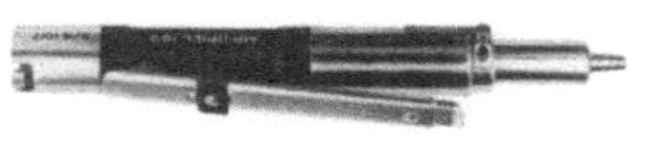

Air drill

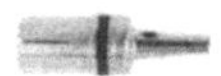

Medium bur guard   04 carbide-tip bur

Excision of an Ossifying Fibroma of the Frontal Bone*

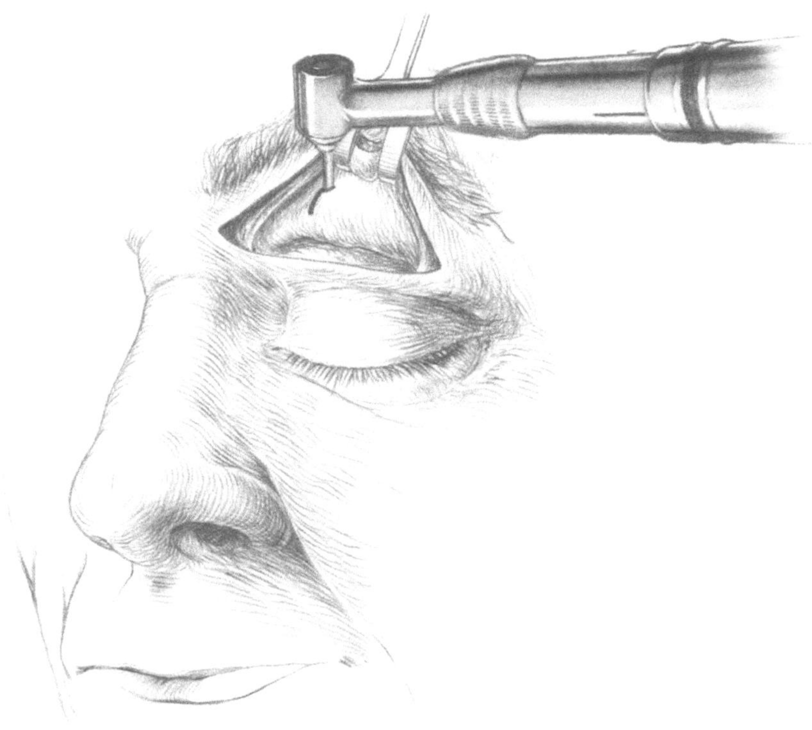

The delicacy and precision attained by use of the drill and bur allows safe penetration of the frontal sinus to expose the fibroma.

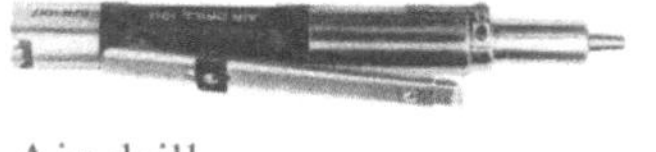

Air drill

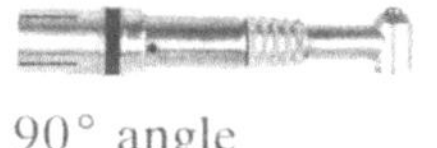

90° angle

02 short carbide-tip bur

* G. K. Thomas, M. D., K. A. Kasper, M. D.: Ossifying Fibroma of the Frontal Bone. **Arch Otolaryn,** 83 : 69 - 72, January 1966.

Dacryocystorhinostomy

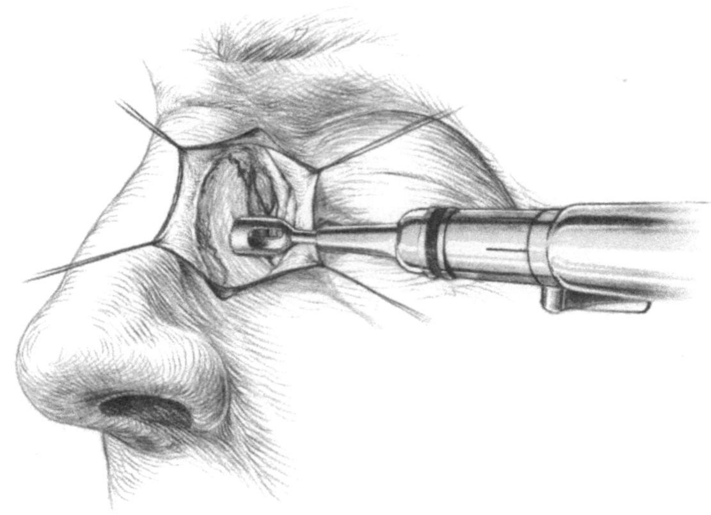

1. With a bone biopsy bur or oval sculpting bur remove the bone at the anterior lacrimal crest to expose the nasal mucosa. Intermittently irrigate the bur tip with isotonic saline to clear the site of bone debris and cool the bone.

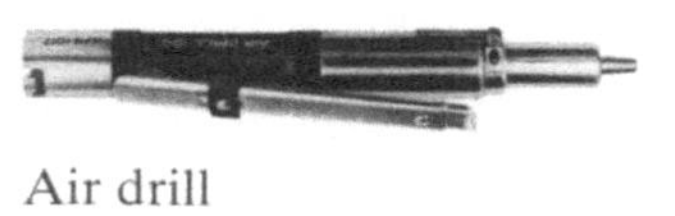

Air drill

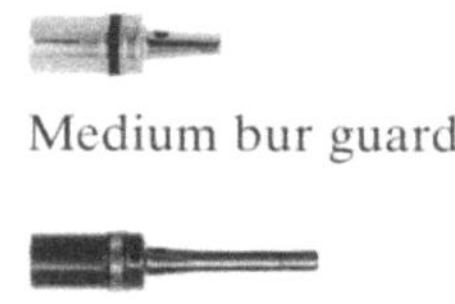

Medium bur guard

Long bur guard

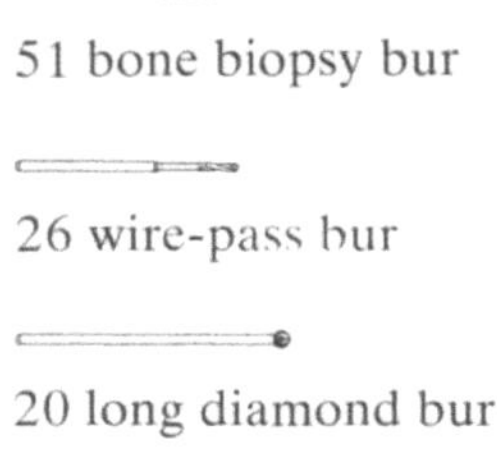

51 bone biopsy bur

26 wire-pass bur

20 long diamond bur

2. If necessary, enlarge the fenestration with the 20 long diamond bur. The diamond bur will not damage the delicate nasal membrane as it is an abrasive rather than a cutting bur.

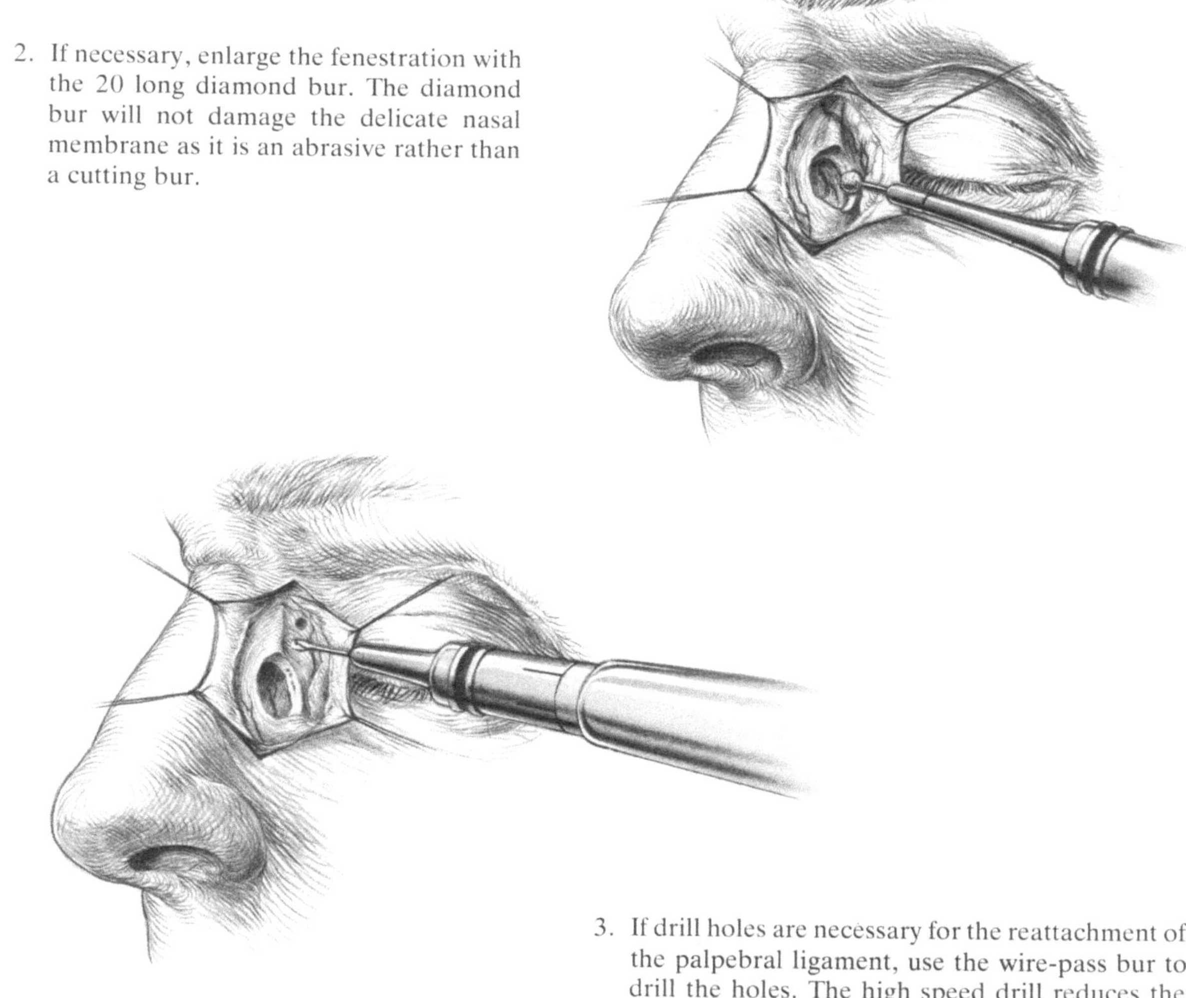

3. If drill holes are necessary for the reattachment of the palpebral ligament, use the wire-pass bur to drill the holes. The high speed drill reduces the possibility of fracture or fragmenting of the bone.

Reconstruction of the Auricle*

Contouring of grafts, both homogeneous and synthetic, is an important function of the air drill. The grafts can be shaped precisely and final polishing of the implants eliminates any rough edges which may erode through the soft tissue.

Assemble the air drill and bur:

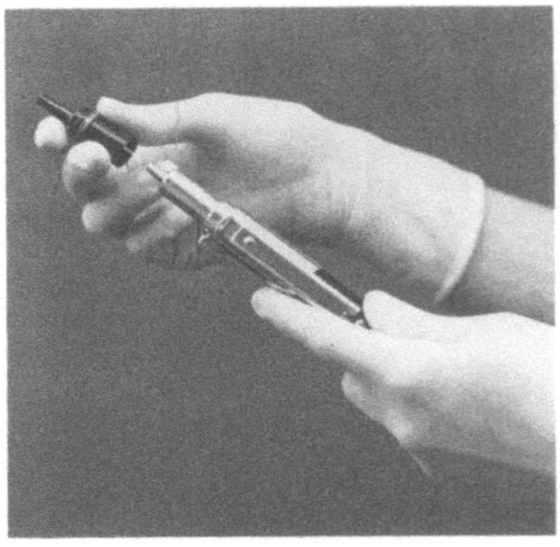

1. Place the bur guard over the drill shoulder.

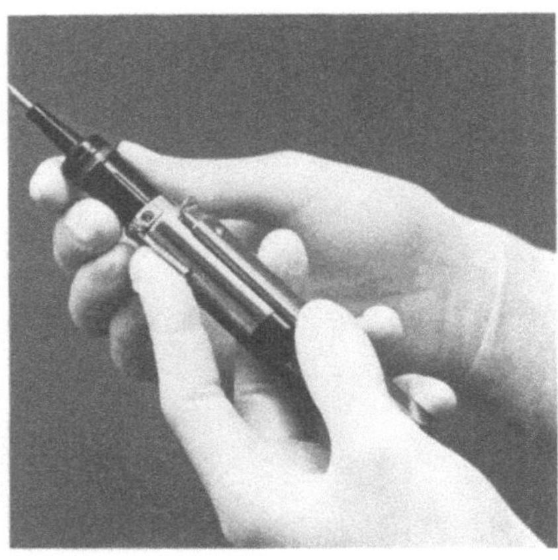

3. Return lever flush against the drill to lock bur.

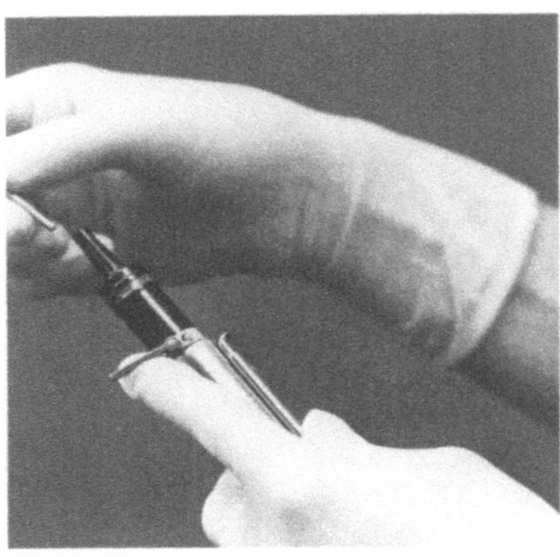

2. Push bur release lever 90° to insert bur.

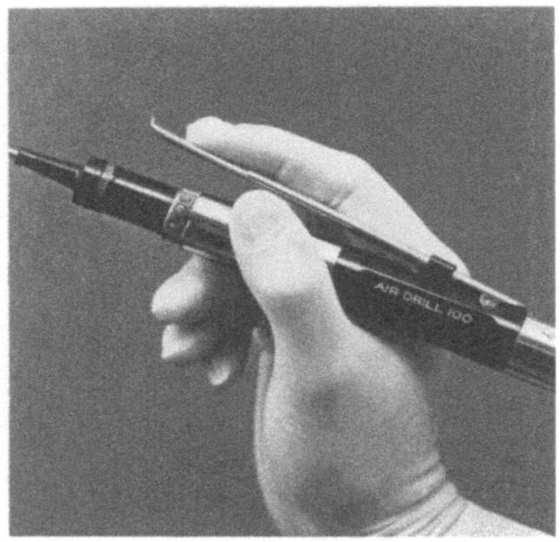

4. Run the instrument at full speed for maximum cutting efficiency.

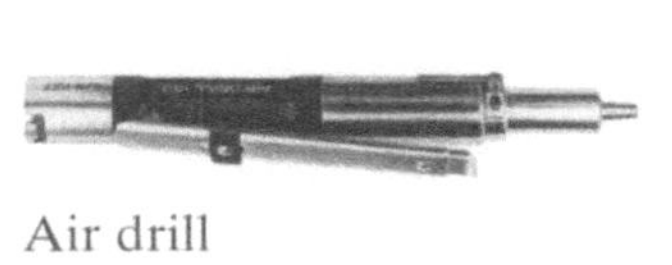

Air drill

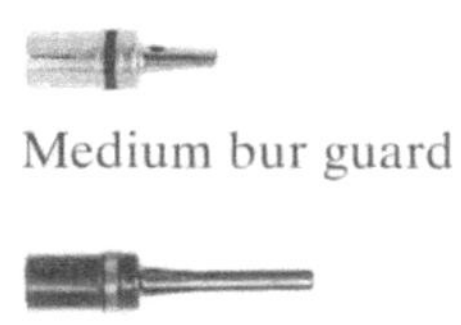

Medium bur guard

Long bur guard

07 steel bur

07 long diamond bur

---

* C. Hansen, D. D. S., M. D. Los Angeles, California, USA 1969 (Personal Communication).

5. Use an 07 steel bur to sculpt a fresh implant of cartilage or bone prior to reconstruction of a congenitally deformed ear.

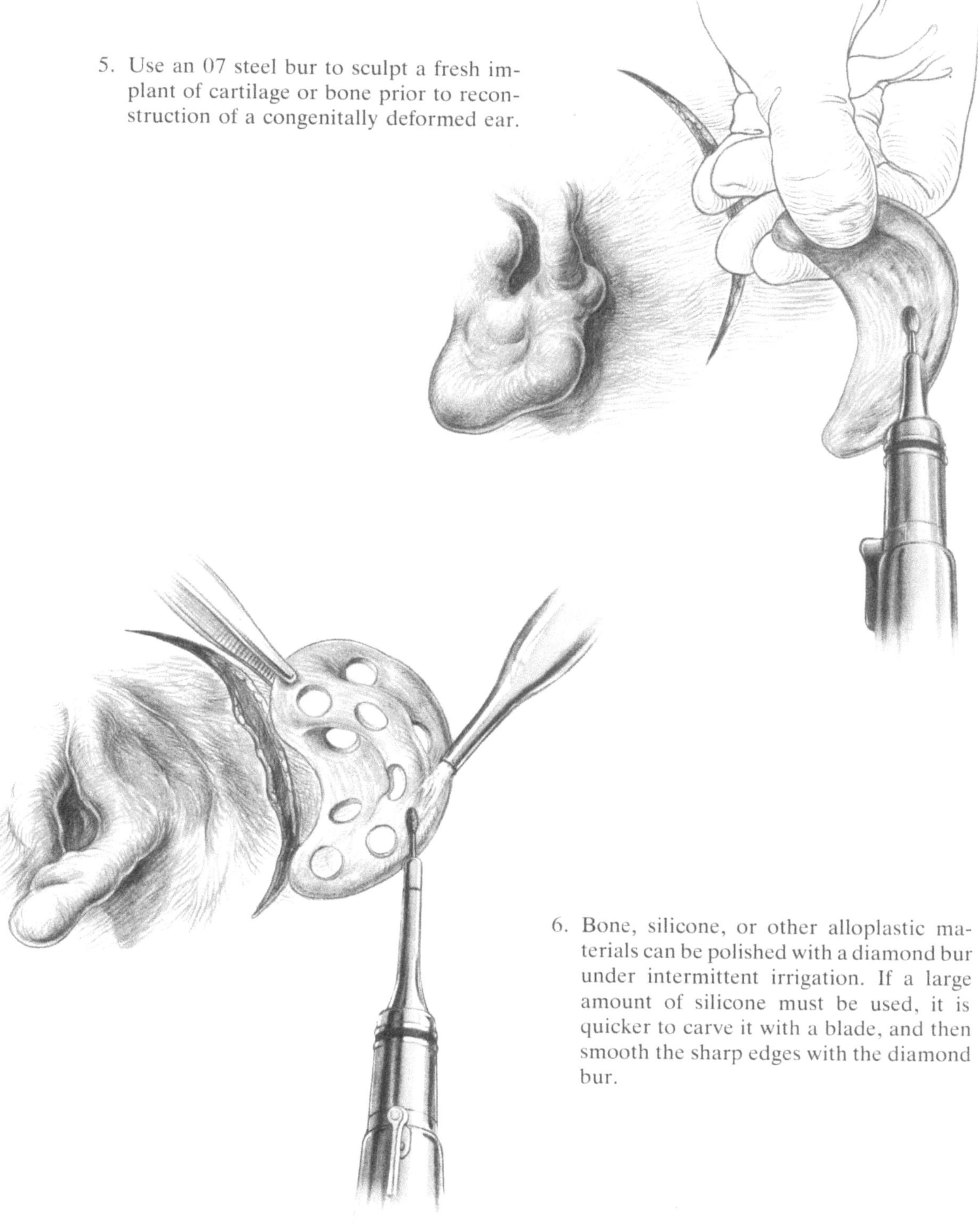

6. Bone, silicone, or other alloplastic materials can be polished with a diamond bur under intermittent irrigation. If a large amount of silicone must be used, it is quicker to carve it with a blade, and then smooth the sharp edges with the diamond bur.

Technique Suggestions

A new steel or carbide-tip bur will quickly remove dense cortical bone. Use a light touch and allow the high-speed rotation and bur to incise the bone.

The rotating speed and torque may be reduced by reducing pressure at the regulator.

The larger steel burs have a tendency to skip, especially if the pressure is reduced, because then more manual pressure is required on the bur. Therefore, use the small headed burs for precision work.

Use a combination of drill irrigation and suction to minimize the amount of bone dust around the operative site.

Do not withdraw or approach the operative site with the bur rotating.

Use Gelfoam to reduce hemorrhage and prevent danger of cottonoids becoming entangled in the bur.

Incise or elevate the periosteum before applying the instrument.

Do not apply pressure against the bur tip. This will cause the bur to slow down and the increase in friction and heat may damage the bone.

The thinnest incision is achieved with the thinnest bur.

Excessive pressure may cause the burs to stall.

Burs must be assembled with the appropriate bur guard.

Running a bur without a bur guard or with a bur guard of incorrect length may cause the bur to whip or break.

Move the bur constantly across the area of resection for a faster, cleaner cut.

The full air return slightly reduces the torque on the drill. If this is a major deterrent to the use of the drill, the drill can be obtained with a single hose.

Bibliography

Adamson, J. E.; Horton, C. E. and Crawford, A. H.: External Pinning of the Unstable Zygomatic Arch Fracture. **Plast. and Reconstr. Surg.,** 36:343-348, September 1965.

Anderson, R. D. and Teague, D. A.: Blowout Fractures of the Orbital Floor. **Amer. J. Ophthal.,** 56:46-50, July 1963.

Bonaccolto, G.: Dacryocystorhinostomy with Polyethylene Tubing: A Simplified Technique. **J. Interna. Coll. Surg.,** 28:789-795, December 1957.

Brown, J. B.; Fryer, M. P. and Morgan, L. R.: Problems in Reconstruction of the Auricle. **Plast. and Reconstr. Surg.,** 43:597-603, June 1969.

Bullard, J. L. and Kingsburg, B. C.: Management of Fractures of Zygomatic Complex. **The Journal,** 214-217, June 1965.

Converse, J. M. and Smith, B.: Reconstruction of the Floor of the Orbit by Bone Grafts. **Arch. Ophthal.,** 44:1-21, July 1950.

Converse, J. M.: Reconstruction of the Auricle, Part 1. **Plast. and Reconstr. Surg.,** 22:150-163, August 1958.

Converse, J. M.: Reconstructive Plastic Surgery, Volume 1, 2 and 3. **W. B. Saunders Co.,** Philadelphia 1964.

Converse, J.M.: Construction of the Auricle in Unilateral Congenital Microtia. **Tr. Am. Acad. Ophth. & Otol.,** 72:995-1013, November/December 1968.

Conway, H.: **Letter** to Dr. Hall refering to "Dish Face Deformity". October 29, 1964.

Denecke, H. J. and Meyer, R.: Plastic Surgery of the Head and Neck. **Springer-Verlag,** Berlin-Heidelberg-New York, 1967.

Dingman, R. O.: Malunited Fractures of the Zygoma: Repair of Deformity. **Tr. Am. Acad. Ophth.,** 57:889-896, 1953.

Dingman, R. O. and Natvig, P.: Surgery of Facial Fractures. **W. B. Saunders Co.,** Philadelphia and London, 1969.

Farrior, R. T.: Implant Materials in Restoration of Facial Contour. **Laryngoscope,** 76:934-954, May 1966.

Foerster, D. W.: Total Reconstruction of the External Ear. **J. Okla. Med. Ass.,** 59:606-608, November 1966.

Gibbings, D. R.: Plastic Reconstruction of Facial Fractures. **J. Amer. Osteopath. Ass.,** 66:836-851, April 1967.

Goldman, J. B.: When is a Rhinoplasty Indicated for Correction of Recent Nasal Fractures? **Laryngoscope,** 74:689-700, May 1964.

Hansen, W. C.: **Letter** to Dr. Hall referring to "Sculpting of Silastic". August, 1969.

Iliff, C. E.: A Simplified Dacryocystorhinostomy. **Tr. Amer. Acad. Ophth. and Otol.,** 590-592, July-August 1954.

Jackson, F. E. et al.: Management of Combined Intracranial Injuries and Extensive Orbital-Facial Fractures. **Military Med.,** 134:7, July 1969.

Bibliography *(continued)*

Lipshutz, H. and Ardizone, R. A.: The Use of Silicone Rubber in Immediate Reconstruction of Fractures of the Orbit. **J. Trauma,** 3:563-568, November 1963.

Obwegeser, H. L.: Surgical Replacement of Small or Retrodisplaced Maxillae. **Plast. and Reconstr. Surg.,** 43:351-365, April 1969.

Pickrell, K. L.: Reconstructive Plastic Surgery of the Face. **Ciba, Clin. Symposia,** 19:71-99, July-August-September 1967.

Rankow, R. M.: An Atlas of Surgery of the Face, Mouth, and Neck. **W. B. Saunders Co.,** Philadelphia-London-Toronto 1968.

Smith, I.: Zygomatic and Orbital Fractures. **S. Afr. Med. J.,** 41:196-199, February 1967.

Stallard, H. B.: Reconstruction of the Socket. **Int. Ophthal. Clin.,** 4:503-521, June 1964.

Thomas, G. K. and Kasper, K. A.: Ossifying Fibroma of the Frontal Bone. **Arch. Otolaryn.,** 83:69-72, January 1966.

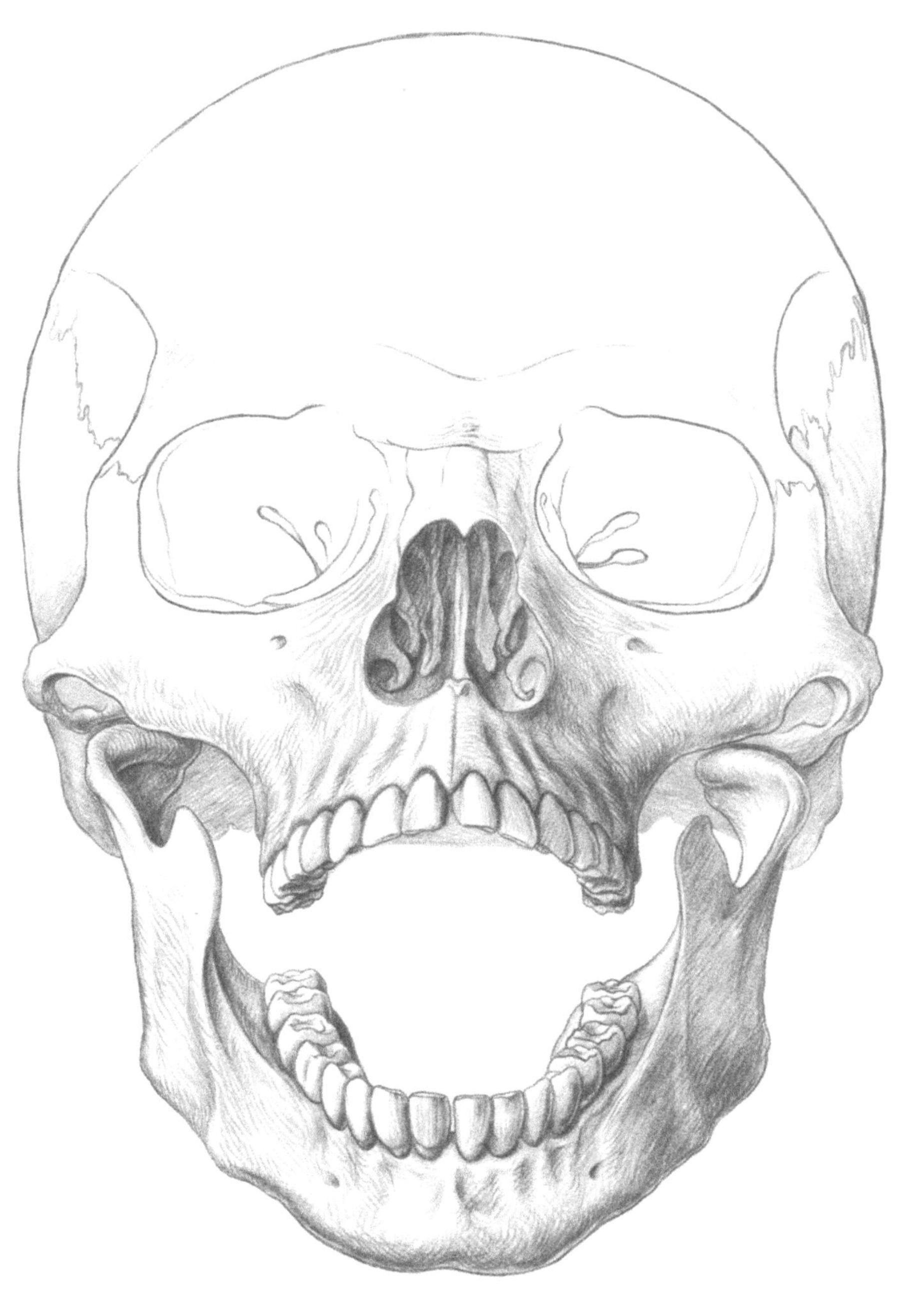

Contents

Contents *(continued)*

Vertical Osteotomy of the Ascending Ramus

1. Via a Risdon approach, elevate the musculature and periosteum; visualize the sigmoid notch and coronoid process. With the air drill and 12 long steel (saw-like) bur, make a vertical bone incision from the sigmoid notch to approximately 0.5 cm superior and posterior to the angle of the mandible. Intermittently irrigate with saline solution.

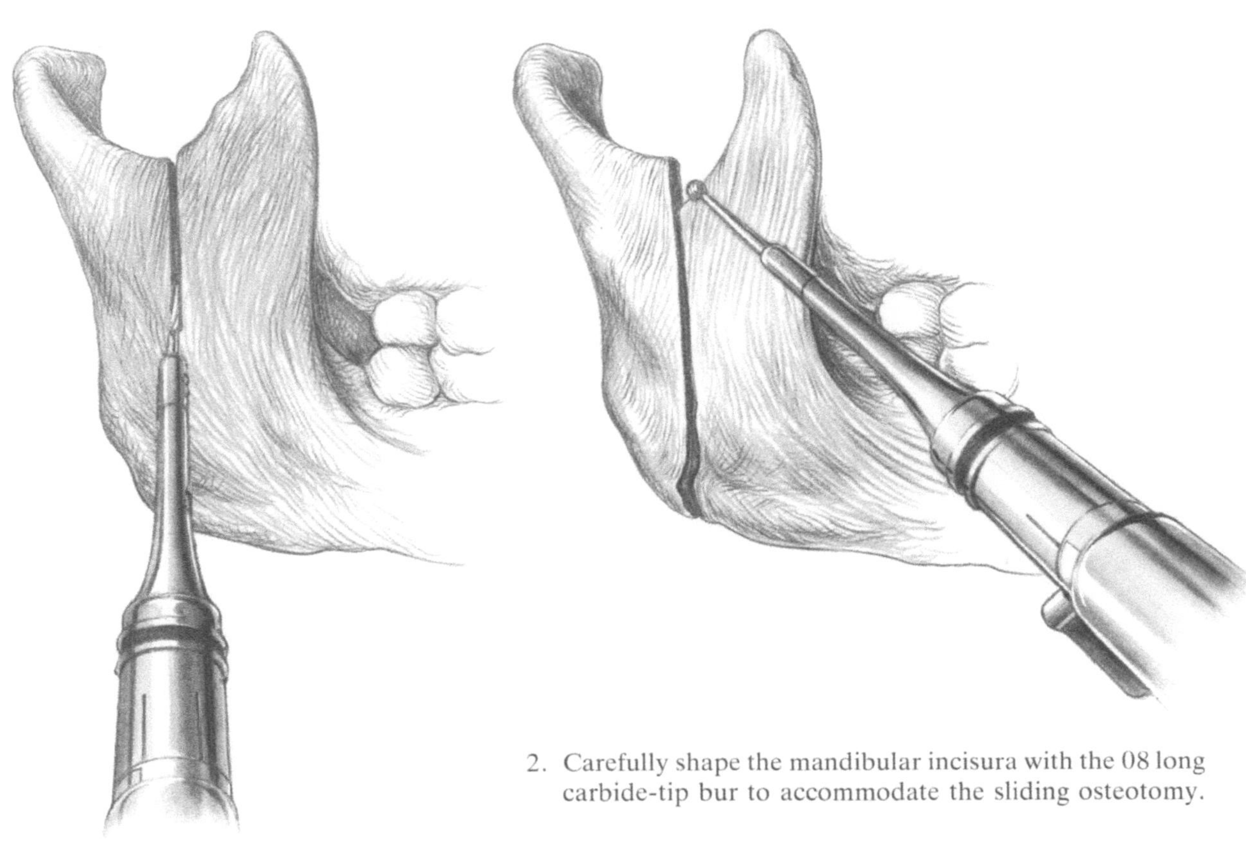

2. Carefully shape the mandibular incisura with the 08 long carbide-tip bur to accommodate the sliding osteotomy.

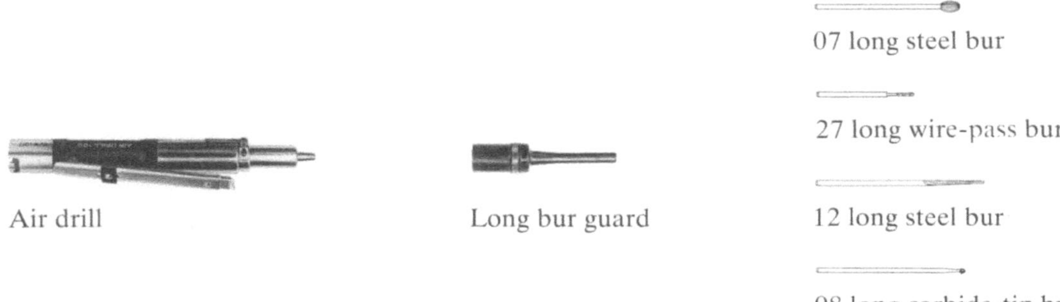

3. With the same bur make a notch in the mandibular angle to imbed and secure the fixation wire.

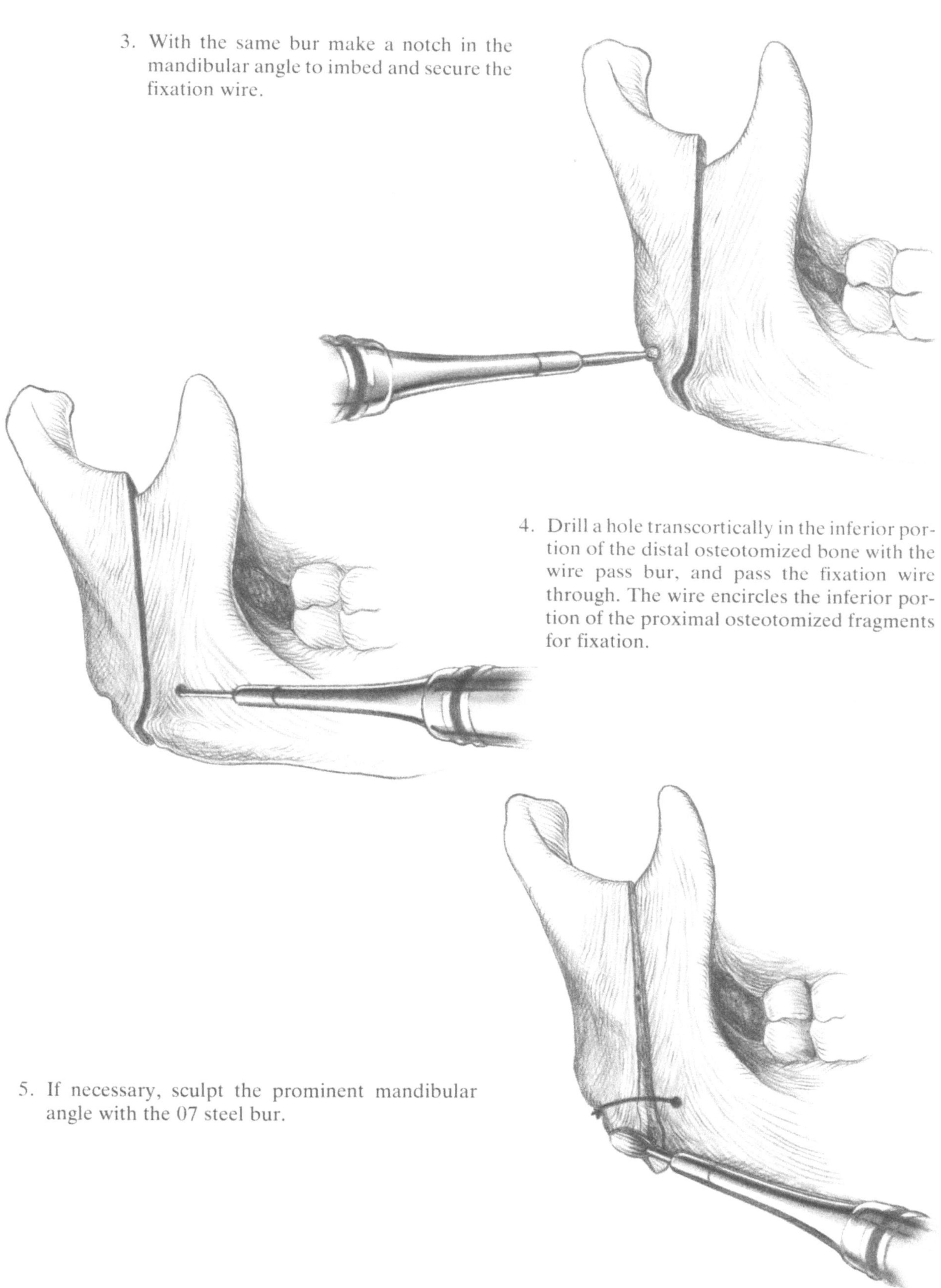

4. Drill a hole transcortically in the inferior portion of the distal osteotomized bone with the wire pass bur, and pass the fixation wire through. The wire encircles the inferior portion of the proximal osteotomized fragments for fixation.

5. If necessary, sculpt the prominent mandibular angle with the 07 steel bur.

Anterior Maxillary Osteotomy*

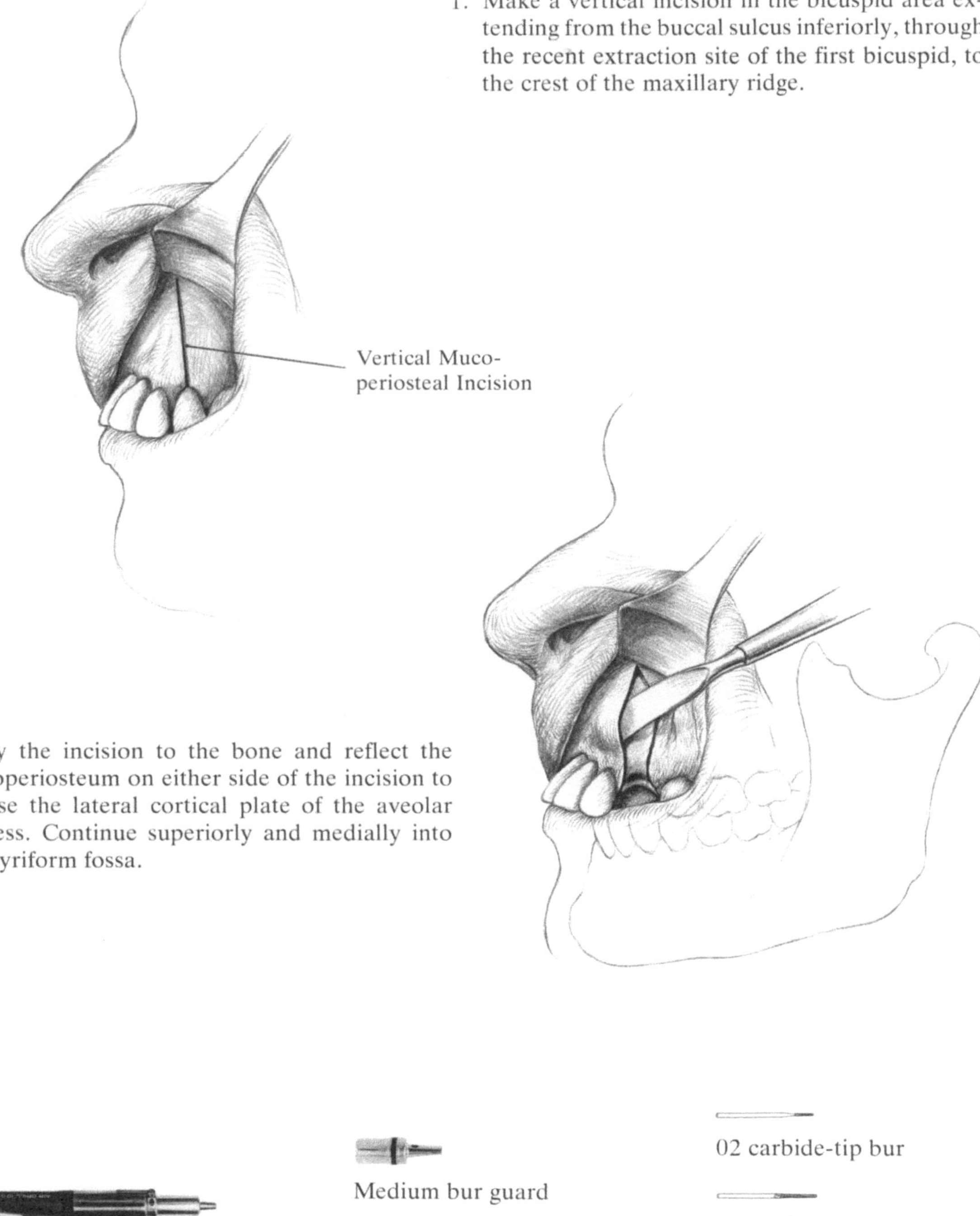

1. Make a vertical incision in the bicuspid area extending from the buccal sulcus inferiorly, through the recent extraction site of the first bicuspid, to the crest of the maxillary ridge.

2. Carry the incision to the bone and reflect the mucoperiosteum on either side of the incision to expose the lateral cortical plate of the aveolar process. Continue superiorly and medially into the pyriform fossa.

---

* Col. Donald C. Osbon, D.C., Chief of Oral Surgery, Letterman General Hospital, San Francisco, California, USA (Personal Communication).

3. With the 02 carbide-tip bur make a vertical incision in the cortical plate in the first biscuspid area. Extend the incision superiorly above the apex of the cuspid root and then angle the incision anteriorly into the lateral portion of the pyriform fossa. Enlarge the groove to obtain the desired space for setback of the premaxilla.

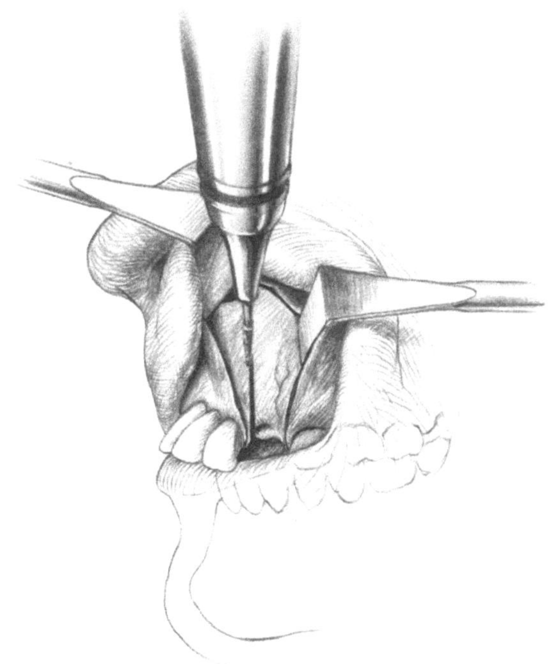

4. Pack the area with gauze sponge. Make a similar incision on the other side of the maxilla and perform the same procedure. Pack this area with gauze sponge and turn the patient's head to expose the palate.

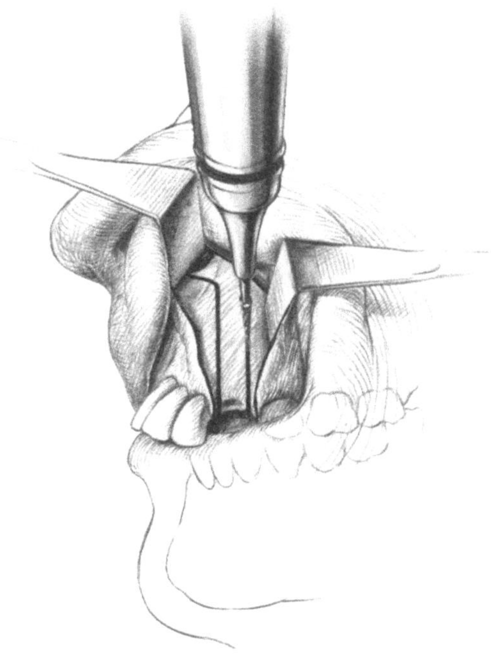

Anterior Maxillary Osteotomy *(continued)*

5. Remove the bone segment on one side.

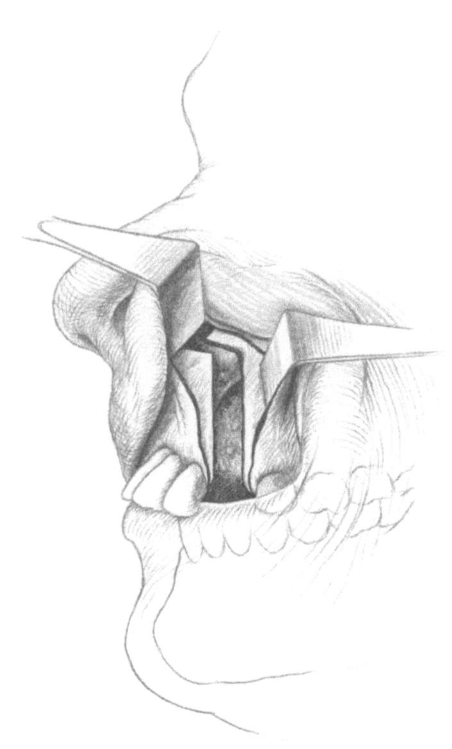

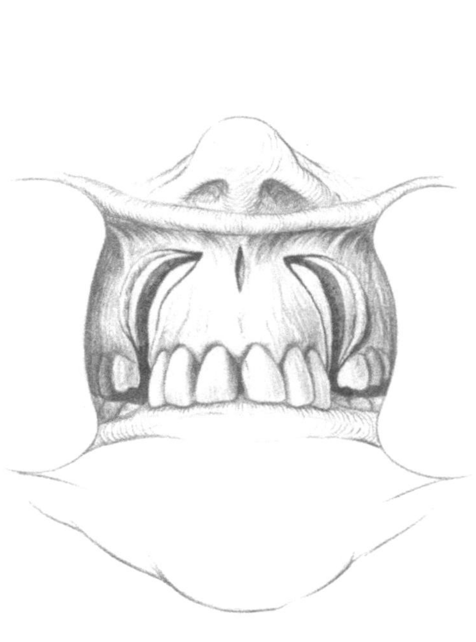

6. Remove the anterior maxillary bone segments. A vertical incision is made over the nasal spine.

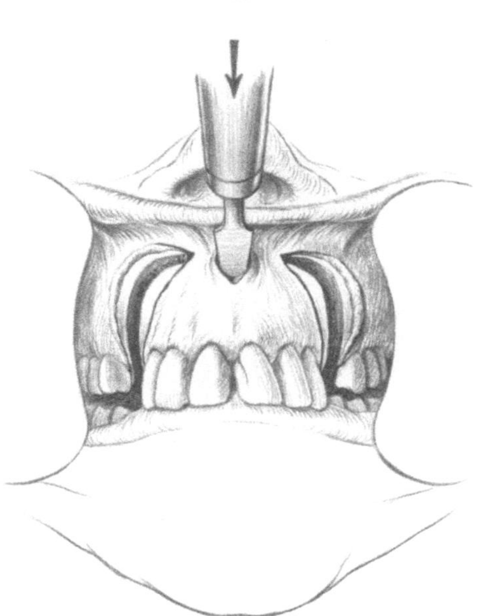

7. With a half-inch bi-bevel chisel tap gently to free the premaxilla and the midline from the nasal septum. Place the chisel just above the nasal spine and direct it posteriorly. It may be necessary to use the chisel on the lateral nasal walls bilaterally if the nasal septum is not completely detached.

8. Turn bilateral palatal mucosal flaps and with the bur and tissue retractor guard tunnel across the palate.

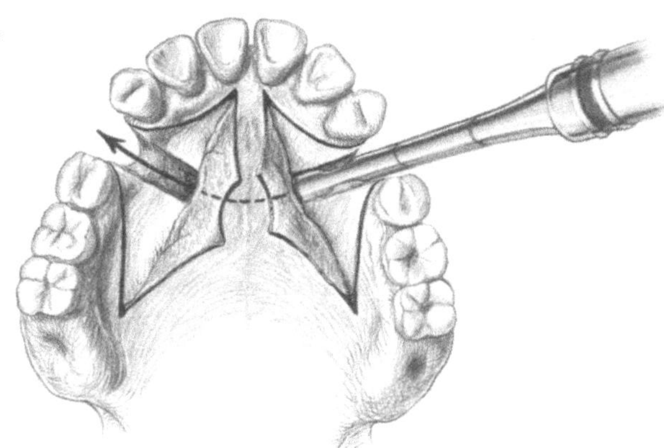

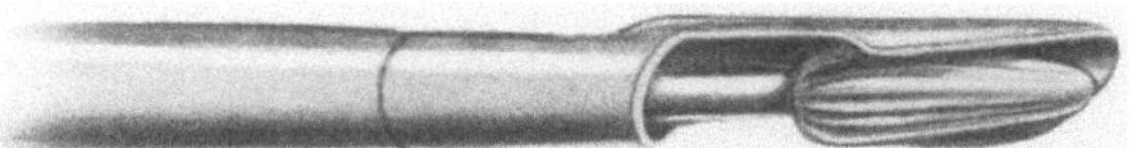

9. The guard (enlarged) covers the bur and prevents tissue trauma.

10. The anterior maxillary push-back is complete.

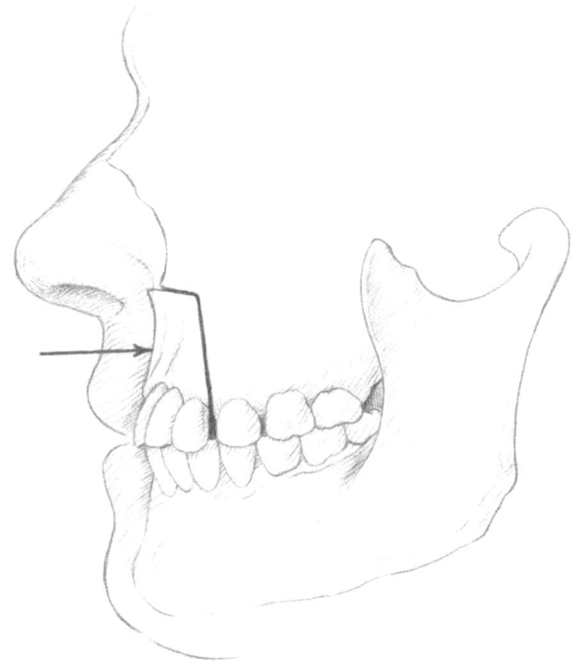

Bilateral Oblique Sliding Osteotomy of the Rami of the Mandible*

With a methylene blue marker indicate the incision line beginning one finger breadth below and behind the angle of the mandible, bisect the angle, and extend the incision for approximately 4.5 cm. Plan the incision to be parallel with the normal skin creases of the neck. Dissect down to the bone in the normal manner. Incise the periosteum and with periosteal elevators elevate the periosteum and the attached masseter muscles and reflect them from the lateral surface of the angle and ramus of the mandible with the internal pterygoid muscle. Also reflect the periosteum from the medial surface of the angle of the mandible.

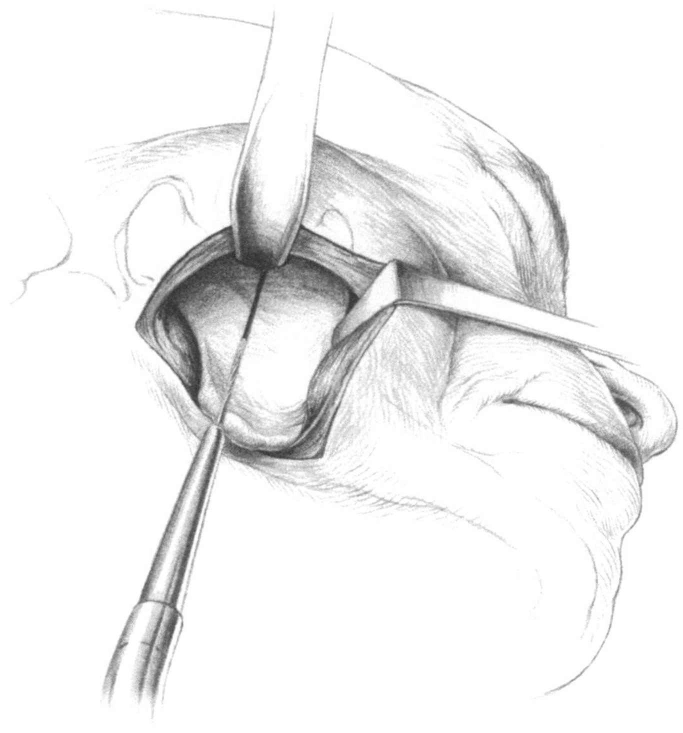

1. Using the 20° angle and 14 steel bur make an incision through the lateral cortical plate of the ramus of the man- dible along the line marked in meth- ylene blue. Do not carry the incision completely through the ramus at this time.

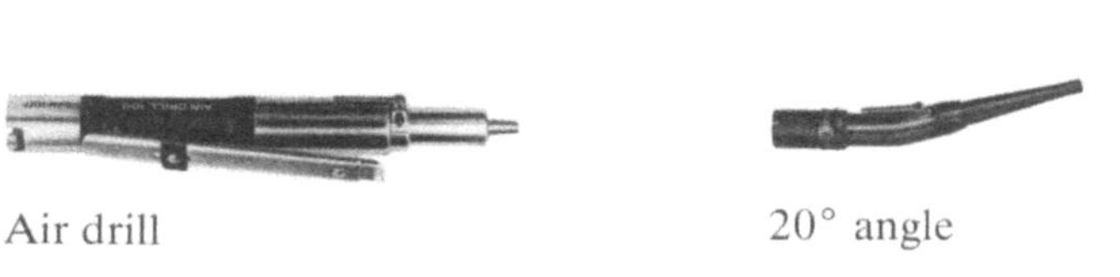

Air drill   20° angle   14 long steel bur

07 long steel bur

04 long carbide-tip bur

27 long wire-pass bur

---

* Col. Donald C. Osbon, D.C., Chief of Oral Surgery, Letterman General Hospital, San Francisco, California, USA (Personal Communication).

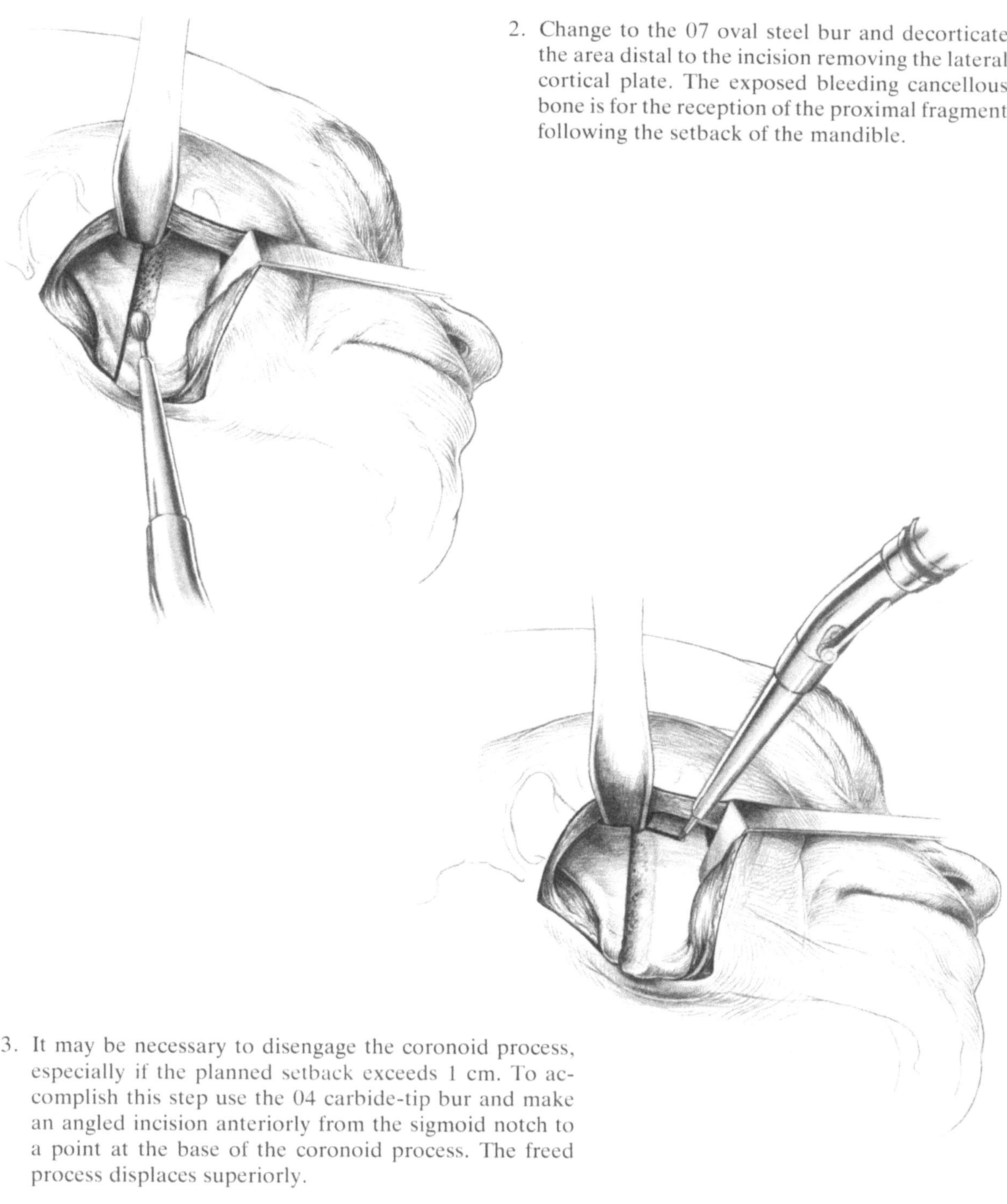

2. Change to the 07 oval steel bur and decorticate the area distal to the incision removing the lateral cortical plate. The exposed bleeding cancellous bone is for the reception of the proximal fragment following the setback of the mandible.

3. It may be necessary to disengage the coronoid process, especially if the planned setback exceeds 1 cm. To accomplish this step use the 04 carbide-tip bur and make an angled incision anteriorly from the sigmoid notch to a point at the base of the coronoid process. The freed process displaces superiorly.

Bilateral Oblique Sliding Osteotomy of the Rami of the Mandible *(continued)*

4. Now, with the same bur, complete the proximal incision through the ramus of the mandible separating the proximal and distal fragments.

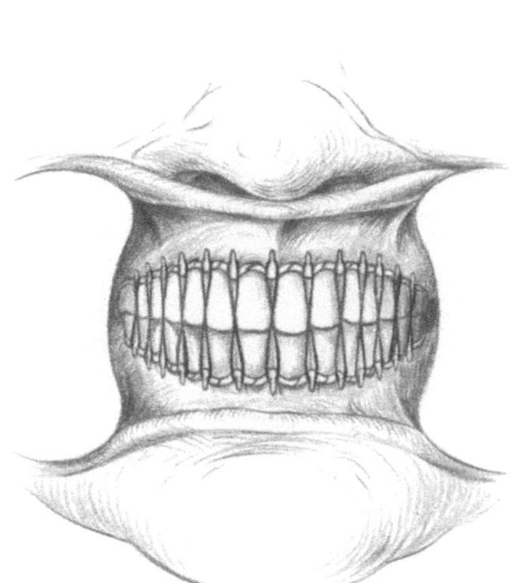

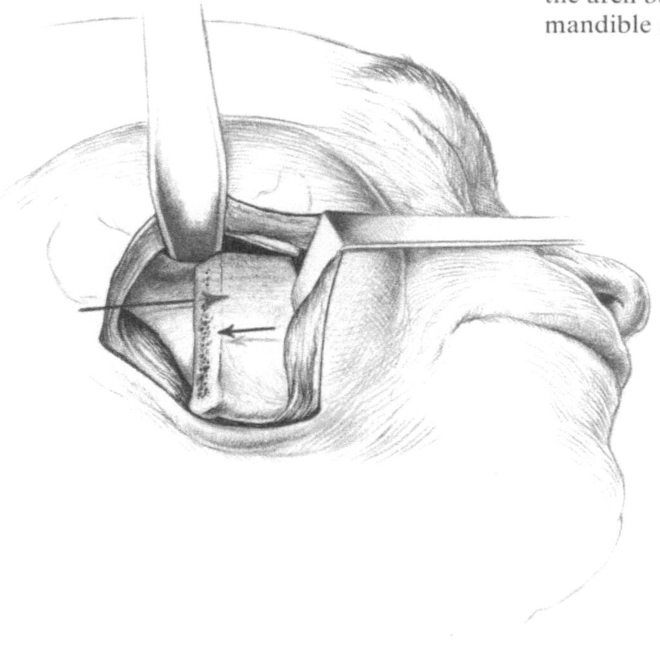

5. Position the proximal fragment laterally and anteriorly to the distal fragment and place a hot laparotomy pack in the wound. Duplicate the procedure on the other side of the mandible. Reposition the patient's mandible and move the mandible back until the teeth are in the predetermined occlusion. Apply intermaxillary elastics to the arch bars inserted preoperatively and immobilize the mandible against the maxilla.

6. The anterior fragment overlies the posterior fragment temporarily after the push-back.

7. Expose once again the submandibular area. With the 27 wire-pass bur drill holes in the distal fragments approximately 1 cm superior to the angle of the mandible and insert a length of .018 wire.

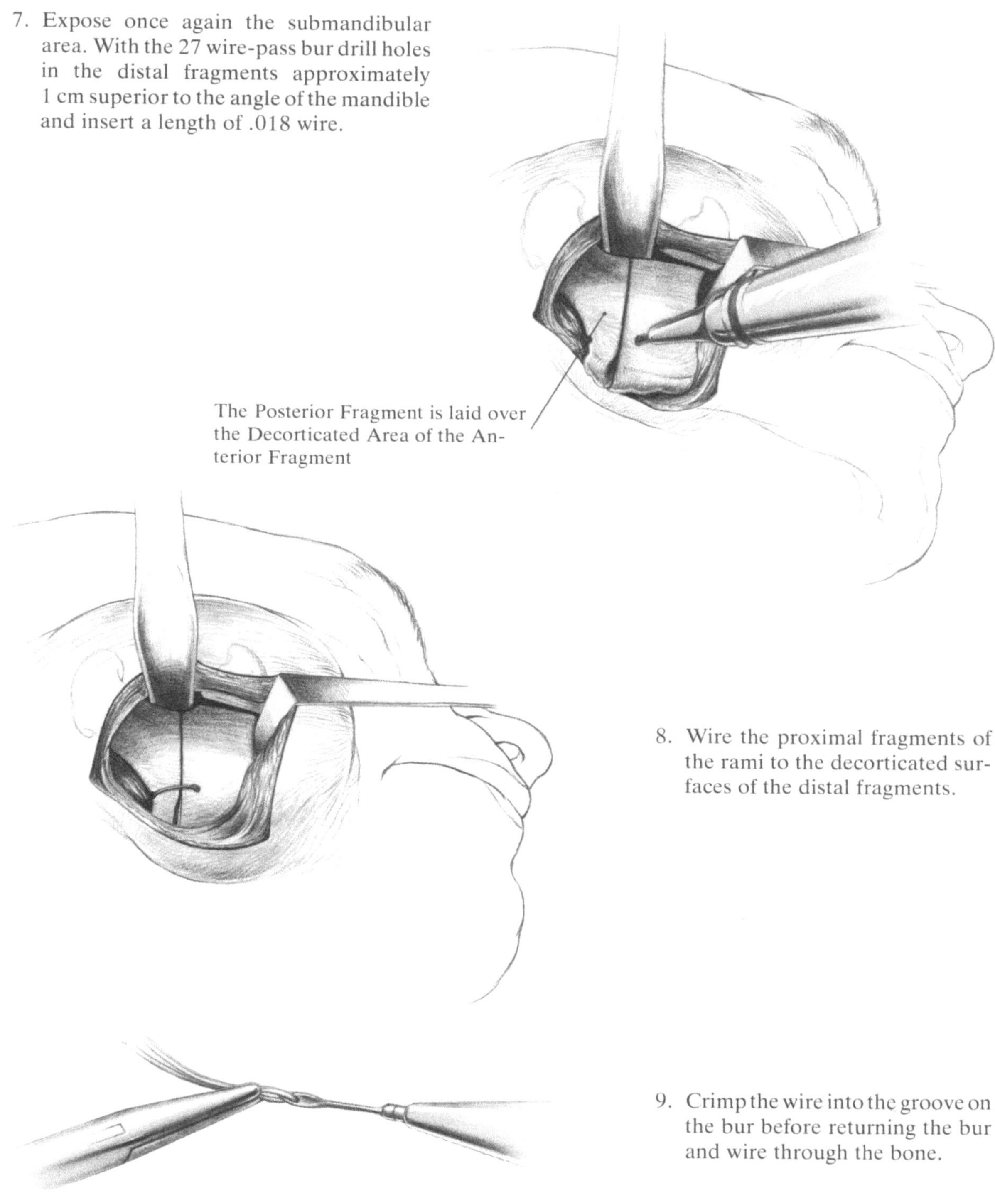

The Posterior Fragment is laid over the Decorticated Area of the Anterior Fragment

8. Wire the proximal fragments of the rami to the decorticated surfaces of the distal fragments.

9. Crimp the wire into the groove on the bur before returning the bur and wire through the bone.

10. Close the wounds in layers with 3-0 Chromic catgut deep, 3-0 catgut subcutaneously and 5-0 dermalon skin sutures. Apply an external pressure dressing to the face and submandibular areas.

Bilateral Midsagittal Osteotomy of the Rami of the Mandible*

1. Begin the incision in the buccal vestibule from a point midway on the anterior surface of the coronoid process of the ramus of the mandible. Extend the incision inferiorly along the external oblique ridge to the buccal surface of the mandible, adjacent to the second molar.

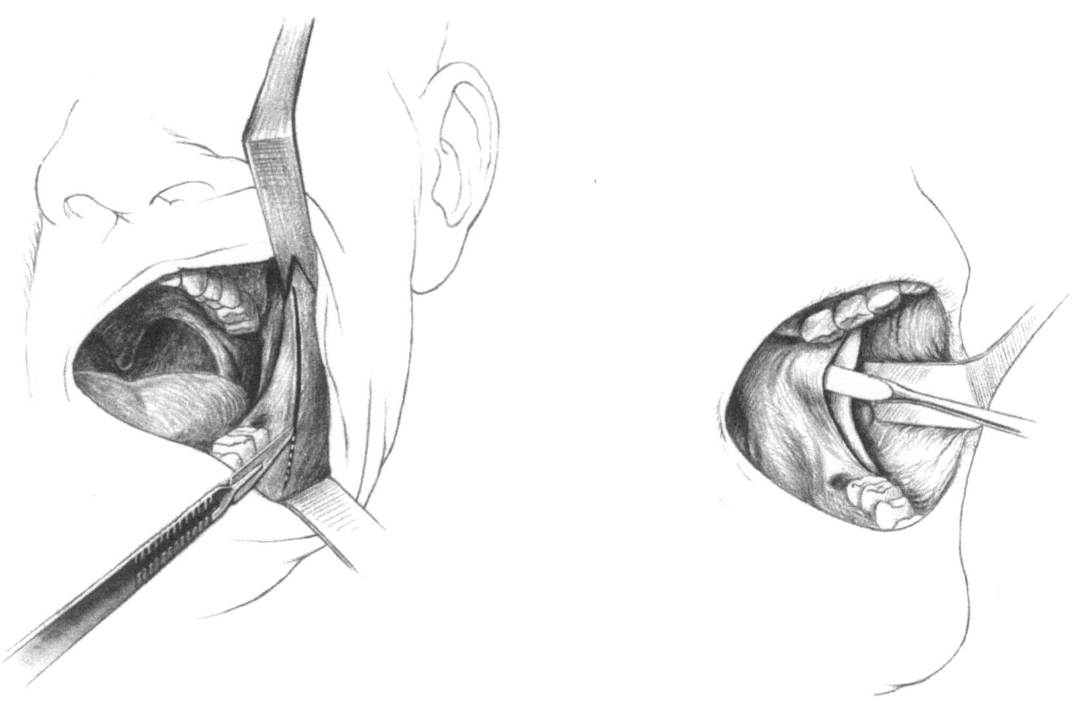

2. With a Obwegeser periosteal elevator reflect the mucoperiosteum from the lateral surface of the mandible from the second molar area to the angle and up the ramus to the level of the sigmoid notch.

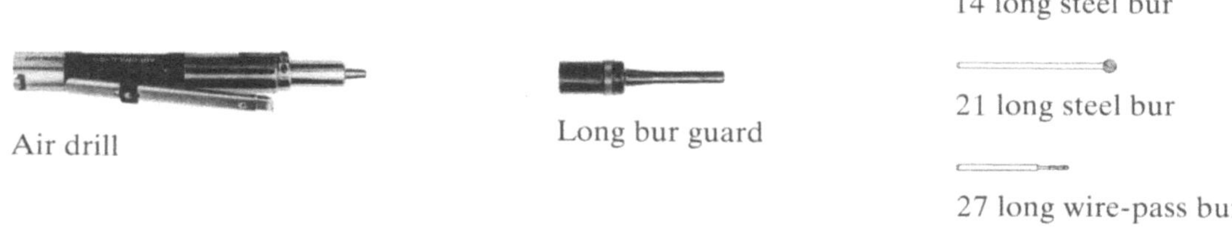

---

* Col. Donald C. Osbon, D.C., Chief or Oral Surgery, Letterman General Hospital, San Francisco, California, USA (Personal Communication).

3. Elevate the mucoperiosteum from the lingual surface of the ramus of the mandible superior to the lingula, and reflect the neurovascular bundle medially. If a third mandibular molar is in position at this time, it is necessary to remove it.

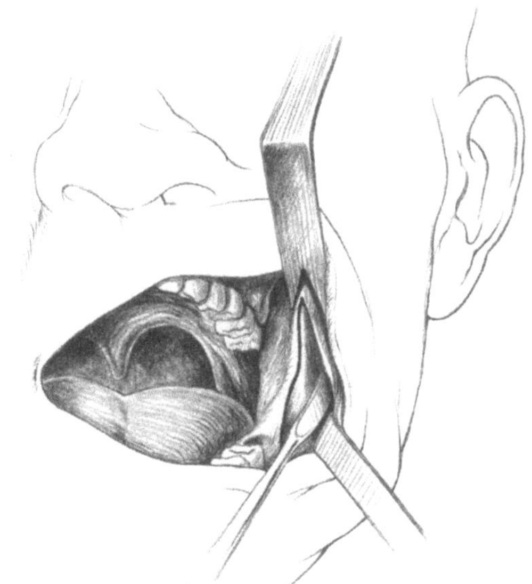

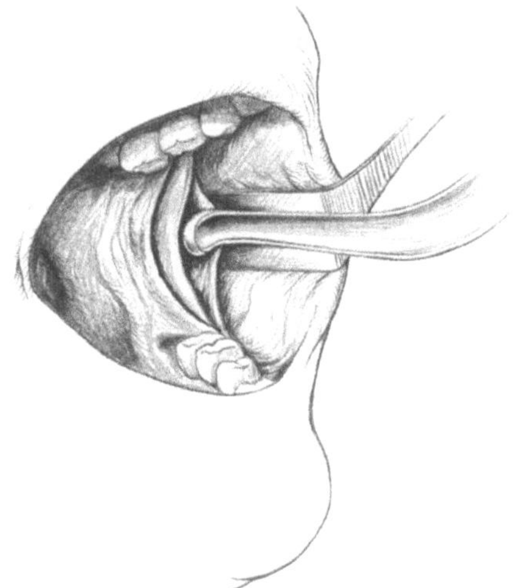

4. Insert the first Obwegeser retractor.

5. Both buccal and lingual cup retractors are inserted to engage the posterior border of the ramus, just below the condylar neck exposing both the lateral and medial surfaces of the ramus of the mandible above the level of the lingula.

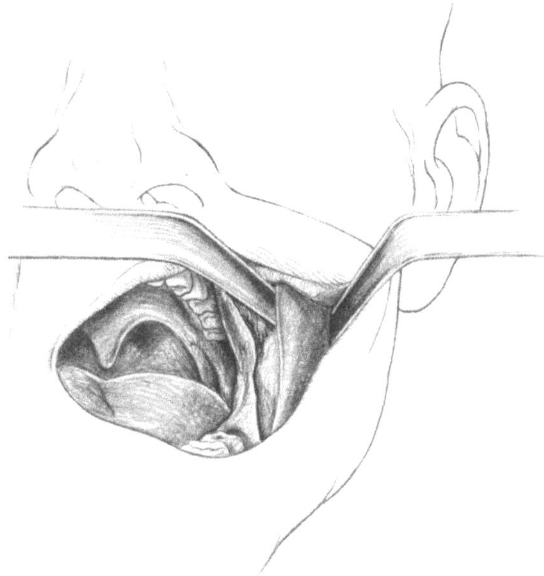

Bilateral Midsagittal Osteotomy of the Rami of the Mandible *(continued)*

6. Using the 20° angle for improved visualization, and the 21 long steel bur, make a horizontal incision on the medial surface of the ramus, just through the cortical plate extending it from the lingual fossa anteriorly, to the external oblique ridge.

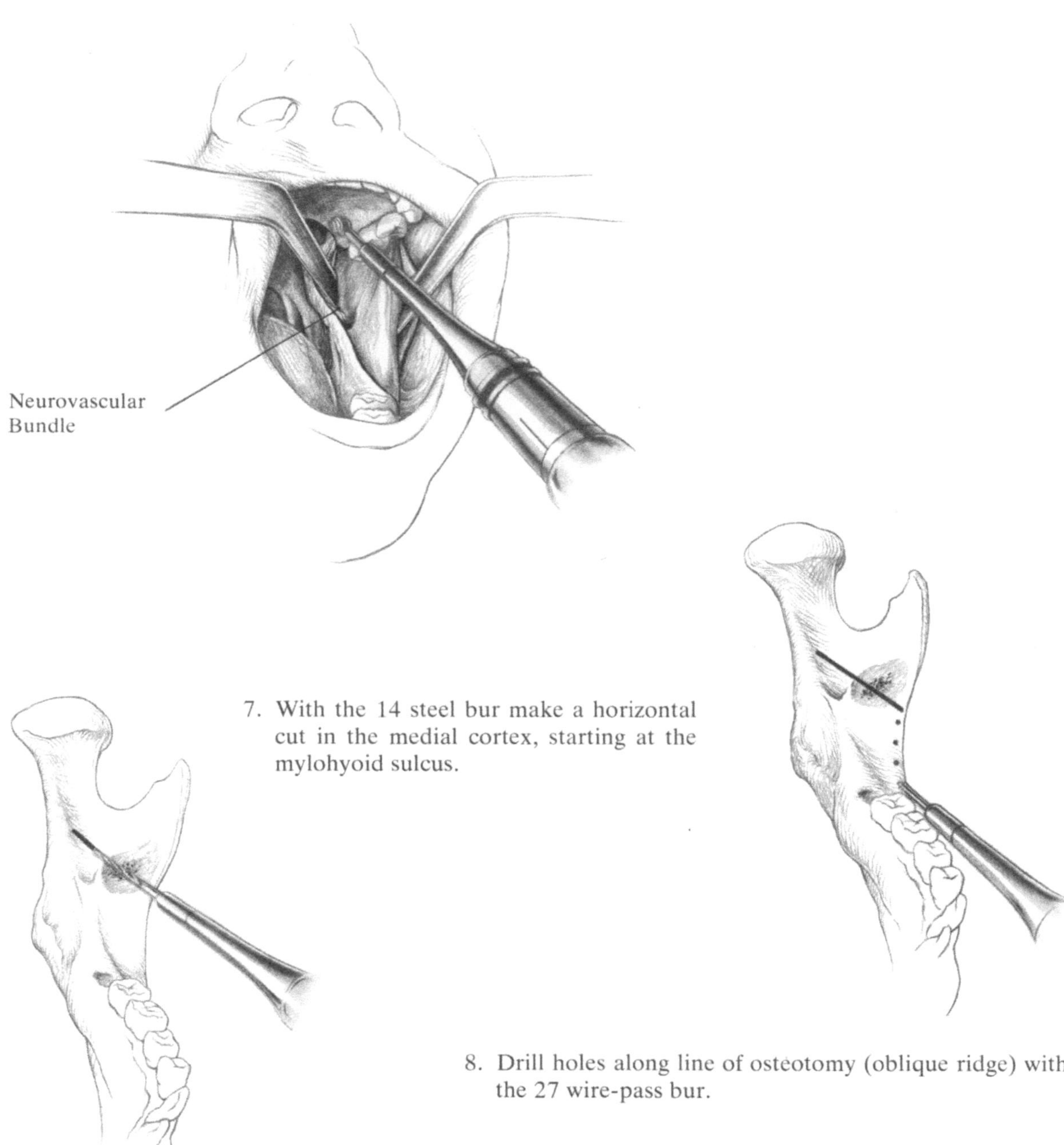

7. With the 14 steel bur make a horizontal cut in the medial cortex, starting at the mylohyoid sulcus.

8. Drill holes along line of osteotomy (oblique ridge) with the 27 wire-pass bur.

9. Drill holes with the same bur on the lateral surface of the ramus to the end of the oblique ridge.

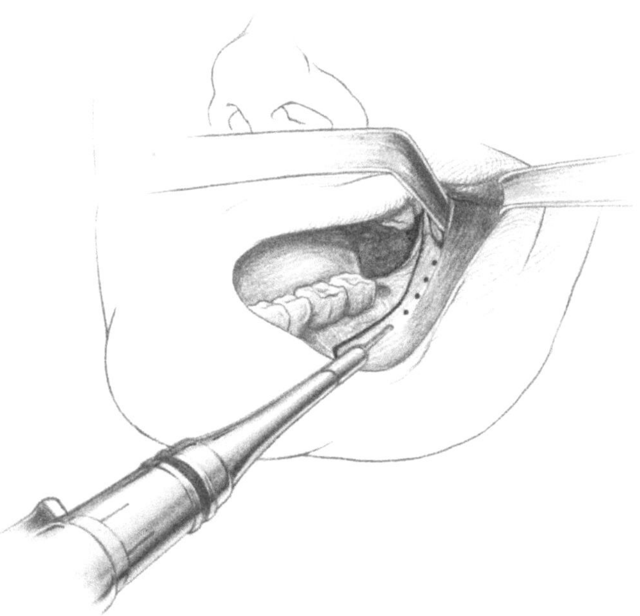

10. Join the drill holes with the 14 steel bur. Do not apply too much pressure to the bur, as it may slow down and then cutting efficiency is reduced.

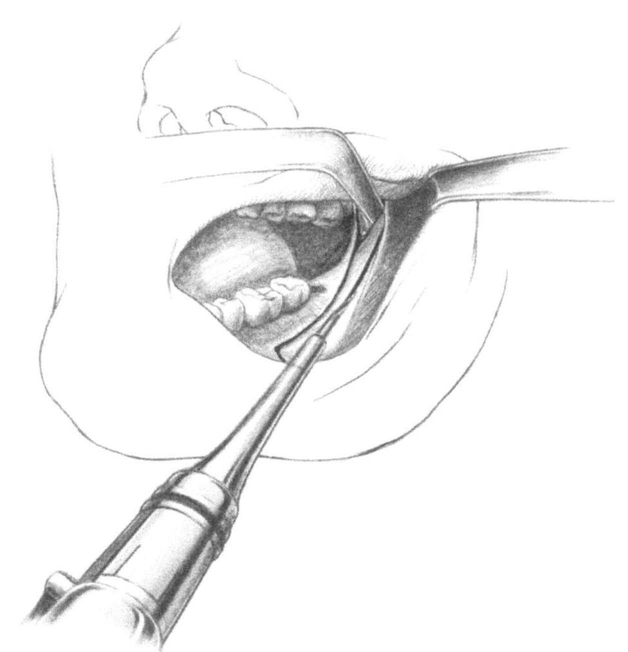

Bilateral Midsagittal Osteotomy of the Rami of the Mandible *(continued)*

11. Make an upward cut to join the incision along the oblique ridge with the 14 steel bur.

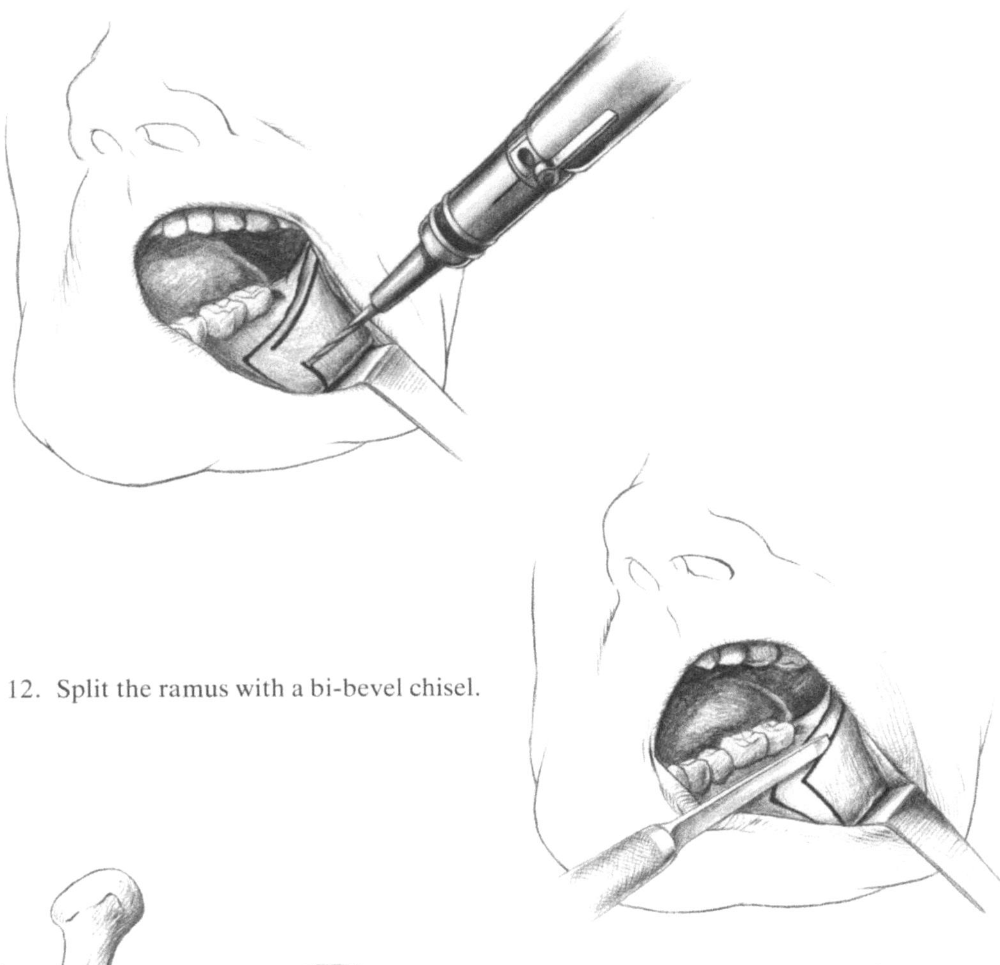

12. Split the ramus with a bi-bevel chisel.

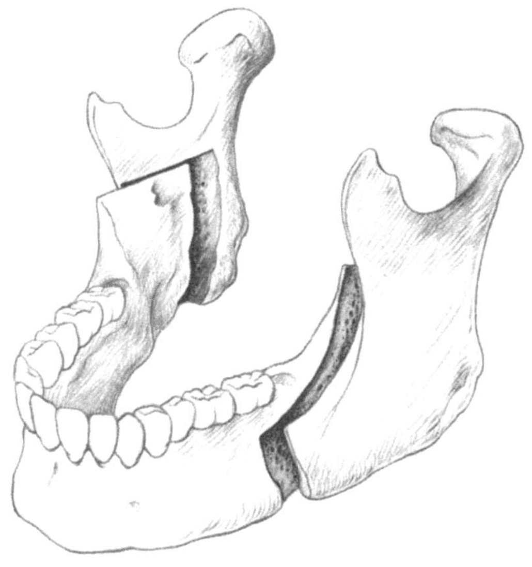

13. Following bilateral osteotomies the mandible is advanced.

Intraoral Step Osteotomy of the Body of the Mandible*

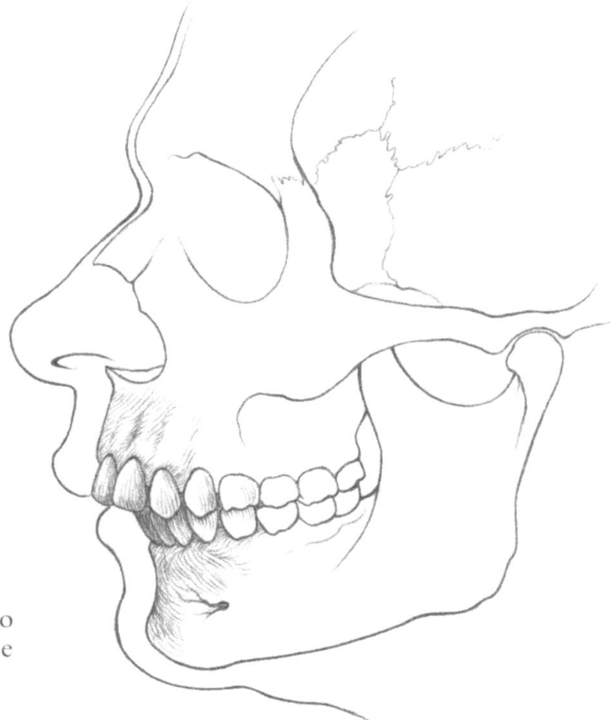

1. Reflect a generous mediolateral flap to expose both cortices of the body of the mandible.

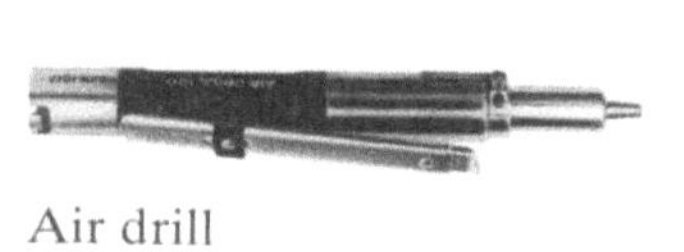

Air drill

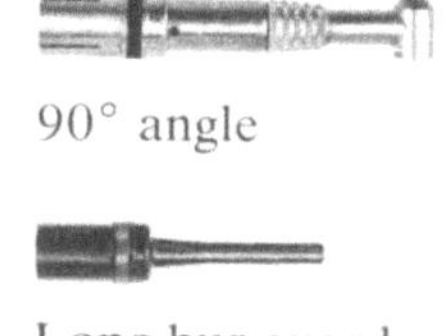

90° angle

Long bur guard

12 short steel bur

22 long diamond bur

21 long steel bur

* J. M. Converse, M.D.: Reconstructive Plastic Surgery. **W. B. Saunders Co.,** 1964.

Intraoral Step Osteotomy of the Body of the Mandible *(continued)*

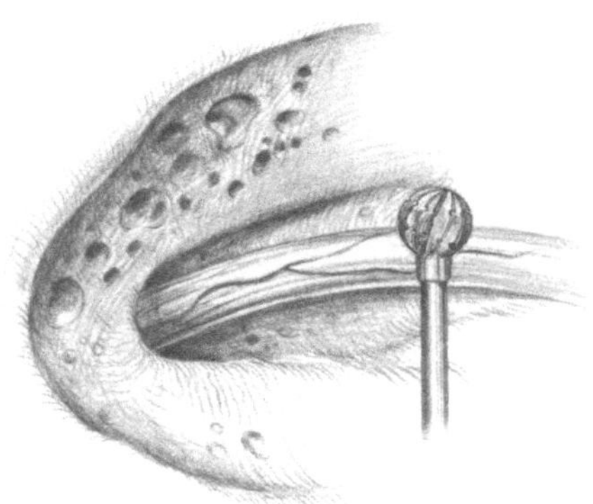

2. Unroof the inferior alveolar nerve with the long bur guard and 21 long steel bur.

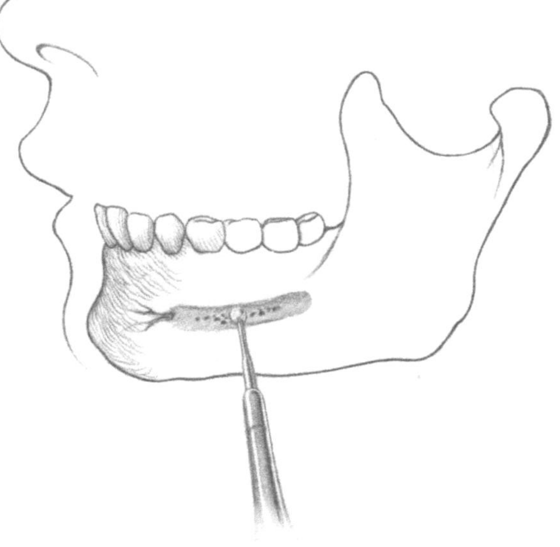

3. During this procedure use constant irrigation and suction. When the nerve sheath is exposed change to the diamond bur.

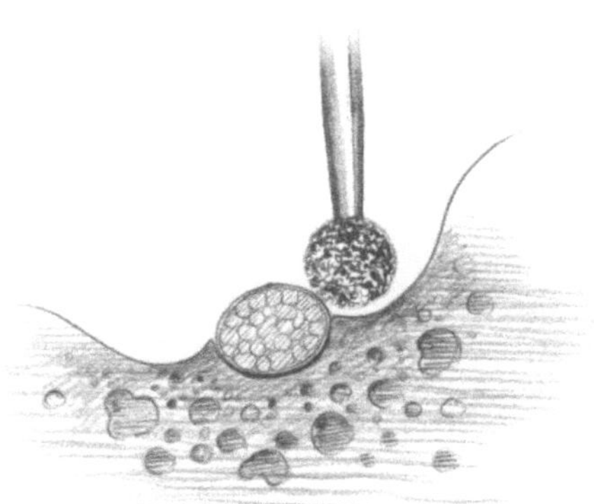

4. Utilize a large diamond bur to remove the bone from around the nerve sheath. To expose a 180° circumference of the nerve sheath, make a trough with the diamond bur along the sides of the nerve*. The use of diamond burs proximal to vital structures is mandatory to prevent surgical laceration or structural damage to this tissue.

---

* J. L. Pulec, M. D.: Facial Nerve Grafting. **Laryngoscope** LXXIX: 1562 - 1582, September 1969.

5. Outline and incise the line of osteotomy with the 90° angle and 12 short steel bur. Hold the nerve gently out of position with a nerve retractor to maintain sensory innervation of the teeth and lower lip.

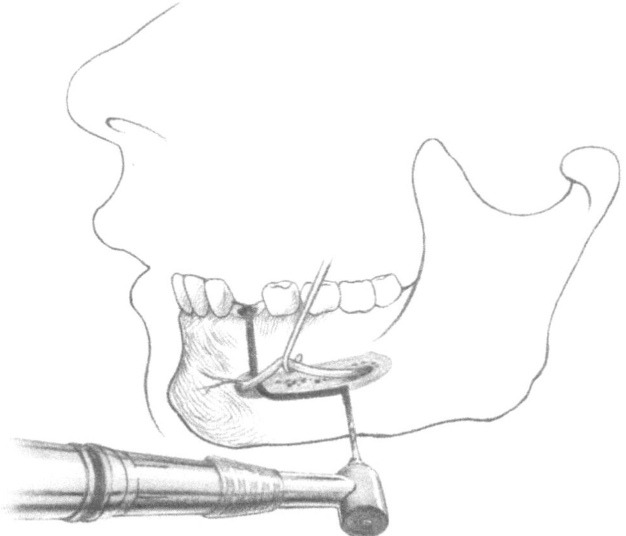

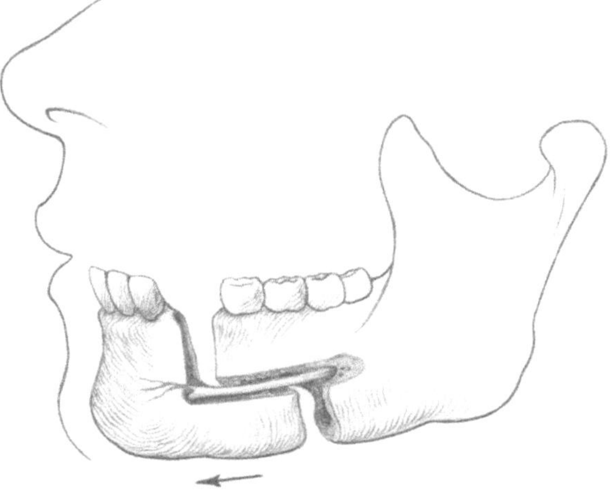

6. A bilateral osteotomy allows repositioning of the mandible with possible insertion of autogenous or heterogenous bone grafts.

Horizontal Mandibular Osteotomy

Some oral procedures, because of the surgical approach or amount of bone to be excised, could benefit from the more traditional powered reciprocating saw. The saw reciprocates at 20,000 times per minute with the air driver at full speed. The speed can be controlled at the throttle or the speed-selector ring. Move the blade slightly in saw-like fashion rather than applying pressure to the blade. This will give a faster, smoother cut. Irrigate with isotonic saline to lubricate the interface of blade and bone.

To assemble the air driver and reciprocating saw:

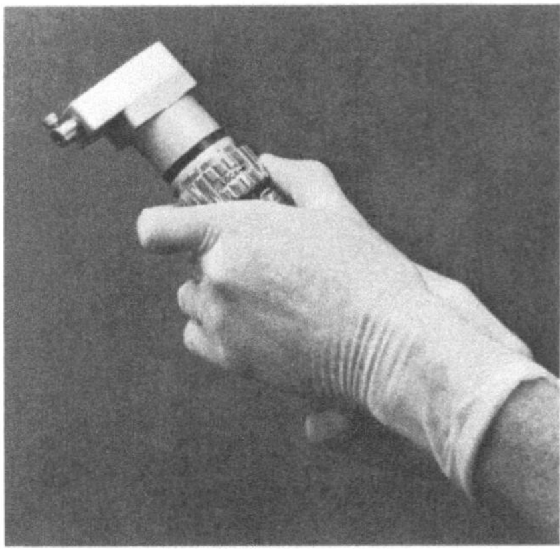

1. Seat attachment securely over the air driver and lock.

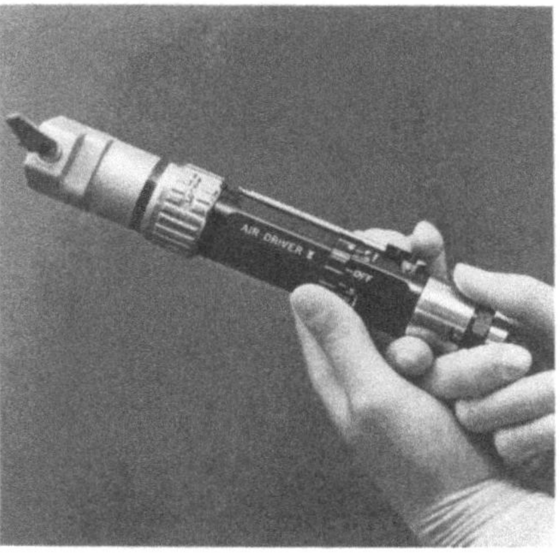

3. For maximum cutting efficiency, run at full speed.

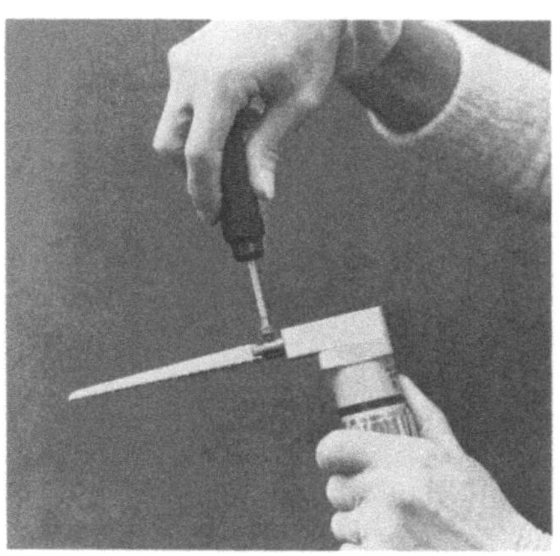

2. Insert reciprocating blade, set at the required angle and secure with the hex wrench.

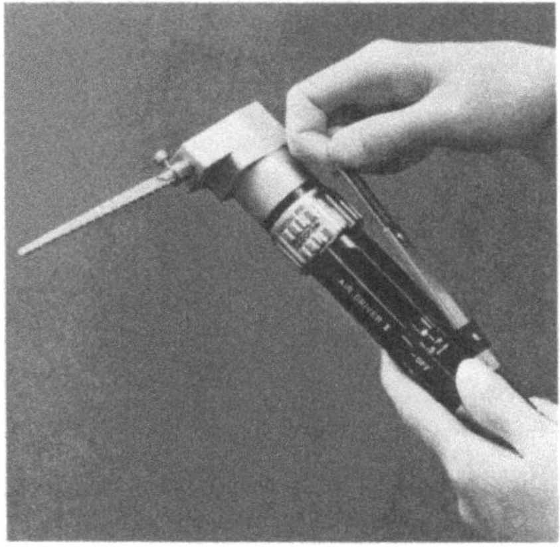

4. The throttle has variable speed and an extension handle.

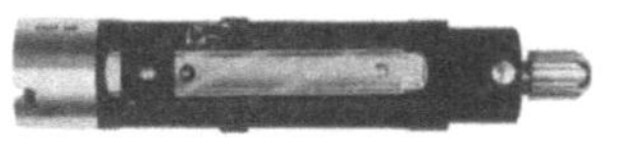

Air driver

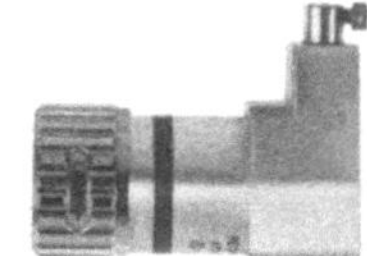

Reciprocating saw attachment

Reciprocating saw blade

5. Make the horizontal incision with the reciprocating blade.

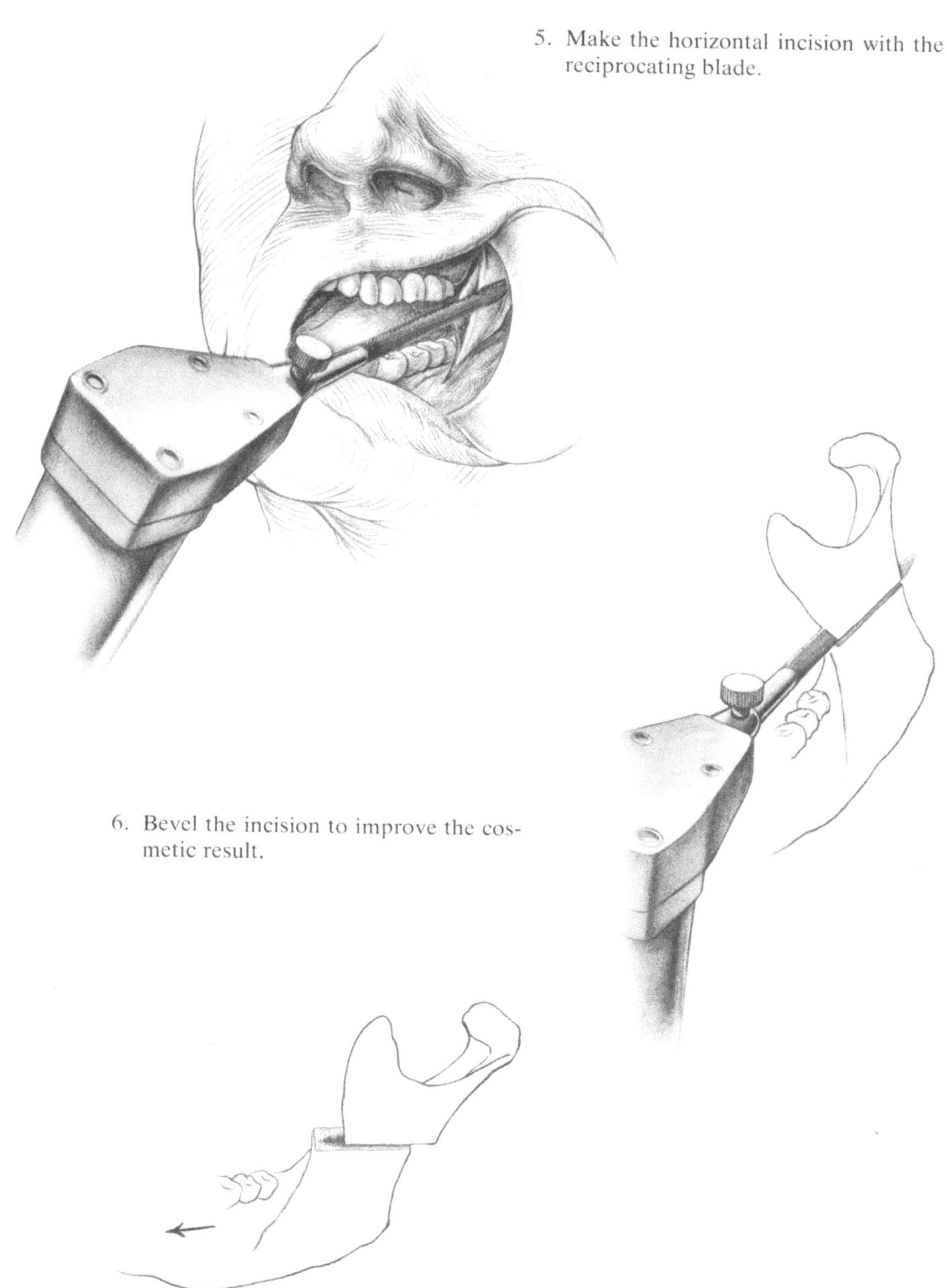

6. Bevel the incision to improve the cosmetic result.

Degloving the Mandible for Mentoplasty

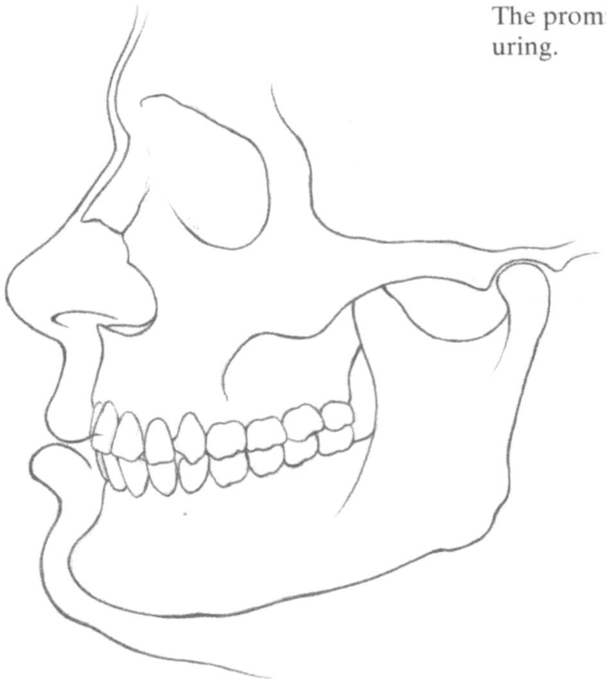

The prominent chin is cosmetically disfiguring.

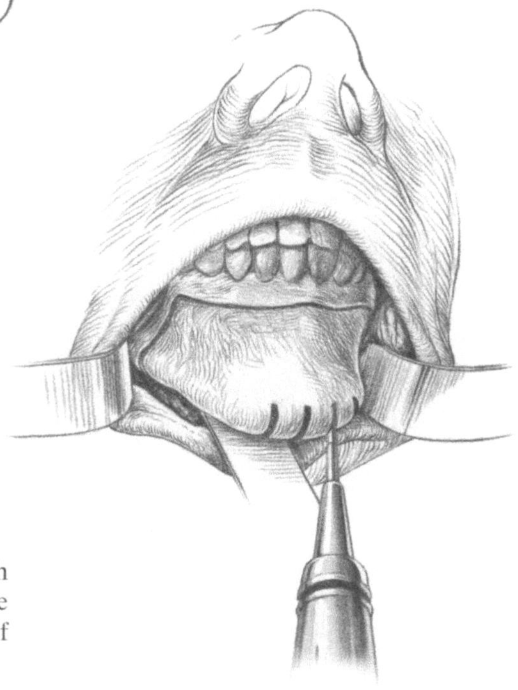

1. Expose the mandibular bone and with the 06 carbide-tip bur make slots in the mandible to determine the amount of bone reduction required.

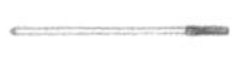

06 carbide-tip bur

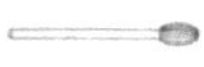

07 steel bur

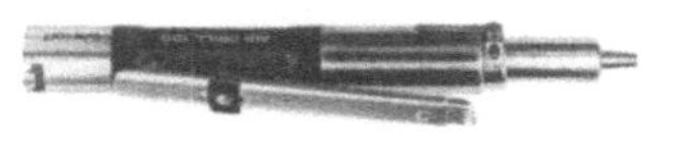

Air drill

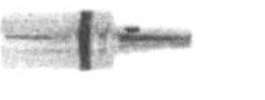

Medium bur guard

2. Sculpt the bone with the 07 oval steel bur down to the required depth.

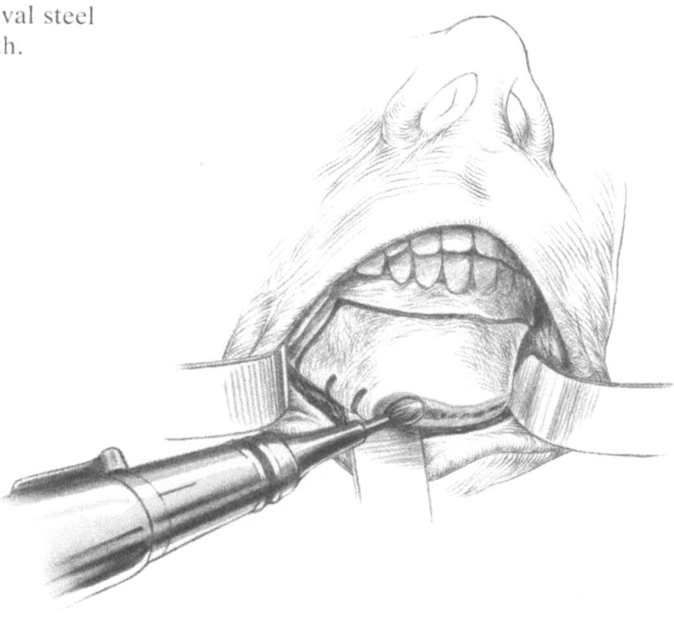

3. The bur produces a smooth contoured reduction.

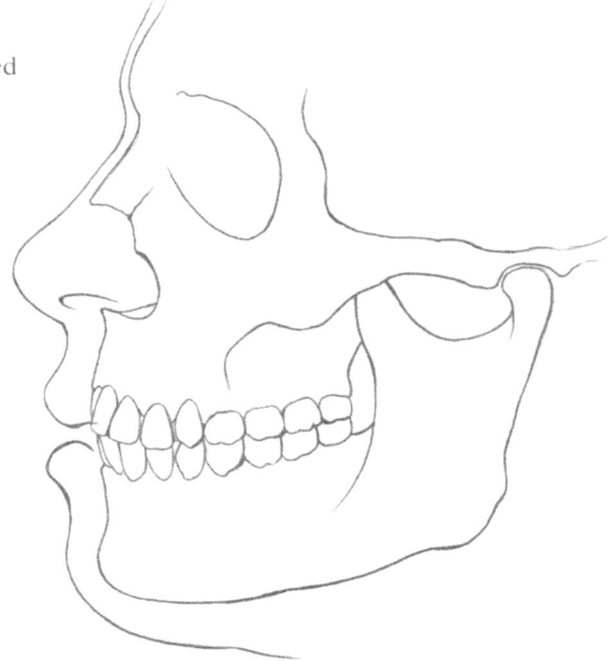

Condylectomy

Assemble the 20° angle and bur:

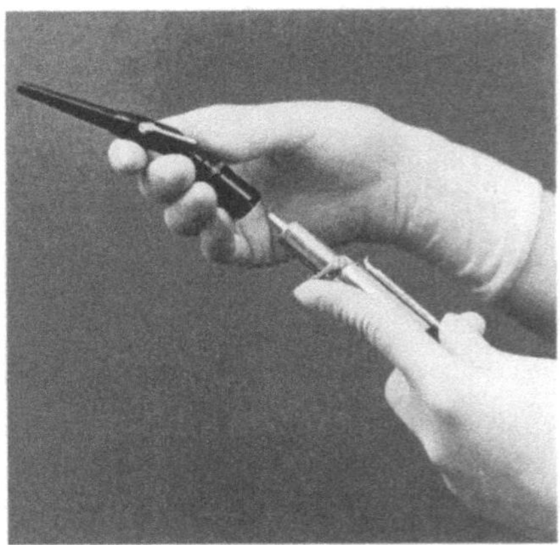

1. Slip 20° angle snugly over the shoulder of the drill, while raising the bur release lever.

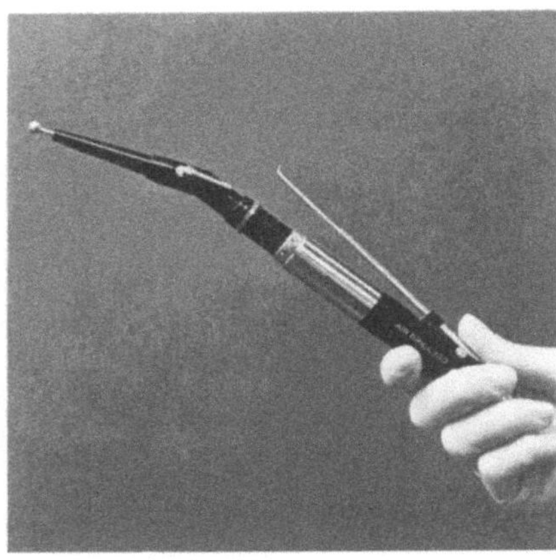

3. Lock bur securely by returning lever flush against attachment.

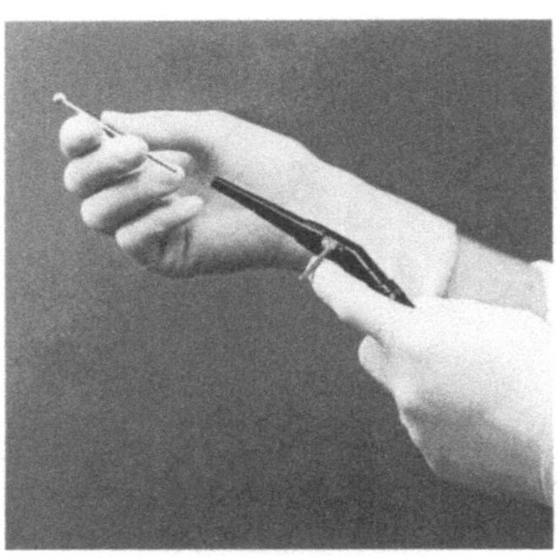

2. Insert a long bur with the release lever raised on the 20° angle.

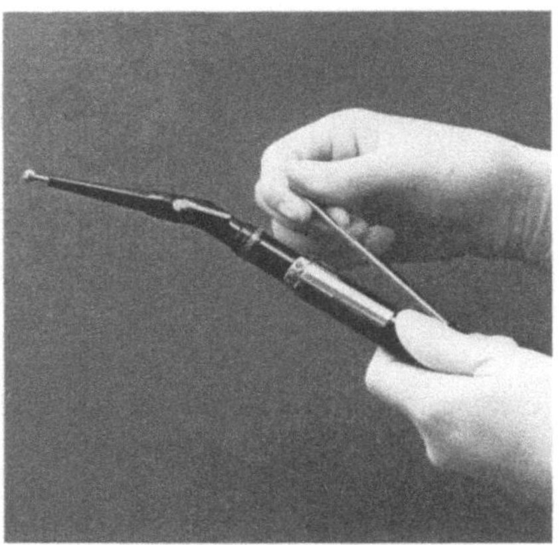

4. Use extension for increased fingertip control.

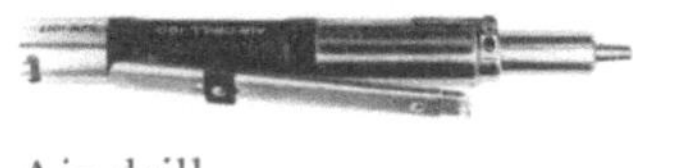

Air drill

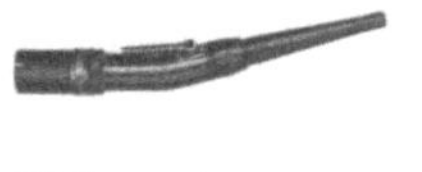

20° angle

06 long carbide-tip bur

19 long steel bur

5. Use the 06 carbide tip bur to section through the neck of the condyle. Excise the bone subperiosteally.

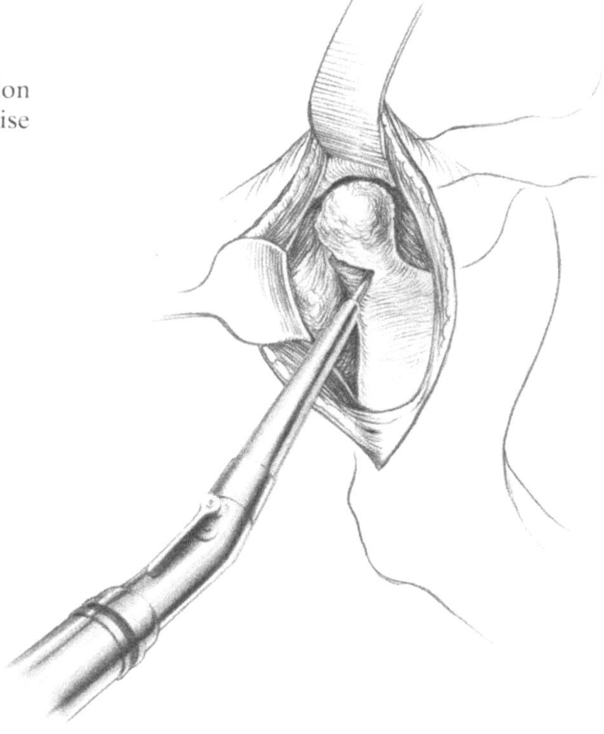

6. Smooth the incised surface of the ascending ramus with the 19 long steel bur. The 20° angle improves visibility at the bur tip but does not eliminate the need for suitable retraction medial to the condylar process.

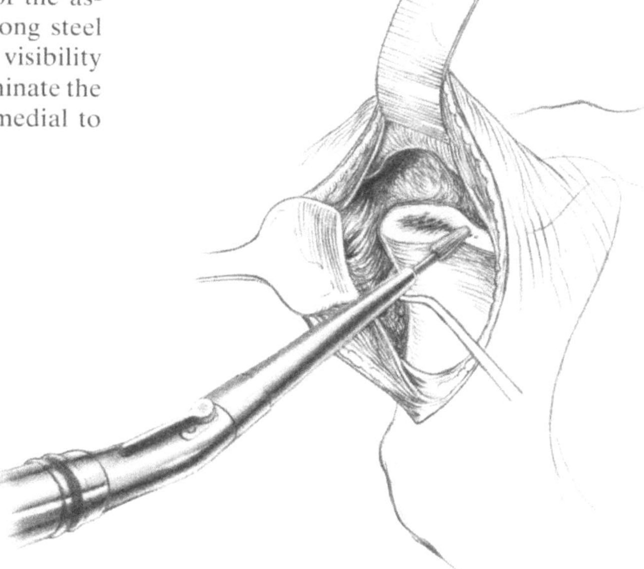

Surgical Orthodontia

Assemble the air drill and 12 steel bur:

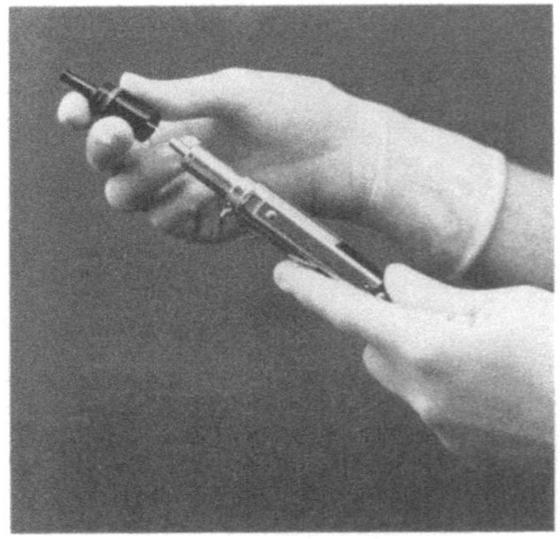

1. Place the medium bur guard firmly over the air drill shoulder.

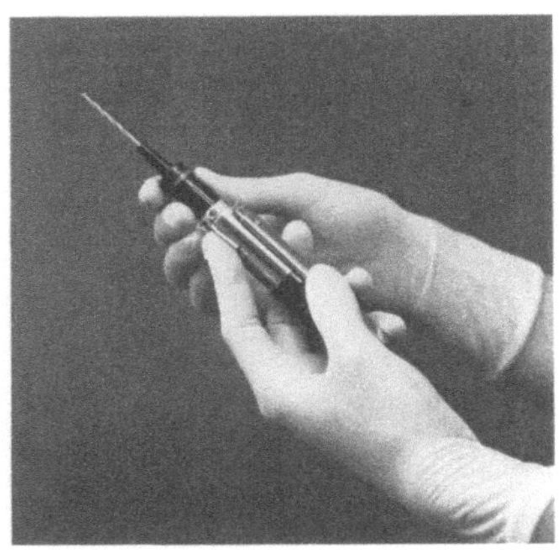

3. Return lever flush against the drill
   to lock bur.

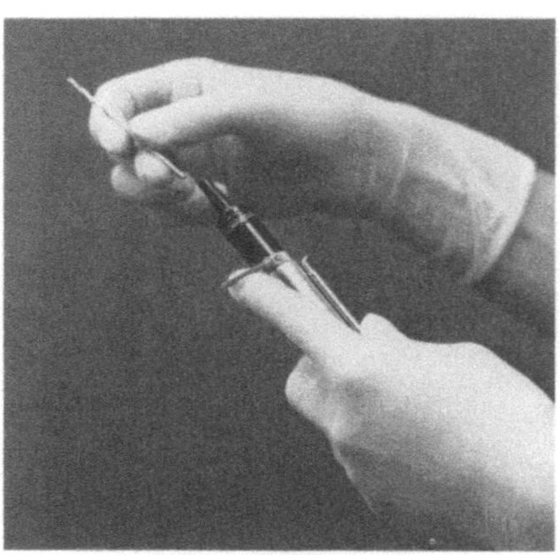

2. Push bur release lever forward 90°
   and insert the bur.

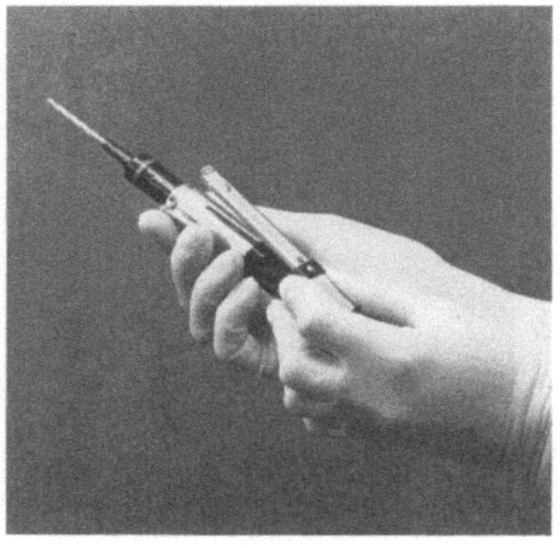

4. Push safety lever on to activate the
   drill.

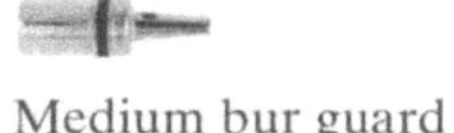

Air drill   Medium bur guard   14 steel bur

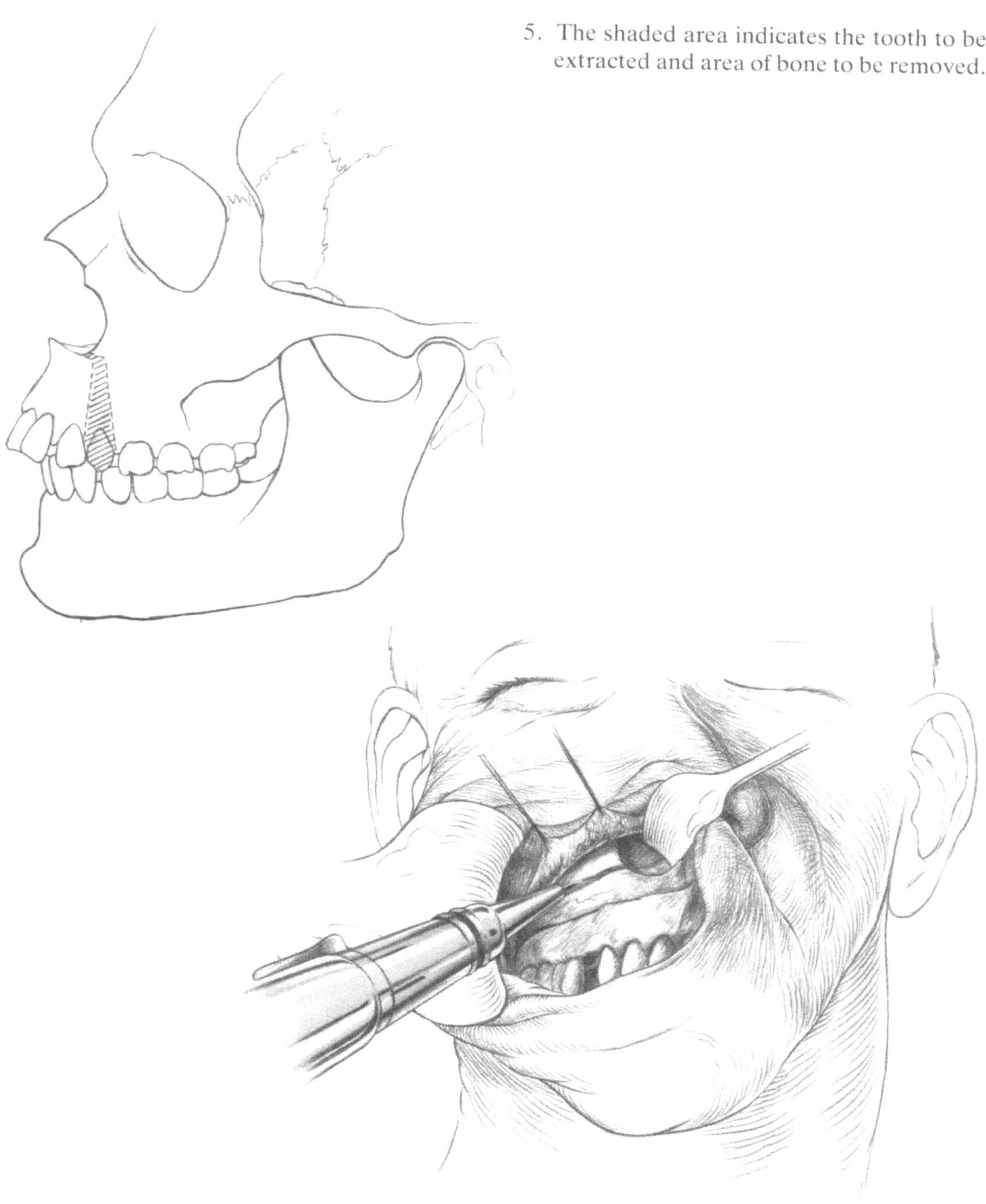

5. The shaded area indicates the tooth to be extracted and area of bone to be removed.

6. With the 12 saw-like steel bur make vertical incisions bilaterally from cuspid to cuspid. Carry the incisions across the hard palate to make one incision. Move the bur slowly in a saw-like fashion to prevent stalling of the bur and to minimize friction and heat to the bone. Irrigate with isotonic saline.

Surgical Orthodontia *(continued)*

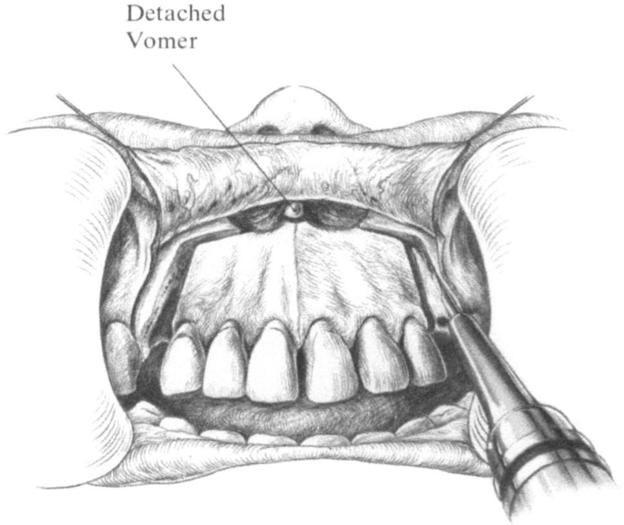

7. Extend the vertical cuts above the apices of the cuspid roots and then medially through the lateral wall of the nasal fossa. Completely free the anterior maxilla by separating the vomer from the nasal fossa with a mallet and chisel.

8. Mucoperiosteal tunnels for the buccal cortical cuts are necessary to ensure maintenance of blood supply. However, the palatal mucosa can be reflected in toto.

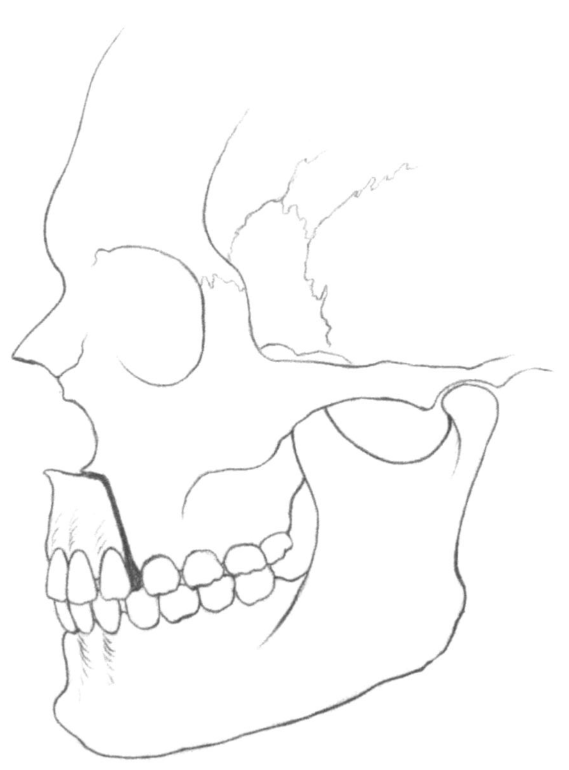

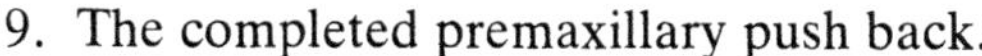

9. The completed premaxillary push back.

Surgical-Orthodontic Treatment of Interincisal Diastematas

A mucoperiosteal flap is reflected buccal to the incisor teeth, implemented by diverging vertical incisions distal to the most posterior interdental osteotomy site.
Bone cuts can be made between most teeth where diastemata are present by osteotomizing the cortical bone with burs and then carefully malletting a small sharp bibevel chisel between the teeth. When, however, there is insufficient space in the central-lateral incisor and cuspid-lateral incisor interspaces, interdental osteotomies may not be feasible*.

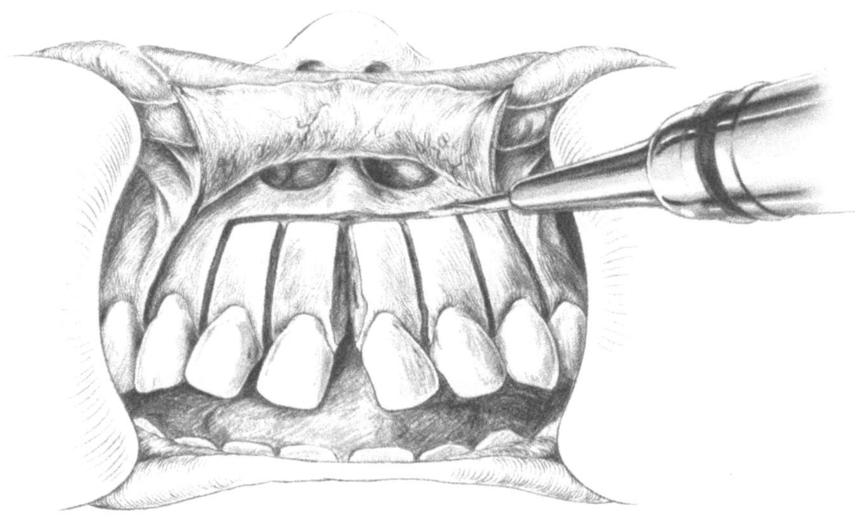

Remove a segment of bone between the central incisor teeth with the air drill and 12 steel bur. The excised bone is in the shape of a trapezoid, the base of which is at the crest of the aveolar ridge and the apex apical to the central incisor teeth. Make other vertical interdental osteotomies in a similar manner, four to five millimeters above the apices of the teeth to be removed. The interdental osteotomies are interconnected with a horizontal bone cut directed palatally above the apices of the teeth.

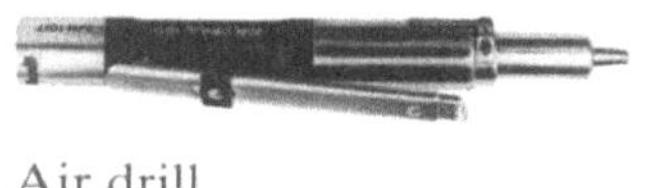

Air drill

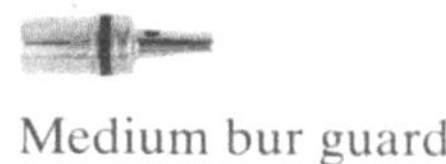

Medium bur guard

12 steel bur

---

* William H. Bell, D.D.S., Dental Science Institute, Houston, Texas, USA. (Personal Communication).

Internal-External Fixation of a Mandibular Fracture

It may be necessary to secure a fractured mandible with threaded or straight pins. The air driver and wire and pin driver are designed specifically for this operation. The cannulated angle of the wire and pin driver allows direct horizontal insertion of the pins. The air driver set at half speed (.5) produces a variable speed of 0-5000 rpm at the throttle. The reverse at the motor makes withdrawal of threaded pins possible without destruction of bone threads.

Assemble the wire and pin driver:

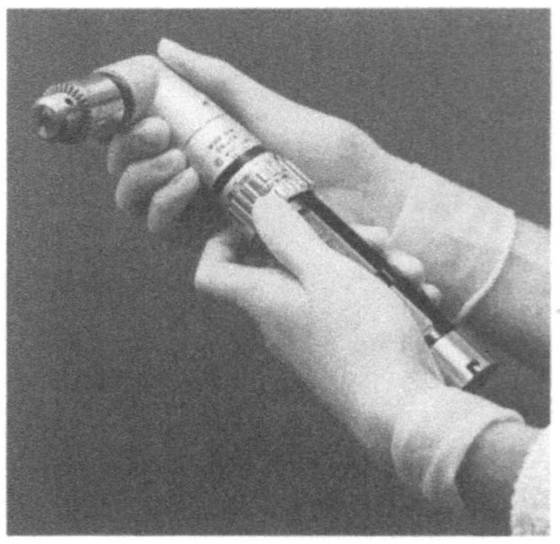

1. Place the attachment over the air driver shoulder. Engage hex drive. Turn ring clockwise to lock.

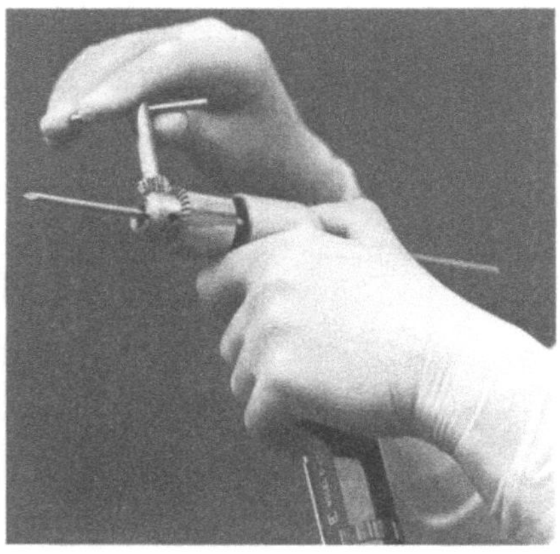

3. Insert fixation pin and lock firmly with key.

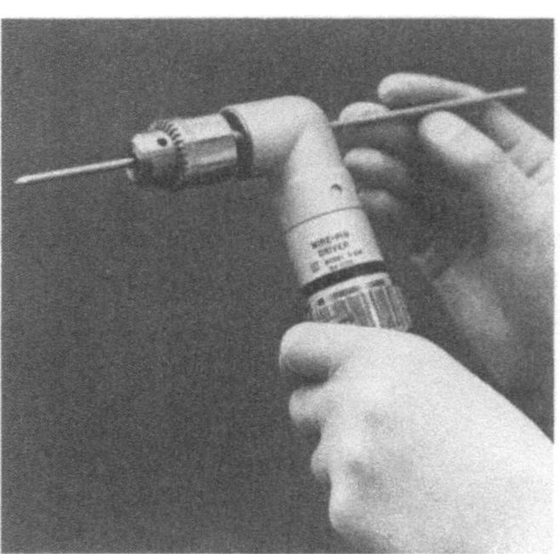

2. Open the chuck with the Jacobs key to fit the fixation pin into the cannulated angle.

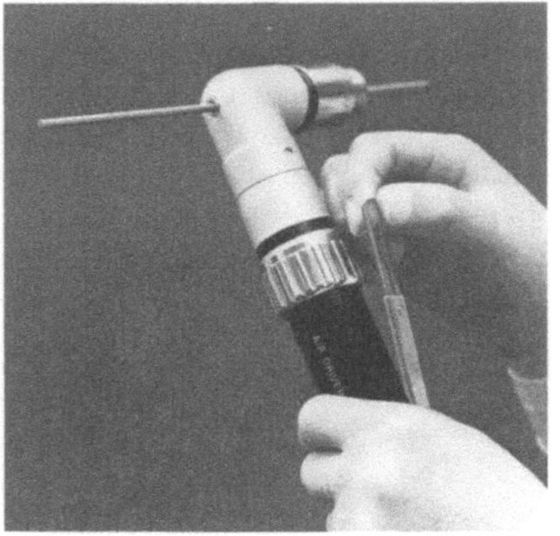

4. Use the extension lever for additional speed control at the throttle.

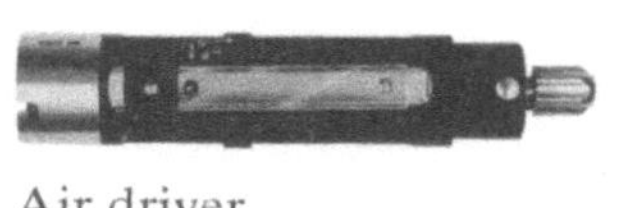

Air driver

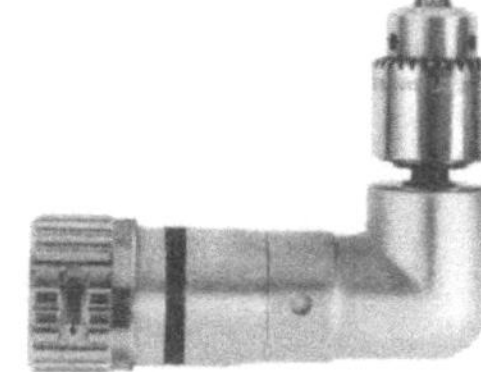

Wire and pin driver

Fixation pins

5. Trauma has caused upward displacement of the proximal fragment of the mandible.

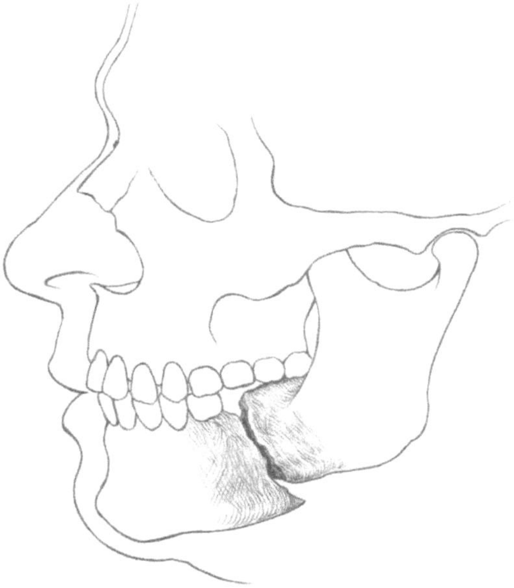

6. Reduce the fracture and direct the threaded pin across the fracture line.

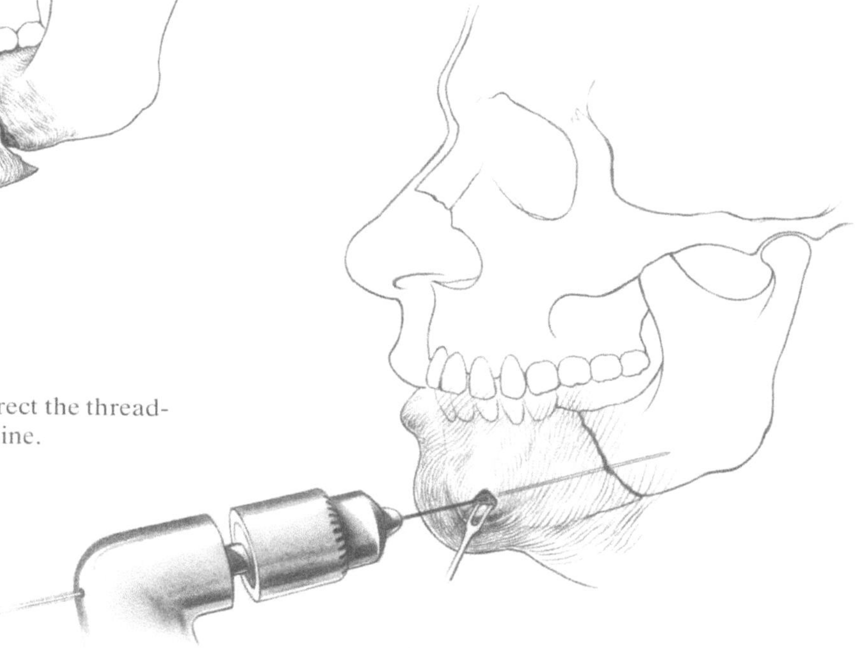

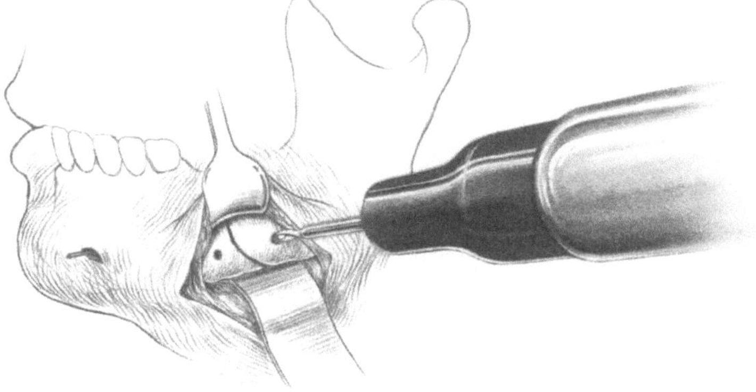

7. Remove the attachment and assemble the wire-pass bur and guard. Through a submandibular incision drill two holes with the bur.

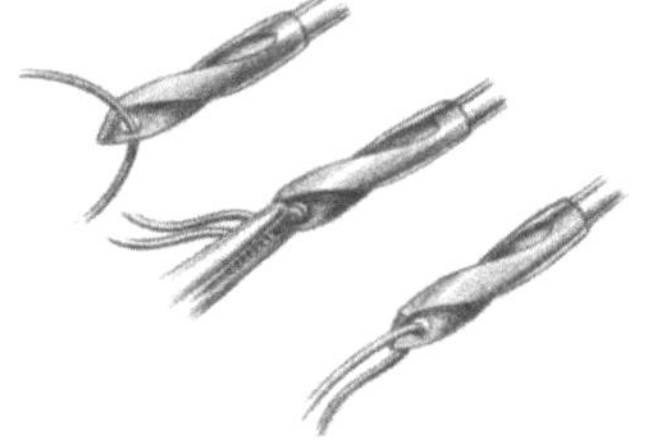

8. Irrigate the bone dust out of the bur tip. Pass the wire through the hole in the bur. Crimp the wire into the groove of the bur tip, and draw the bur and one end of the wire through the drill hole.

Simple Fixation of a Fracture of the Mandibular Symphysis

Assemble the wire and pin driver:

Align the fractured segments of the mandible. Only one hand is necessary to regulate the speed and direct the pin. A powered pin driver minimizes the lateral drift experienced with hand operated drills, reducing the possibility of insecure fixation.

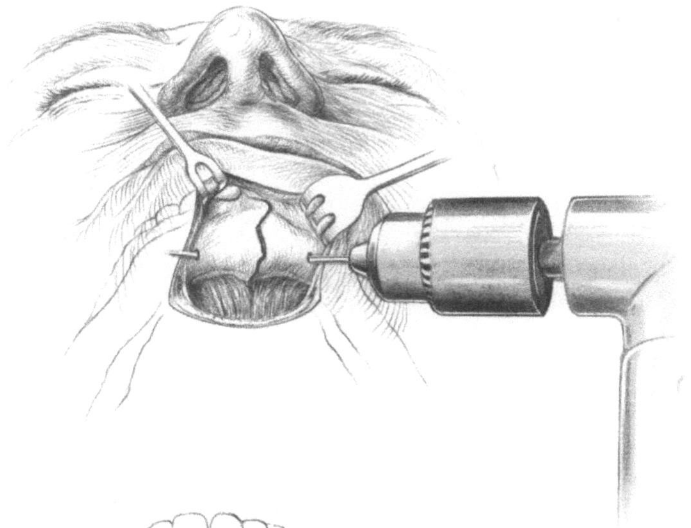

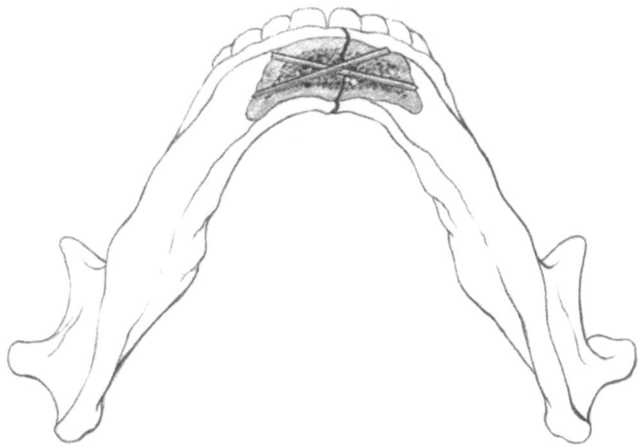

Direct two threaded pins diagonally across the fracture line to hold the segments in positive position.

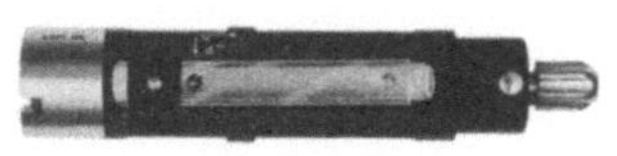

Air driver

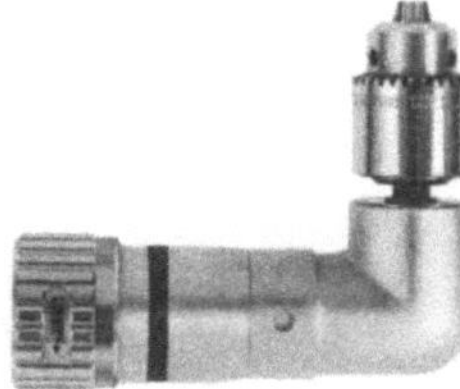

Wire and pin driver

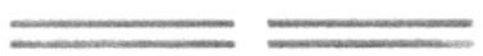

Fixation pins

Figure Eight Wiring of a Mandibular Symphysis Fracture

It is possible to drill wire fixation holes with air driver and bur or the air drill and bur. The air drill with the 90° angle provides the same right-angle drive with a selection of three drilling burs for various wire strengths. The high speed of the drill (100,000 rpm) minimizes further fracture to the bone fragments. Have the drill running before placing the bur on the bone. Placing the bur against the bone without the drill running may cause the bur to skid across the smooth moist bone.

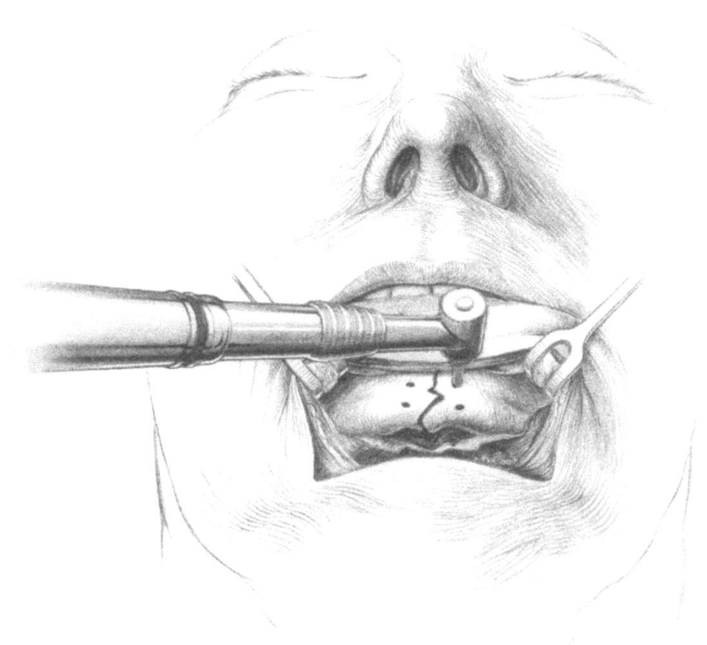

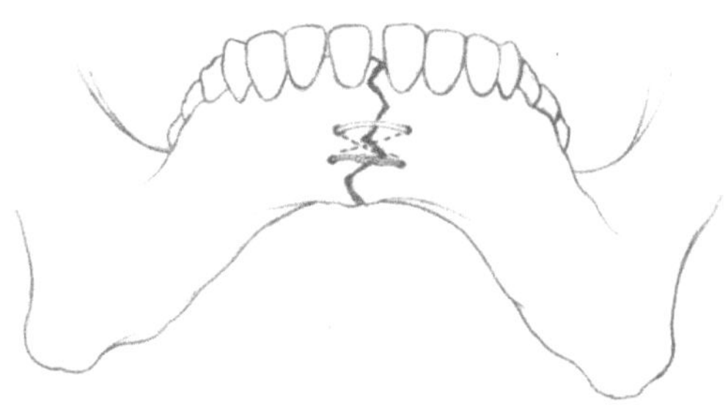

Reduce the fracture and drill the holes for wiring the mandibular fracture.

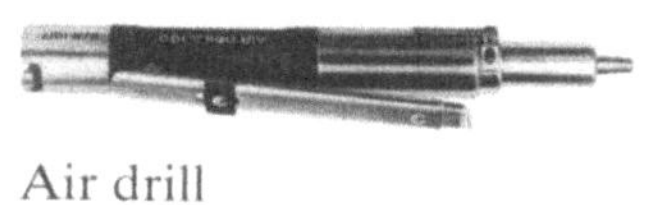

Air drill

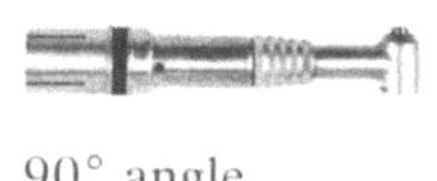

90° angle

26 short wire-pass bur

27 short wire-pass bur

28 short wire-pass bur

Intraoral Mandibular Reduction

Assemble the 90° angle and wire-pass bur:

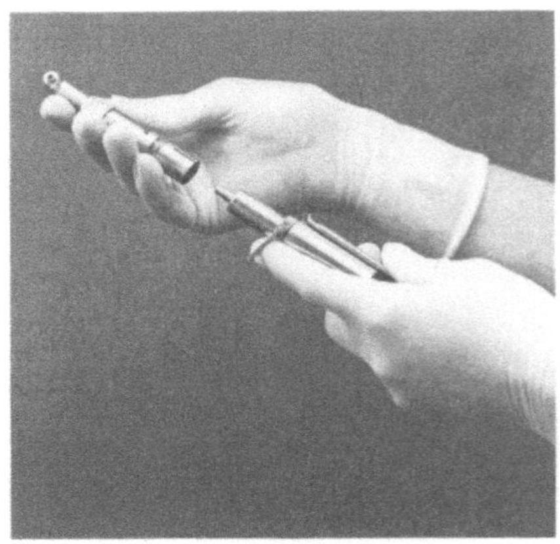

1. Push the bur release lever forward on the air drill to assemble attachment. Completely seat.

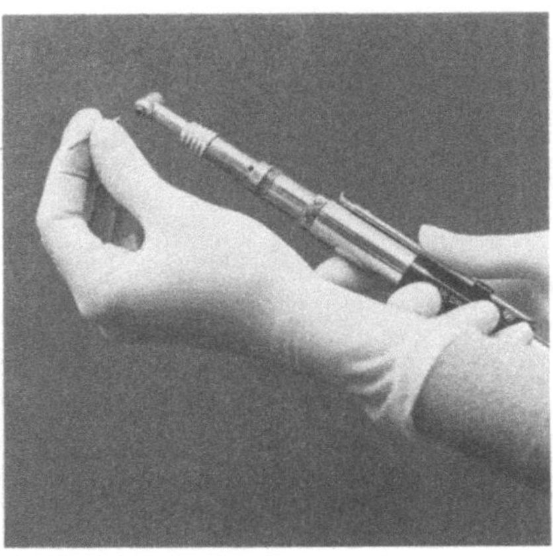

3. Place wire-pass bur into the collet.

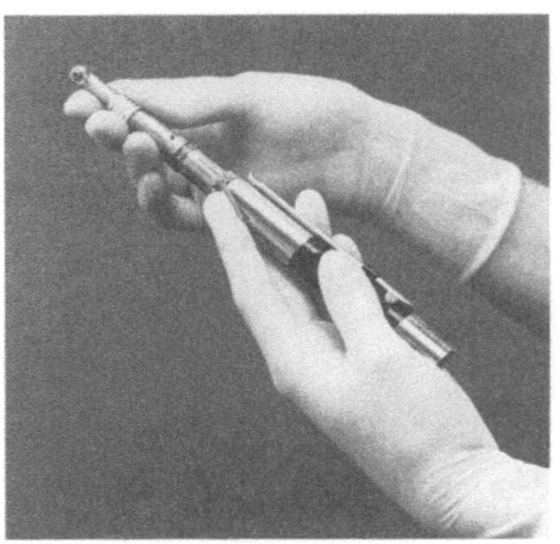

2. Return lever flush against the drill to lock attachment.

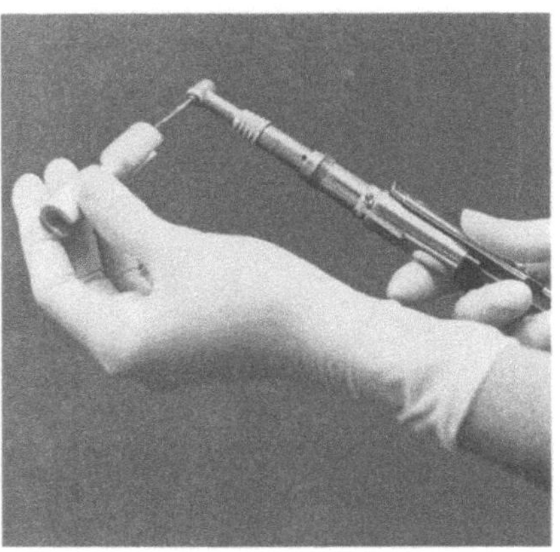

4. Slide hollow side of bur changer over bur. Press the bur firmly into the collet.

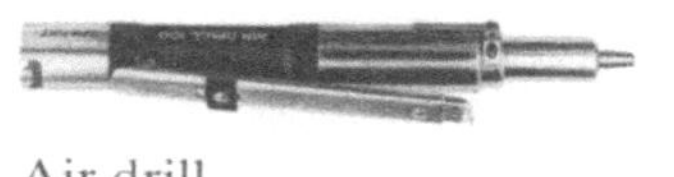

Air drill

90° angle

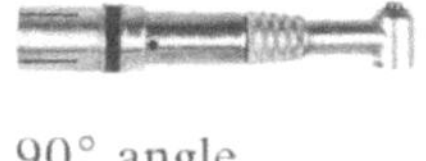

26 short wire-pass bur

27 short wire-pass bur

28 short wire-pass bur

5. For transosseous fixation remove the tooth in the fracture line and penetrate the buccal plate in the area of the lateral oblique ridge through the molar alveolus with the bur.

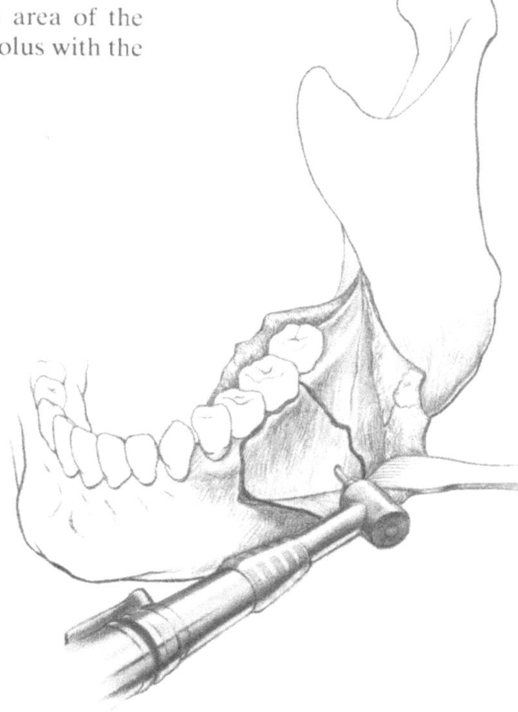

6. Drill the wire fixation holes with the 90° angle and 27 wire-pass bur.

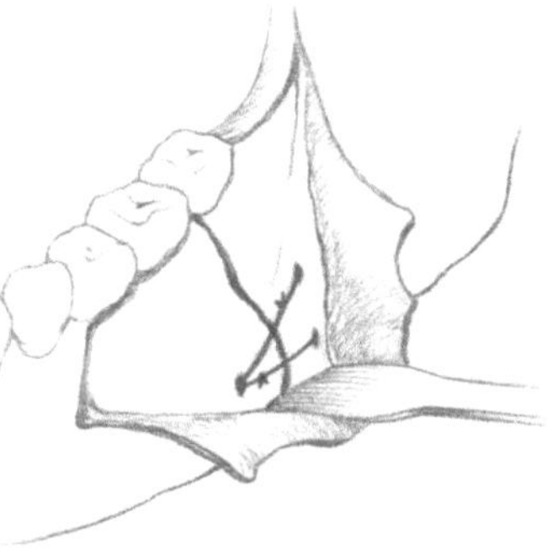

7. Secure both ends of the wire and bury the knot in the drill hole.

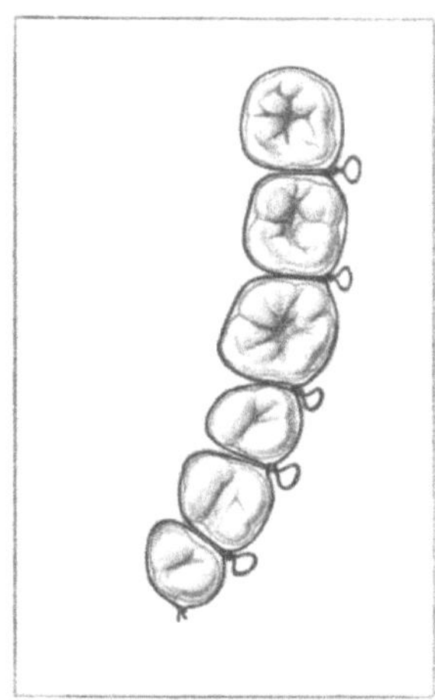

8. It is only necessary to penetrate the buccal plate and secure, since some method of arch ligation usually accompanies this procedure.

Interseptal Wiring

When a very thin portion of bone must be penetrated with accuracy, for example penetration of the nasal spine, the air drill with bur is the instrument of choice.

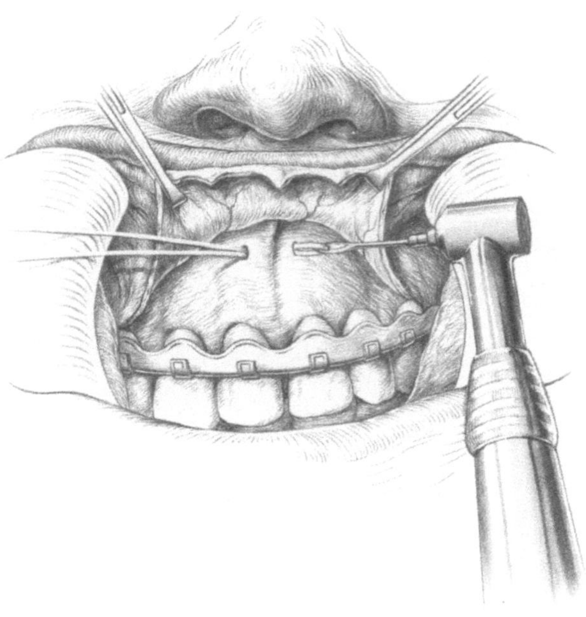

With the 90° angle and 26 wire-pass bur drill through the nasal spine for anterior fixation.

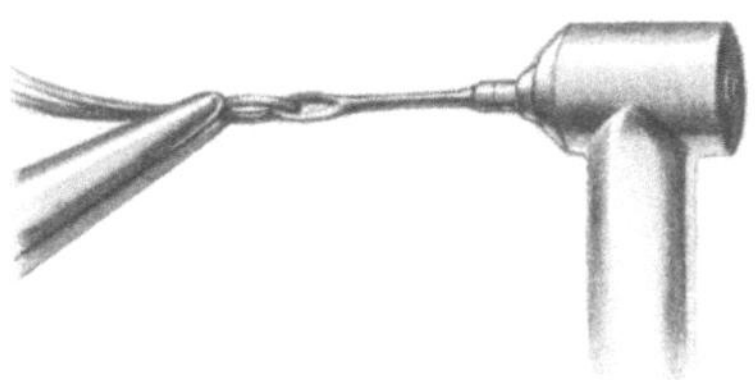

Irrigate the bone dust out of the hole in the bur tip. Pass the wire through the hole in the bur tip. Crimp the wire into the grooves of the bur tip, and draw the bur and one end of the wire back through the drill hole.

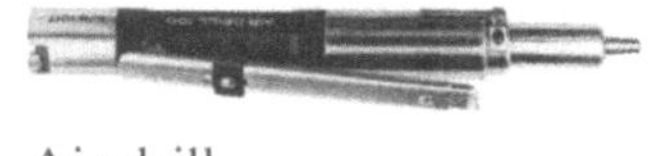

Air drill

90° angle

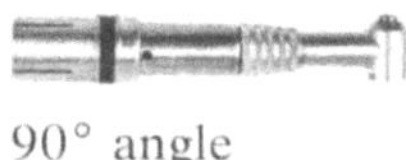

26 short wire-pass bur

The "L" Splint for Immobilization of Iliac Grafts to the Mandible*

The "L" splint, used for immobilization of iliac bone grafts, is a method of replacement of lost mandibular bone. Make a submandibular incision and divide the tissues down to the bone of the proximal and distal fragments.

Assemble the air drill and 20° angle:

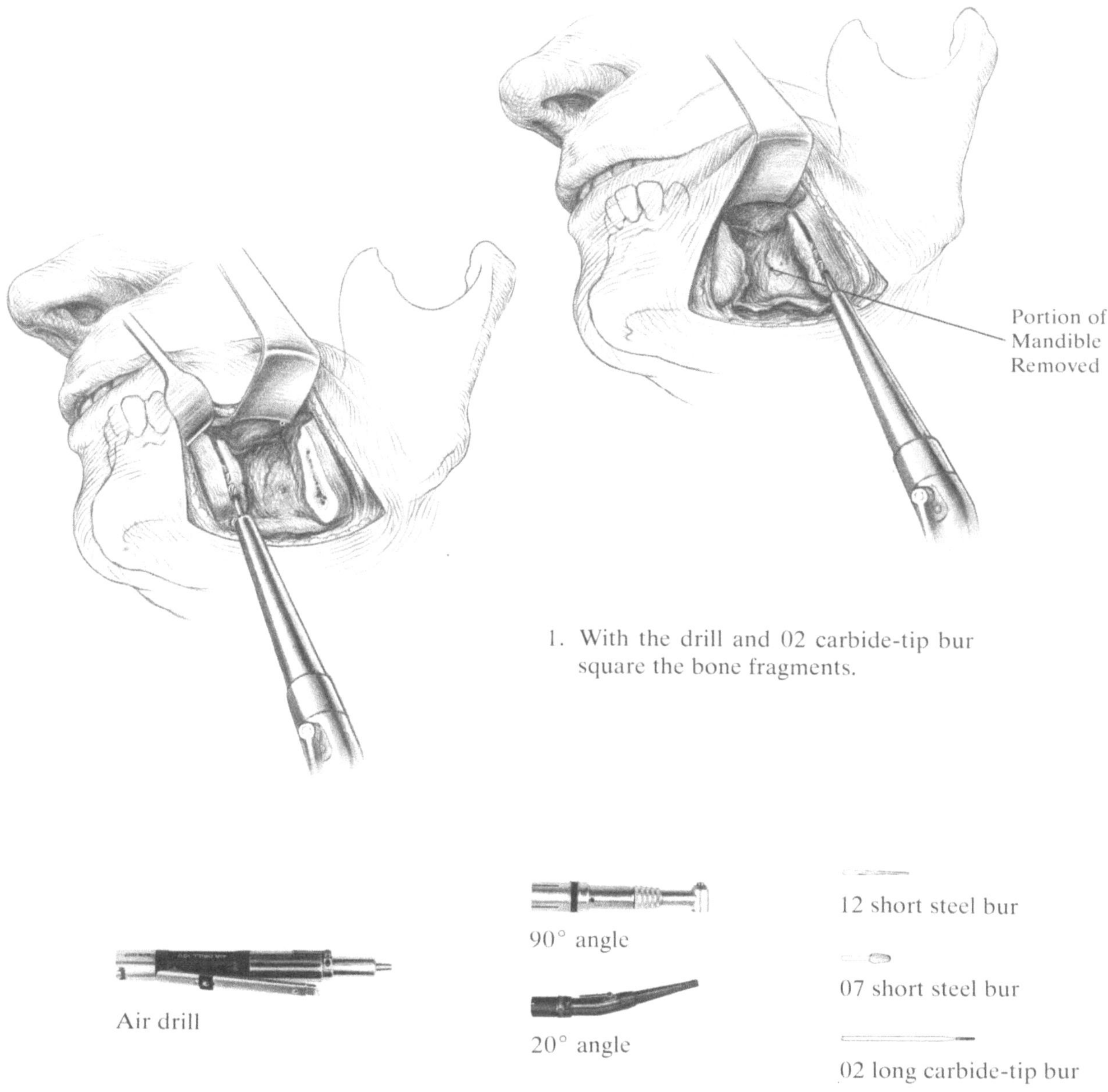

---

* M. Robinson, D.D.S., M.D., and R. Shuken, D.D.S.: The "L" splint for immobilization of Iliac Bone Grafts of the Mandible. **J of Oral Surg** 24:10-14, January 1966.

The "L" Splint for Immobilization of Iliac Grafts to the Mandible *(continued)*

2. Enter the oral cavity and place an intraoral acrylic splint between the arches of the teeth in a correct, almost normal position. Immobilize the acrylic splint with five stainless steel intermaxillary wires attached to previously placed arch bars.

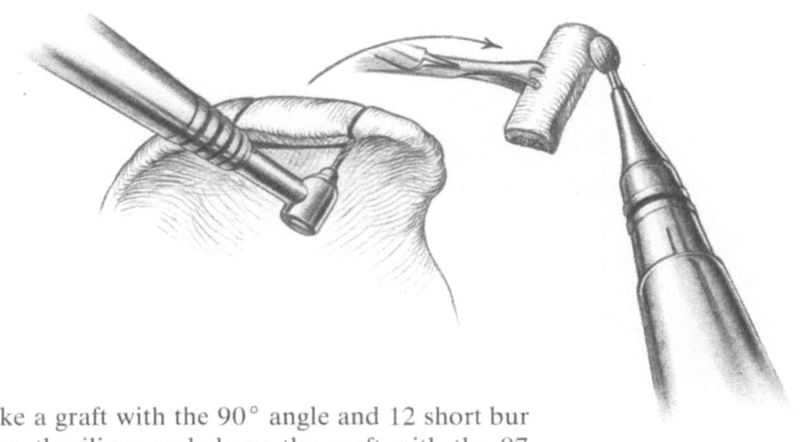

3. Take a graft with the 90° angle and 12 short bur from the ilium and shape the graft with the 07 short steel bur.

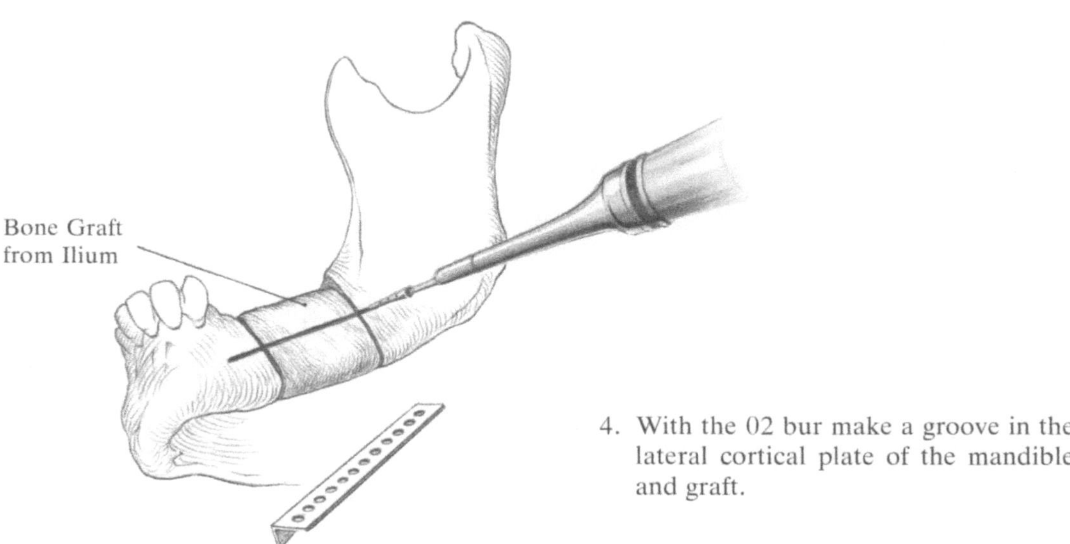

4. With the 02 bur make a groove in the lateral cortical plate of the mandible and graft.

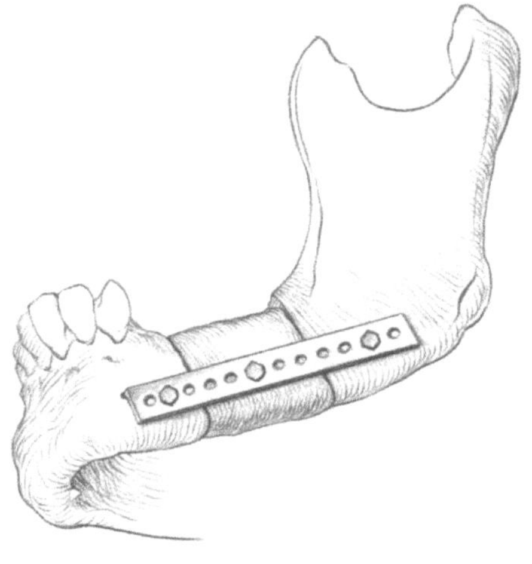

5. Place the "L" splint within the groove across the lateral surface of the mandible and graft.

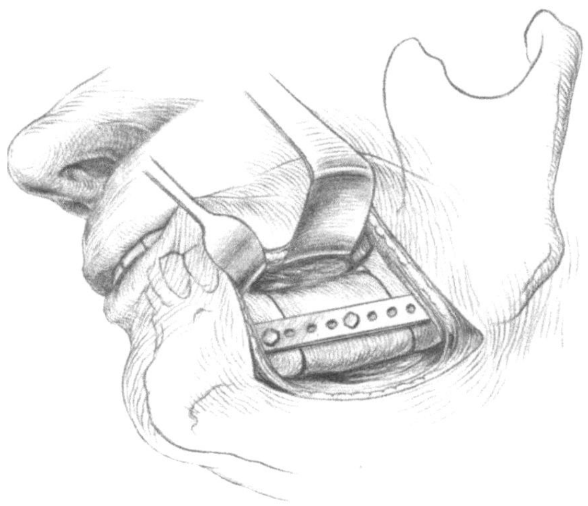

6. Secure the splint with three screws at the distal and proximal fragments, and the graft. Close the wound and apply a pressure dressing.

Ostectomy of a Mandibular Ameloblastoma

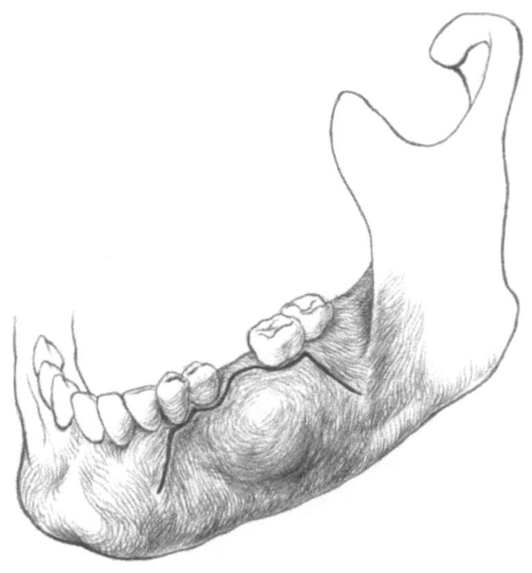

1. Design the mucoperiosteal incision to permit a good bony base under the suture line upon closure of the wound.

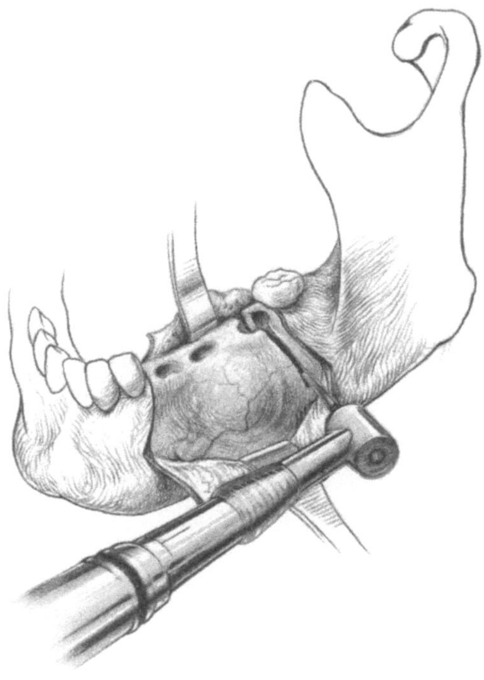

2. Extract the involved teeth. With the drill, 90° angle and side-cutting 12 steel bur begin the ostectomy.

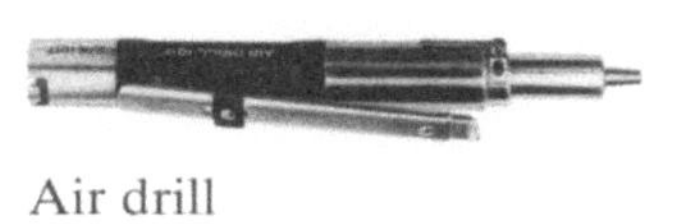

Air drill

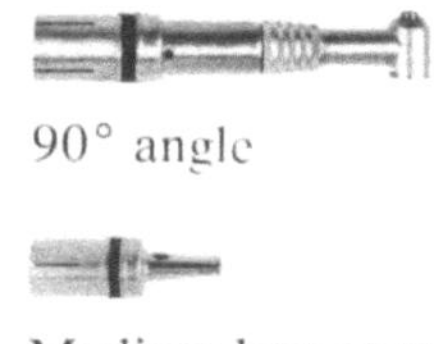

90° angle

Medium bur guard

12 short steel bur

07 steel bur

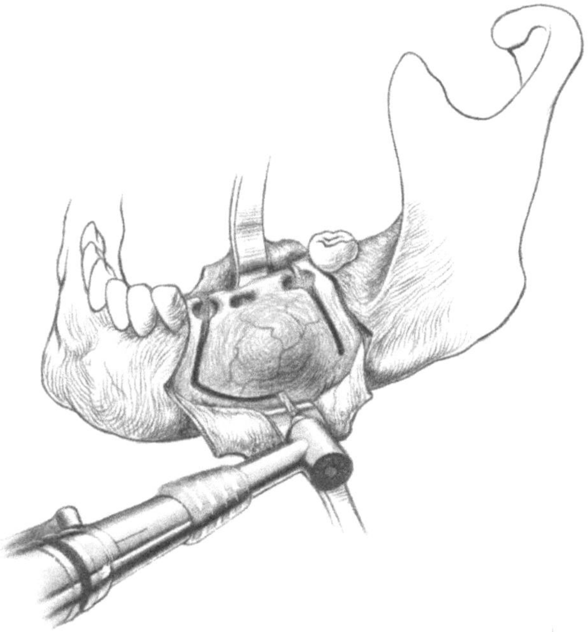

3. Complete the ostectomy, and remove the full thickness of the mandible.

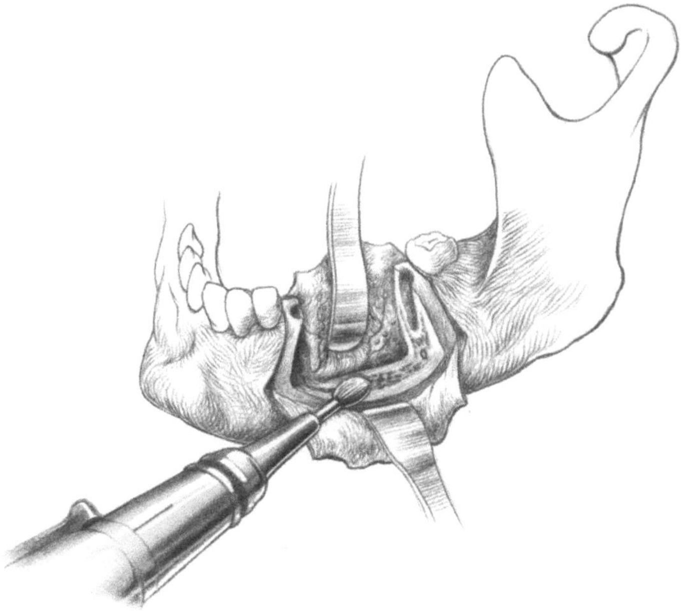

4. Smooth the rough bony margins with the 07 steel bur.

5. Pack the defect and loosely close the flap.

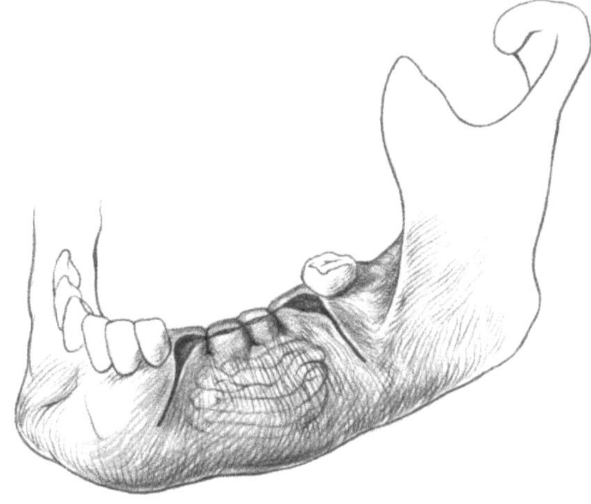

Unroofing of a Mandibular Dentigerous Cyst

It is possible to expose cysts and nerve roots and excise bone tumors of the oral cavity with the air drill and burs. The gradual removal of bone and accuracy of excision minimizes bone and tissue trauma.

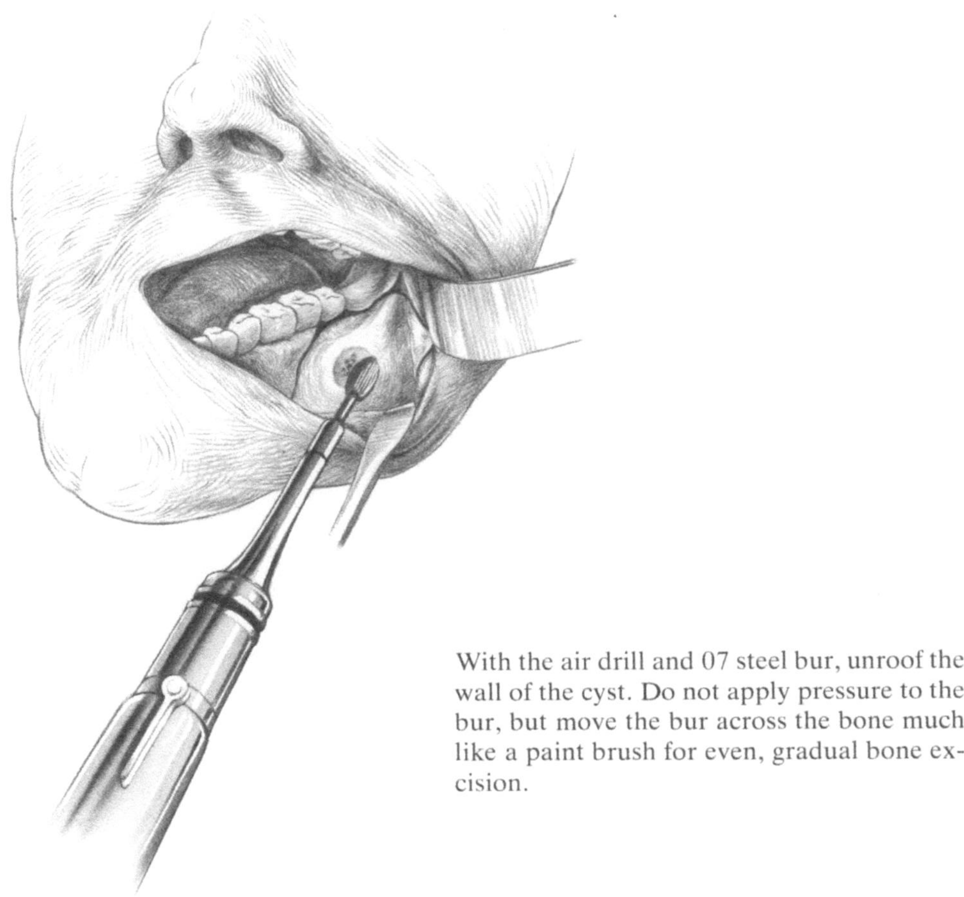

With the air drill and 07 steel bur, unroof the wall of the cyst. Do not apply pressure to the bur, but move the bur across the bone much like a paint brush for even, gradual bone excision.

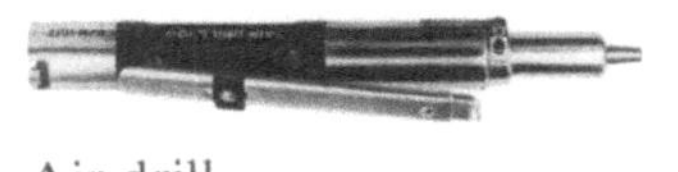

Air drill

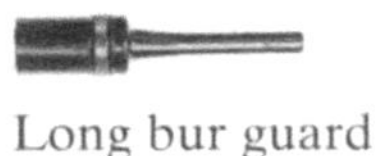

Long bur guard

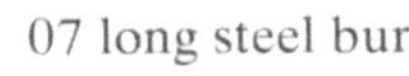

07 long steel bur

Marsupialization of a Globulomaxillary Cyst

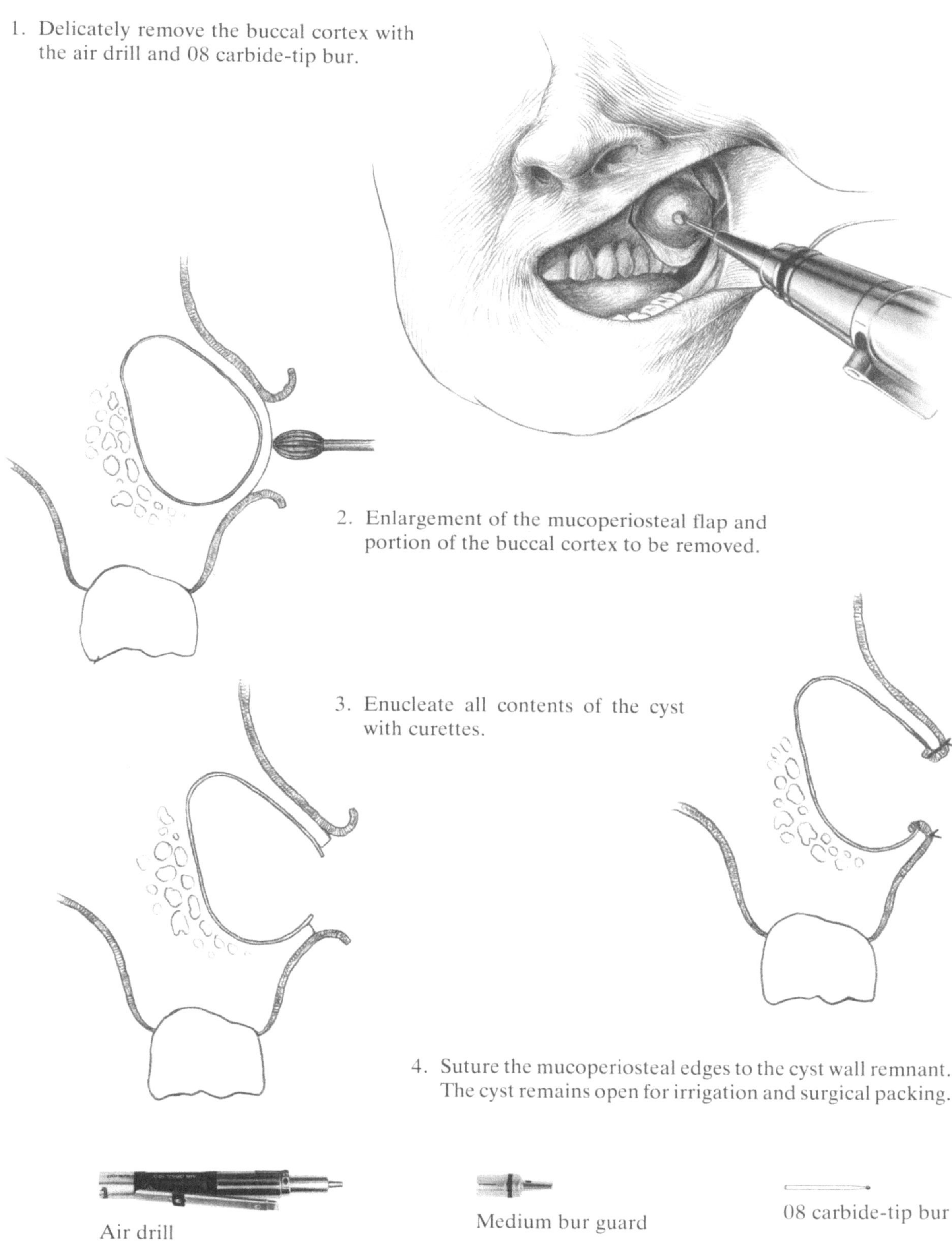

1. Delicately remove the buccal cortex with the air drill and 08 carbide-tip bur.

2. Enlargement of the mucoperiosteal flap and portion of the buccal cortex to be removed.

3. Enucleate all contents of the cyst with curettes.

4. Suture the mucoperiosteal edges to the cyst wall remnant. The cyst remains open for irrigation and surgical packing.

Removal of Torus Palatinus

This technique of bone removal prevents accidental fracture and perforation of the nasal floor and possible formation of an oronasal fistula. It assures an even, concave surface that will serve as a maxillary palatal denture base. Conclude the bone removal with a diamond bur. The diamond burs polish bone, thus preparing a smooth surface for replacement of tissue.

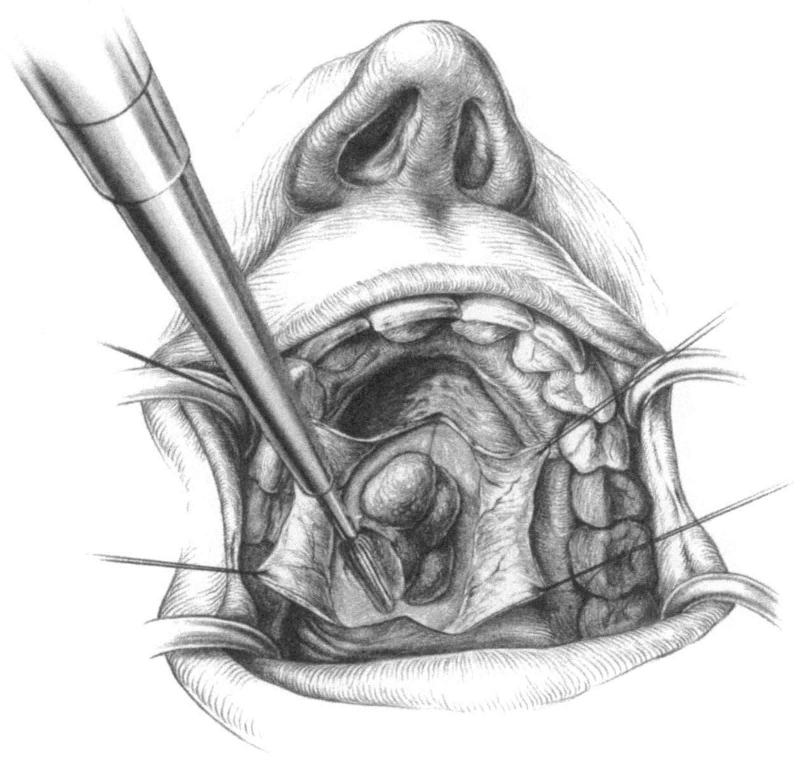

The 20° angle provides the best visualization of the bur.
Sculpt away the torus palatinus.

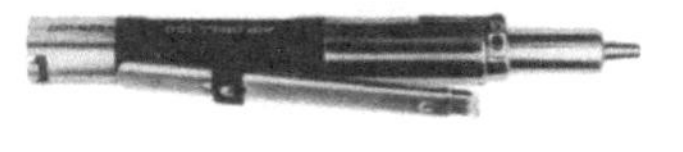

Air drill

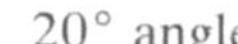

20° angle

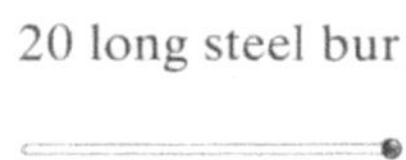

20 long steel bur

19 long diamond bur

Removal of Torus Mandibularis

Excise the torus mandibularis with the 19 long steel bur and tissue retractor guard. During sculpture of the exostosis the tissue retractor guard obliterates all lingual undercuts and protects the lingual mucosa.

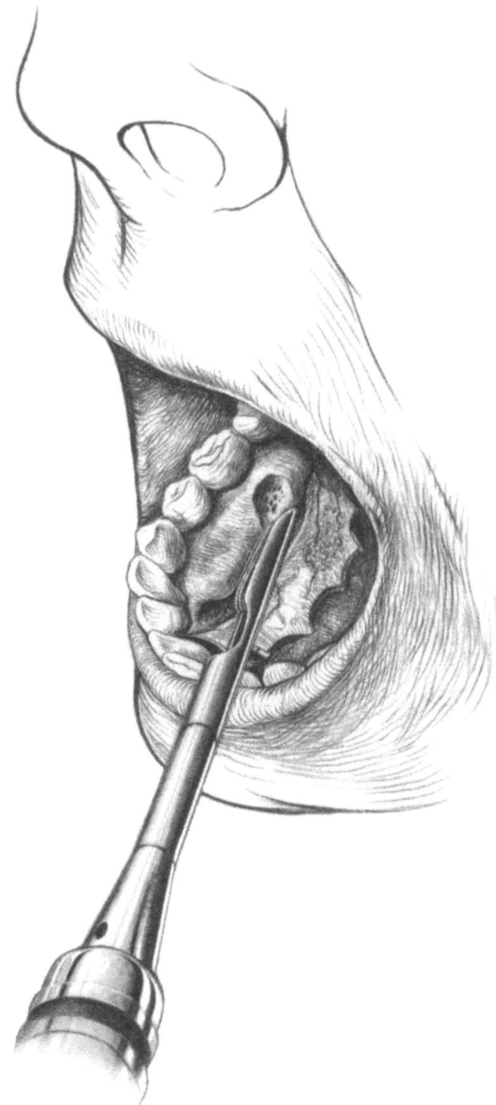

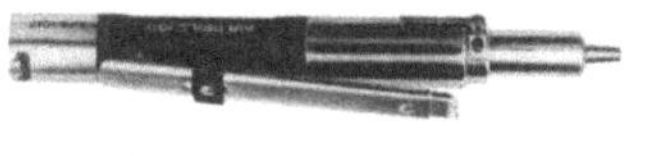

Air drill

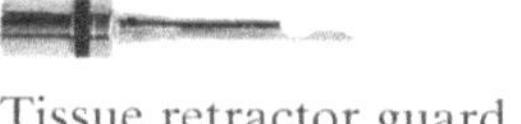

Tissue retractor guard

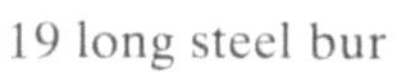

19 long steel bur

Maxillary Alveolectomy

Remove the bony undercuts and smooth the remaining alveolar ridge with the 19 long steel bur. The tissue retractor guard will retract and protect the surrounding soft tissue. In fact, this guard and bur can be used while bone is removed in any area where preservation of the overlying soft tissue is mandatory.

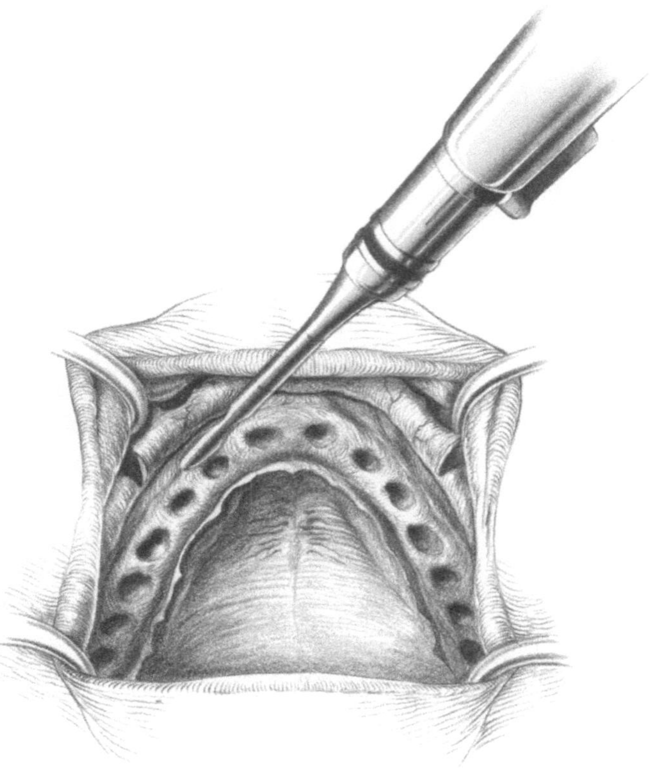

Sculpt the alveolar ridge with the 19 long steel bur. Irrigate intermittently with isotonic saline.

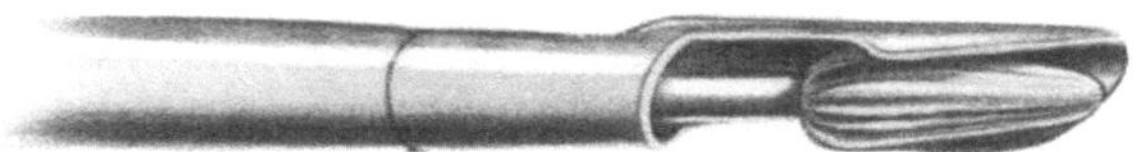

Enlargement of tissue retractor guard

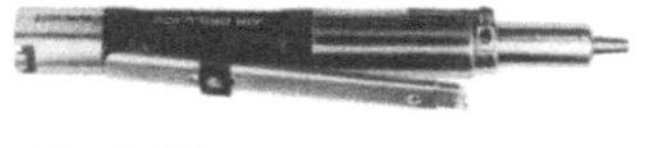

Air drill

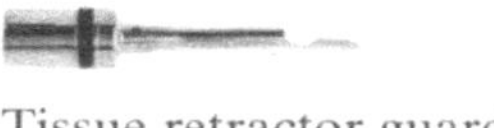

Tissue retractor guard

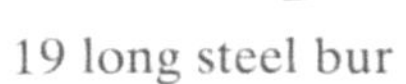

19 long steel bur

Removal of a Palatal Root from an Edentulous Maxilla

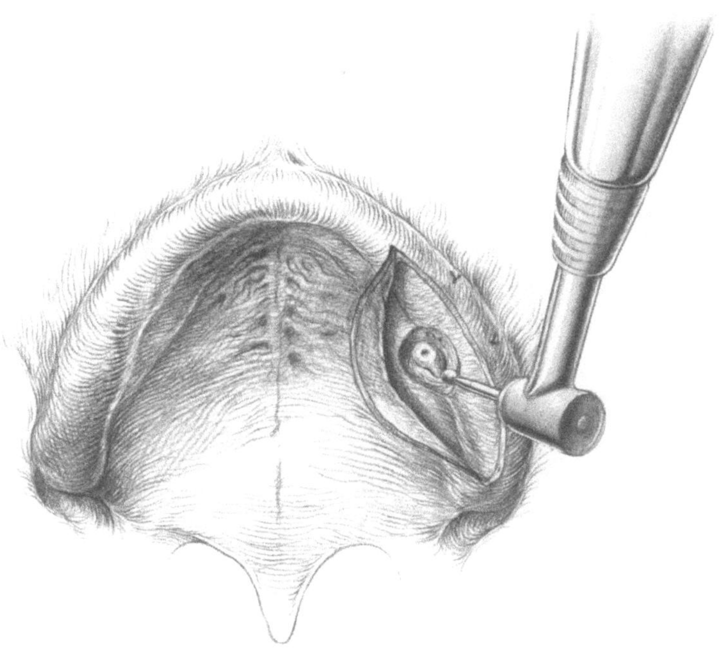

The proximity of the root tip to the maxillary sinus demands a delicate approach. Use the 08 short carbide-tip bur to erase the overlying bone so that the root can be luxated and removed.

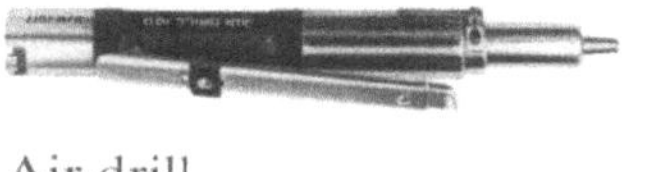

Air drill

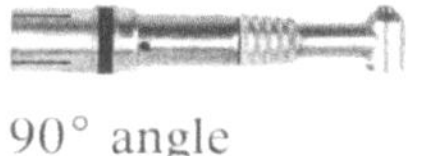

90° angle

08 short carbide-tip bur

Surgical Removal of a Partially Impacted Wisdom Tooth*

The close proximity of the multiple dilacerated roots to the maxillary sinus necessitates surgical removal of the tooth.

Assemble the 90° angle and 08 carbide-tip bur:

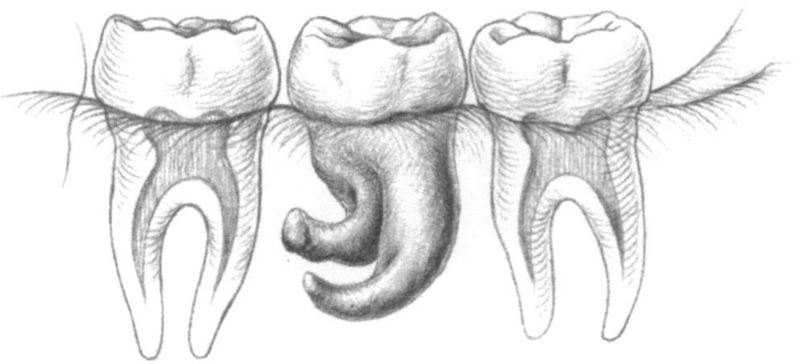

Dilacerated roots.

1. Reflect a small mucoperiosteal flap. Access to the buccal bone is simplified with the 90° angle. Erase the bone to expose the bifurcation.

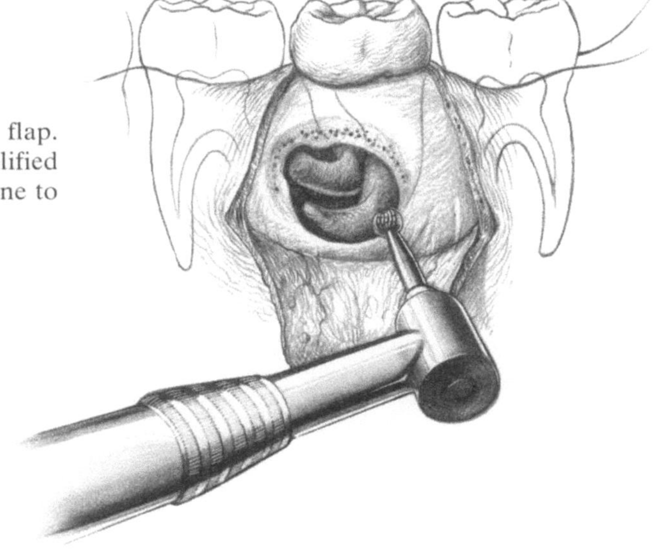

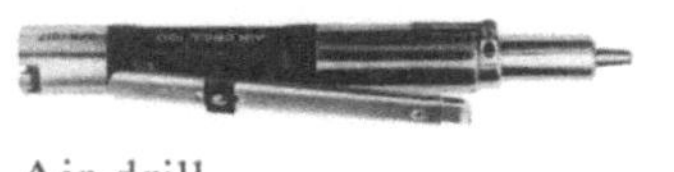

Air drill

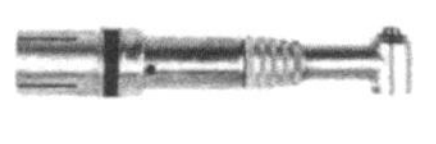

90° angle

08 short carbide-tip bur

04 short carbide-tip bur

---

* Theodore E. Trebowski, D. D. S. San Francisco, California, USA (Personal Communication).

2. Excise the deformed distal portions of the dilacerated roots with the 04 carbide-tip bur.

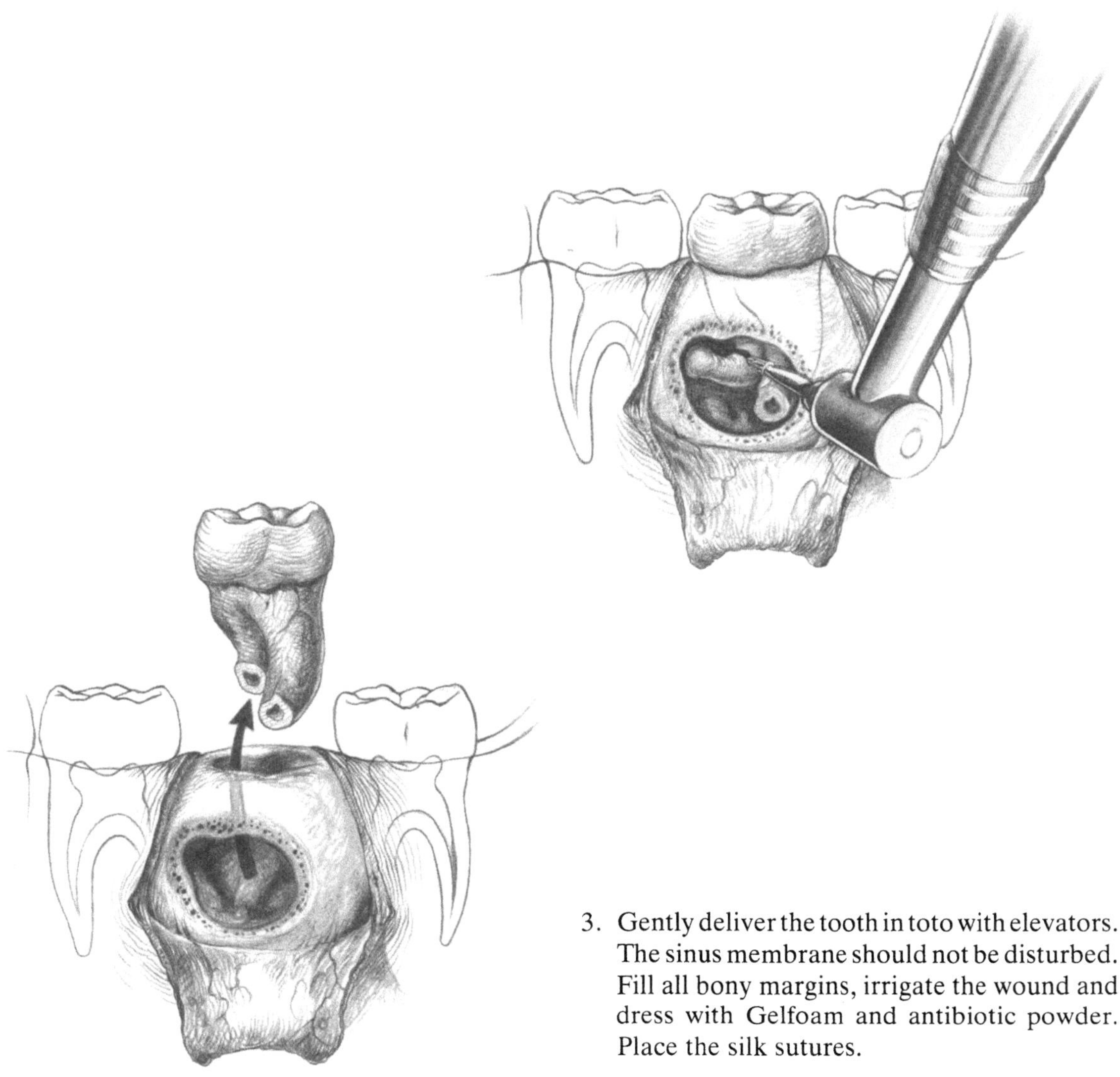

3. Gently deliver the tooth in toto with elevators. The sinus membrane should not be disturbed. Fill all bony margins, irrigate the wound and dress with Gelfoam and antibiotic powder. Place the silk sutures.

Sectioning of a Horizontal Impacted Mandibular Third Molar*

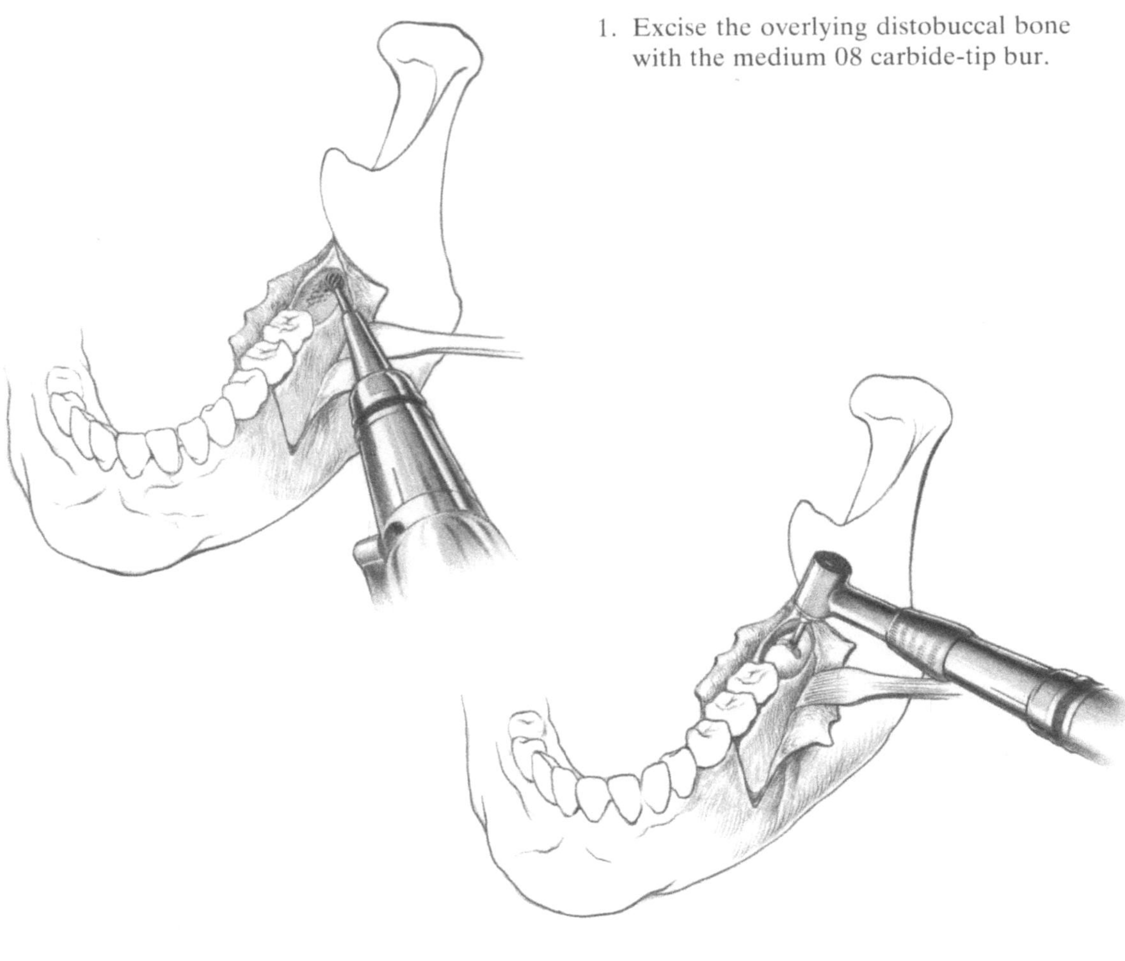

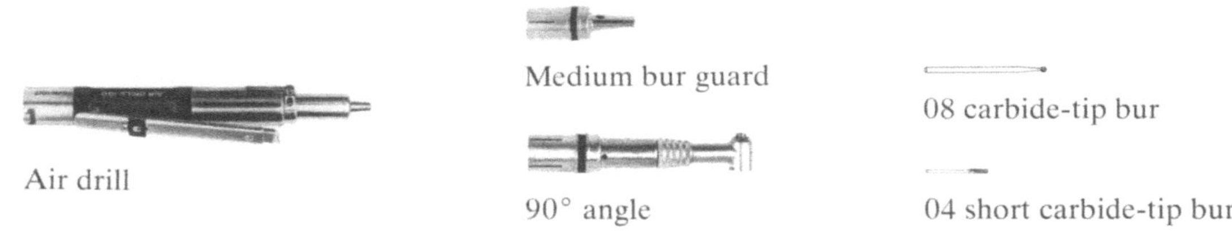

* E. Ågren.: High-Speed or Conventional Dental Engines for Removal of Bone in Oral Surgery. 1. A Study of the Reactions
  Following Removal of Bilateral Impacted Lower Third Molars. **Acta Odont Scandinav** 21:585-625, December 1963.

Removal of an Unerupted Mandibular Second Bicuspid*

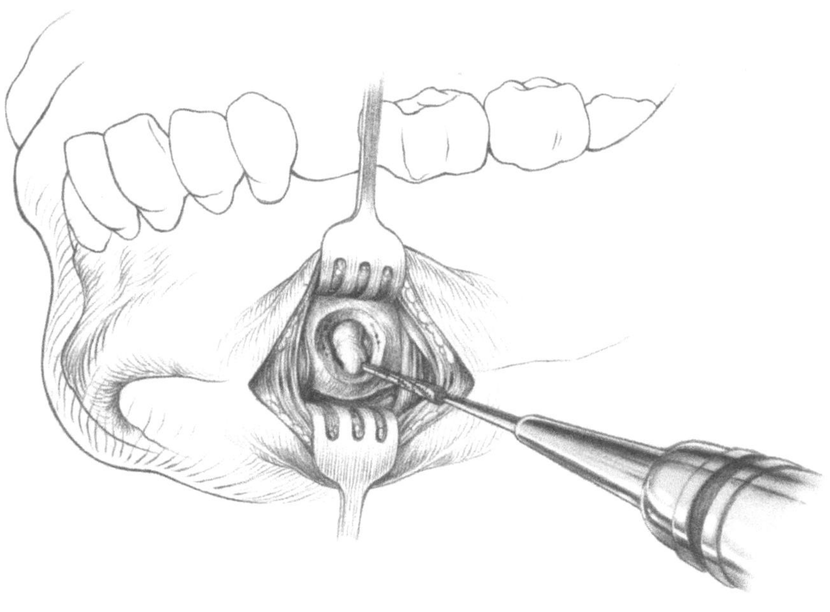

Use the 06 carbide-tip bur to gently excise the inferior border of the mandible; then carefully elevate the tooth from the bony crypt and remove it.

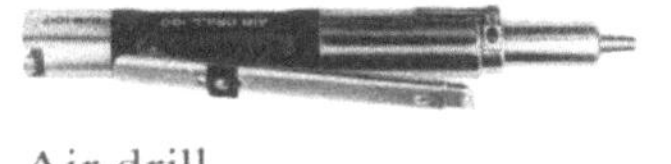

Air drill

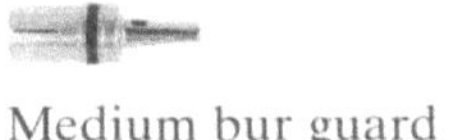

Medium bur guard

06 carbide-tip bur

---

* H. M. Goldman, D.M.D., et al.: Current Therapy in Dentistry, Volume 3. **The C. V. Mosby Co.,** St Louis, Missouri, USA 1968.

Excision of an Ankylosed Deciduous Mandibular Molar*

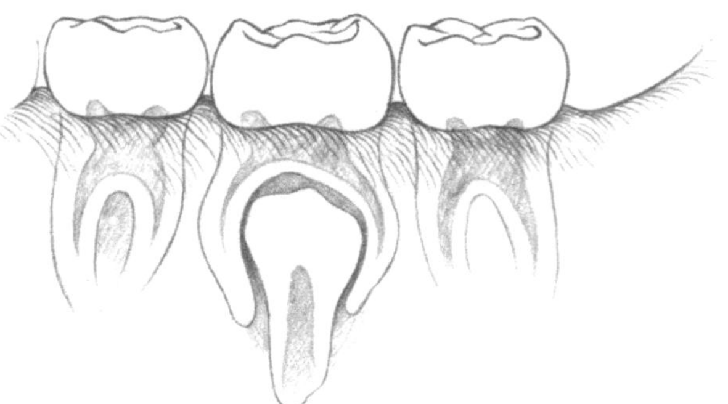

The deciduous mandibular molar roots encompass the crown of the unerupted bicuspid.

1. Make a flap which extends around the neck of the tooth, then onto the buccal mucosa both mesially and distally at a 45° angle.

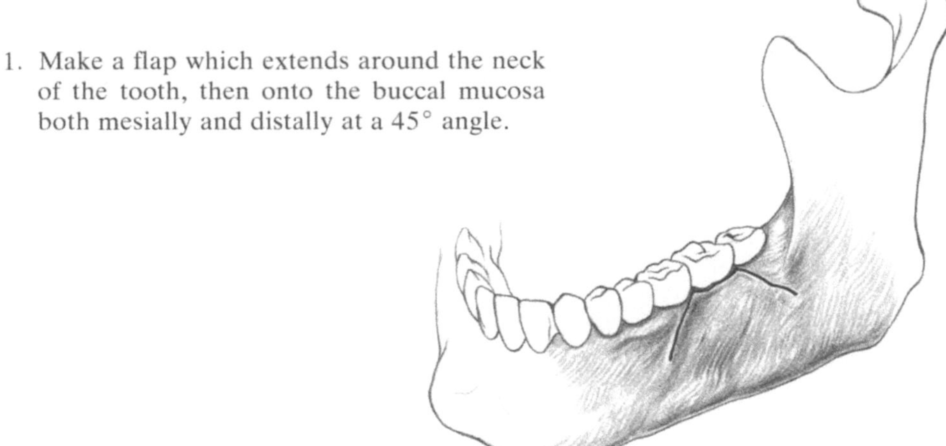

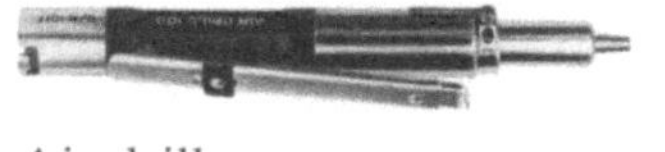

Air drill

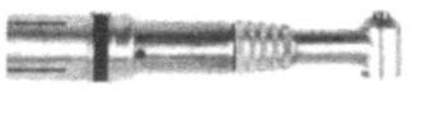

90° angle

08 short carbide-tip bur

04 short carbide-tip bur

---

* W. Harry Archer, B.S., M.A., D.D.S. A Manual of Oral Surgery, Third Edition. **W. B. Saunders Company**, Philadelphia, Pennsylvania, USA 1961.

2. Excise the gingival third of the supporting cortical bone with the 90° angle and 08 carbide-tip bur. Do not apply pressure on the bur tip, or the small head on the bur may drill a hole in the bone, rather than evenly excising it.

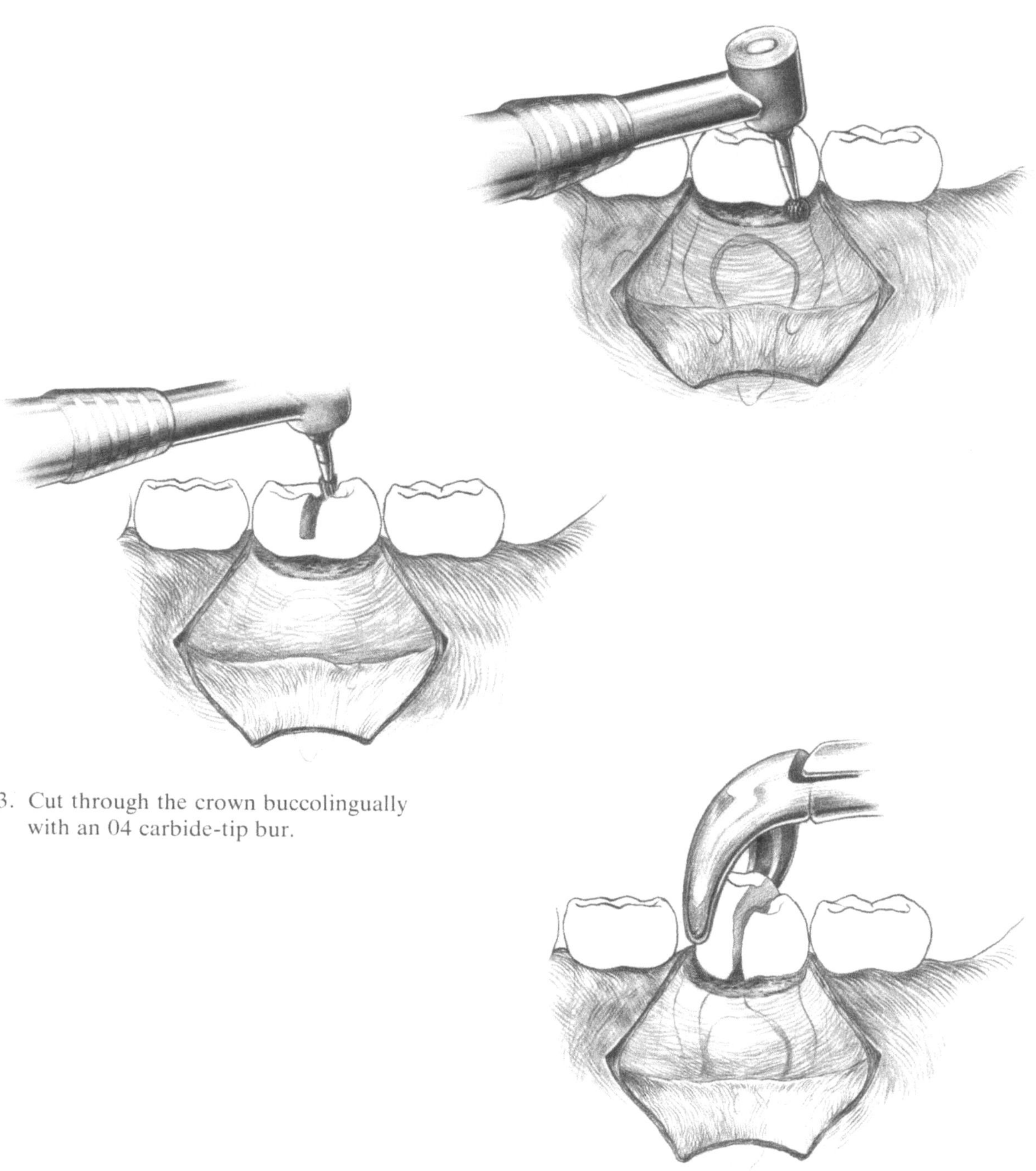

3. Cut through the crown buccolingually with an 04 carbide-tip bur.

4. Lift the distal fragment mesially with forceps. The mesial fragment is removed distally. Approximate and suture the flap.

Removal of an Impacted Maxillary Third Molar

Access to this impaction must be made with care to avoid forcing the tooth into the maxillary sinus or the pterygomaxillary fossa. Remove the bone with the 06 carbide-tip bur. Irrigate intermittently with isotonic saline.

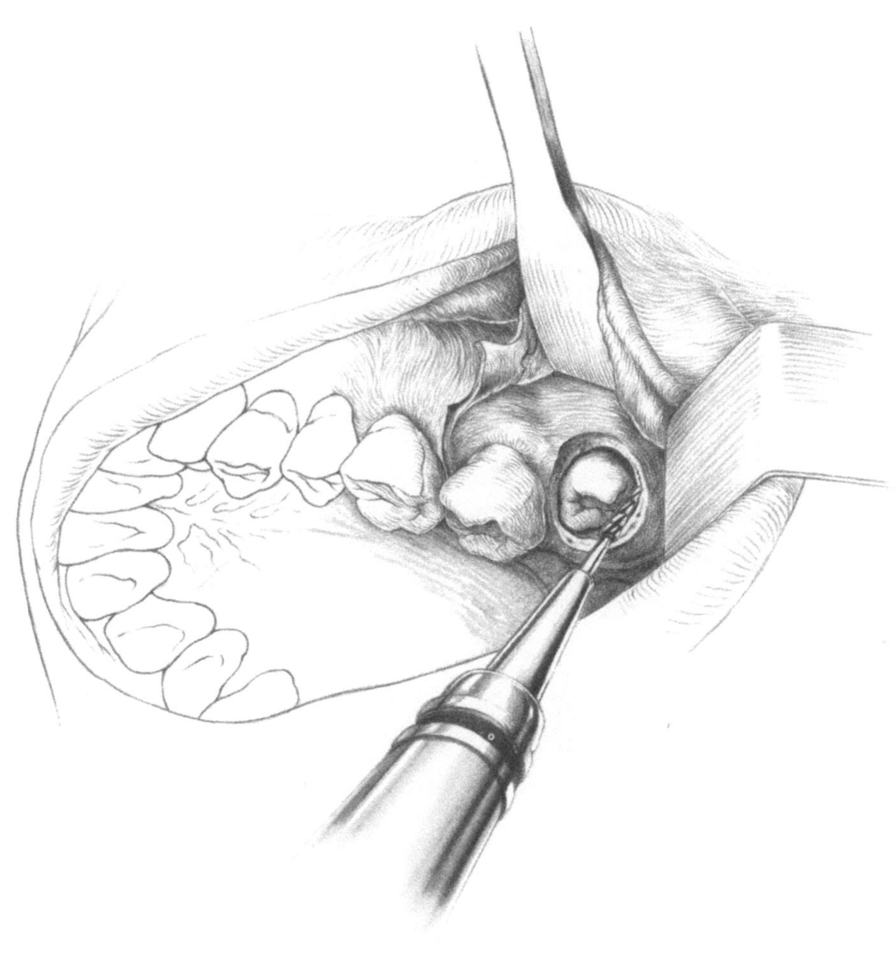

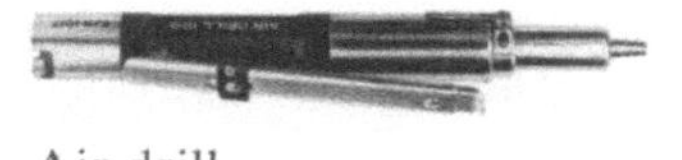

Air drill

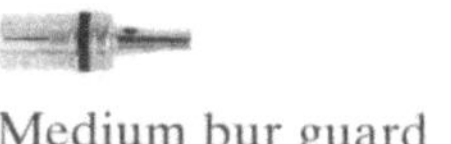

Medium bur guard

06 carbide-tip bur

Removal of an Impacted Palatal Maxillary Cuspid

1. Gently uncover the impacted cuspid with the 20° angle and 08 carbide-tip bur.

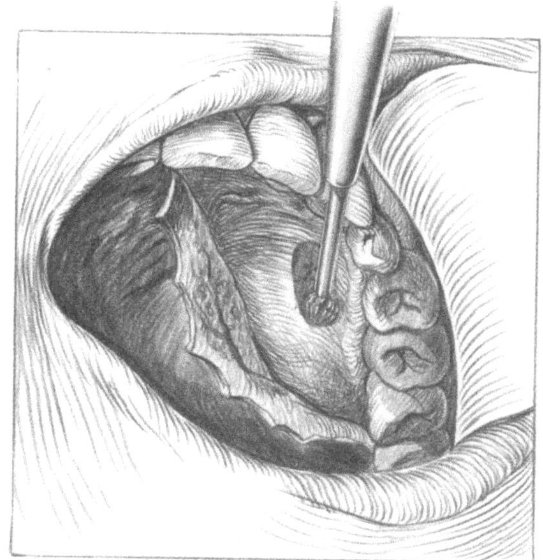

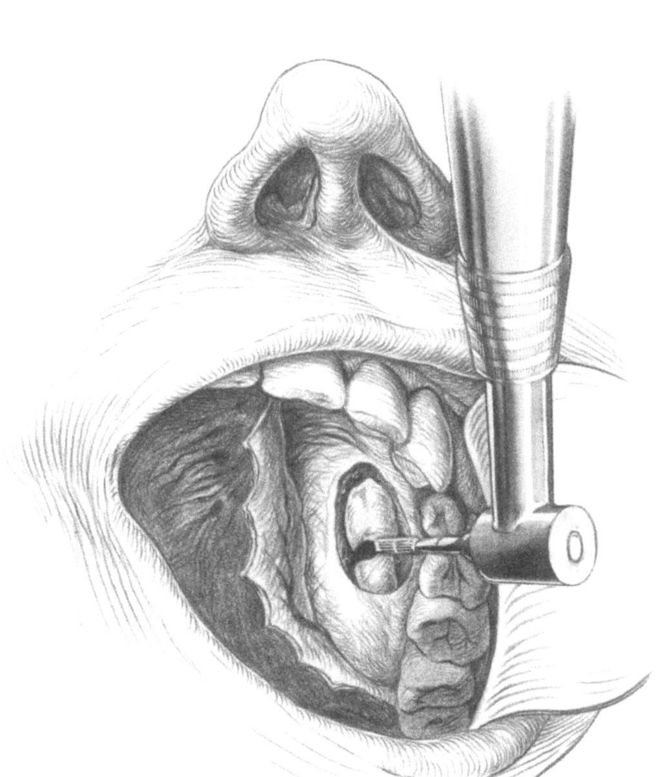

2. Section the tooth with the 90° angle and 04 carbide-tip bur. Luxate to remove the sectioned portions of the tooth.

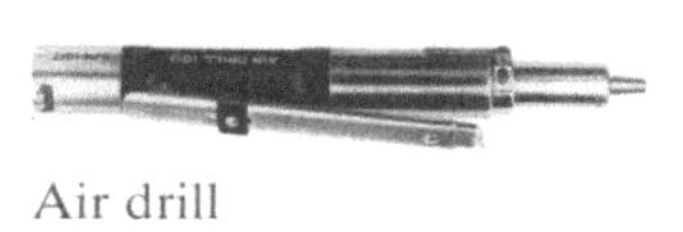

Air drill

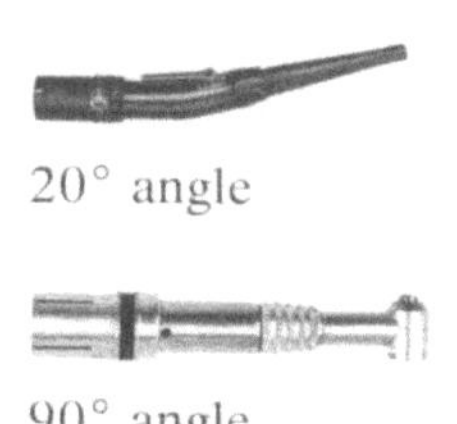

20° angle

90° angle

08 long carbide-tip bur

04 short carbide-tip bur

Apicoectomy of a Maxillary Incisor

Make a semilunar incision beginning in the region of the apex of the mesial tooth.
Extend the incision down to a point two thirds of the distance between the apex of
the root and the gingival line of the infected tooth. Then continue the incision back
up to the apex of the distal tooth.

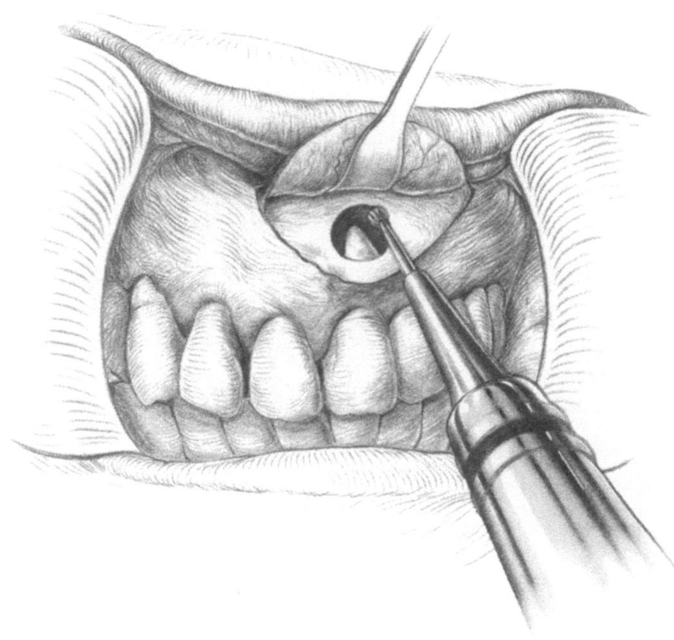

1. Following assembly of the air drill, retract the flap upward and hold it with a samll
   retractor. Excise the bone plate with the 08 carbide-tip bur. Extreme care should
   be taken not to expose or cut into the roots of the adjacent teeth.

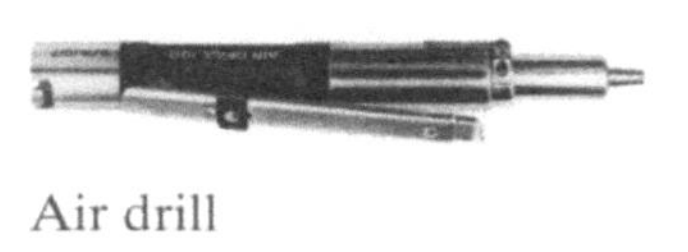

Air drill

Medium bur guard

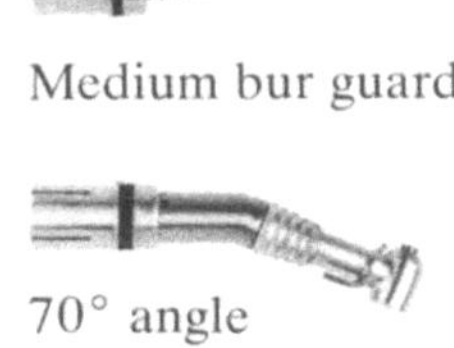

70° angle

08 carbide-tip bur

57 friction-grip bur

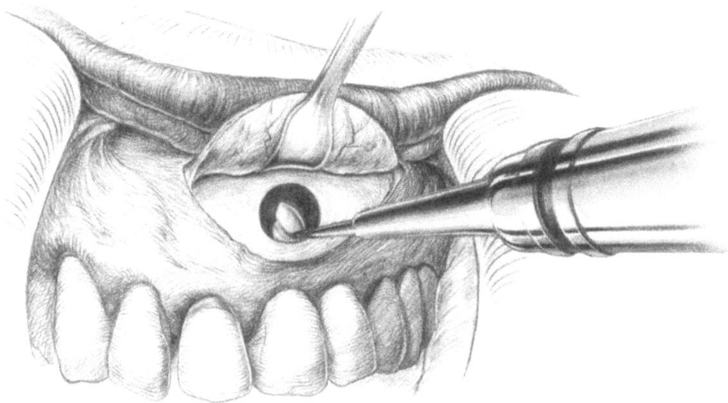

2. Make a beveled cut at the root apex with an 02 carbide-tip bur. Do not excise more than one third of the tooth.

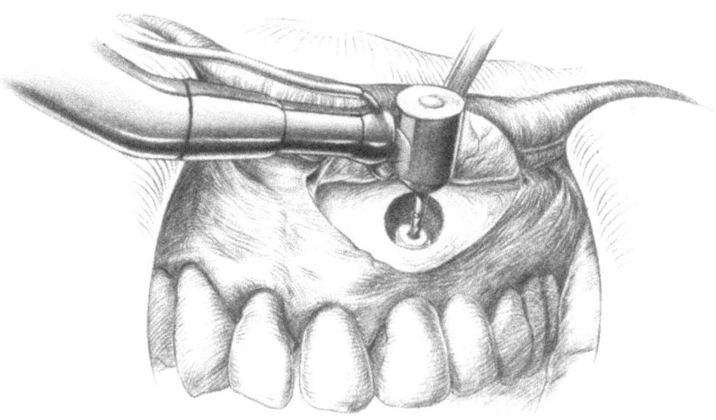

3. Change attachments. With the 70° angle and 57 friction-grip bur, enlarge the root canal. Fill the cavity before replacing the flap.

Periodontal Alveoloplasty

When surgery is performed to eliminate periodontal disease, most periodontists believe it is necessary to contour the alveolar bone. This resculpting is necessary when the bone contour presents ledges, interproximal craters, inconsistent margins, hemisepta, and intrabony pockets.

All bone removal can be successfully performed with the 70° dental angle and friction-grip burs.

Assemble the 70° angle and bur:

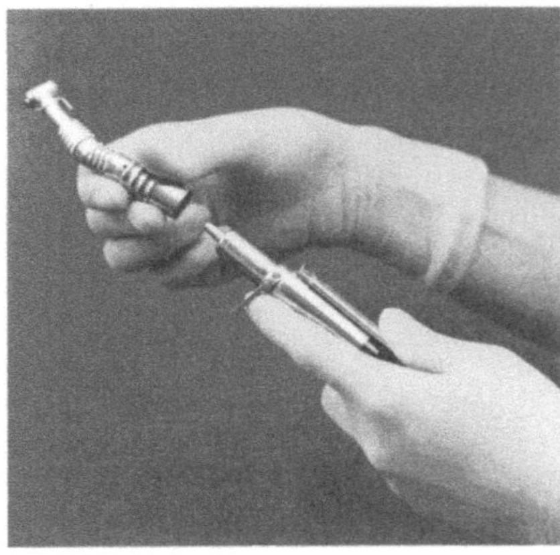

1. Push bur release lever forward 90° to assemble attachment. Completely seat.

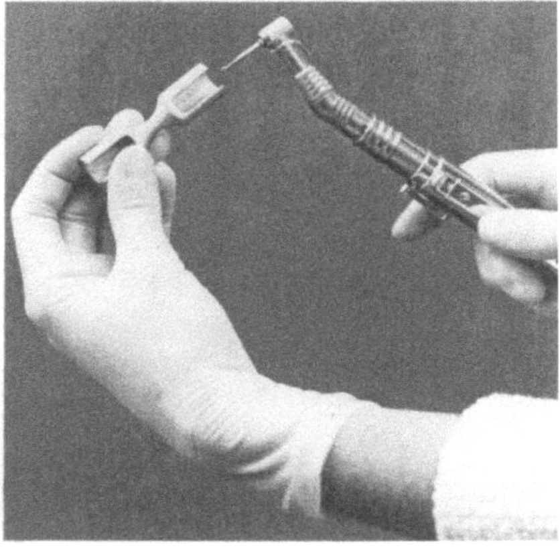

3. Place bur into collet. Slide hollow side of bur changer over bur.

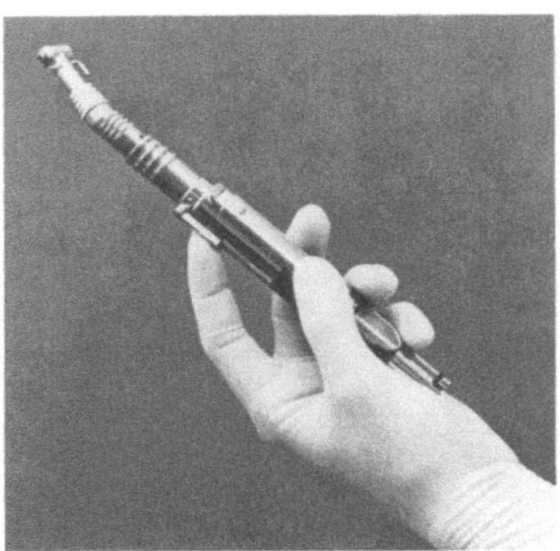

2. Return lever flush against drill to lock attachment.

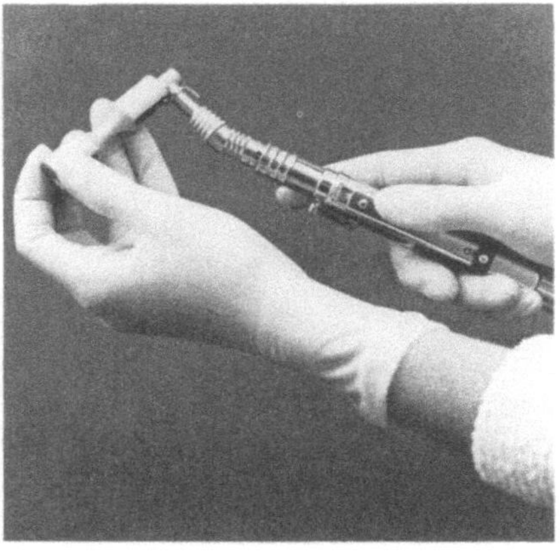

4. Press the bur firmly into place.

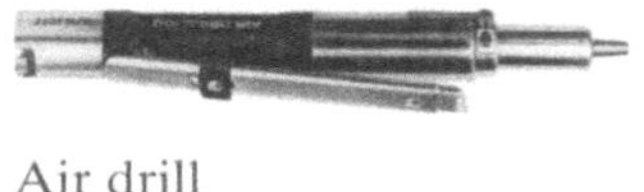

Air drill

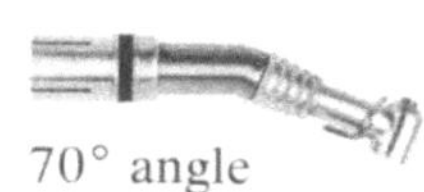

70° angle

Friction-grip dental burs

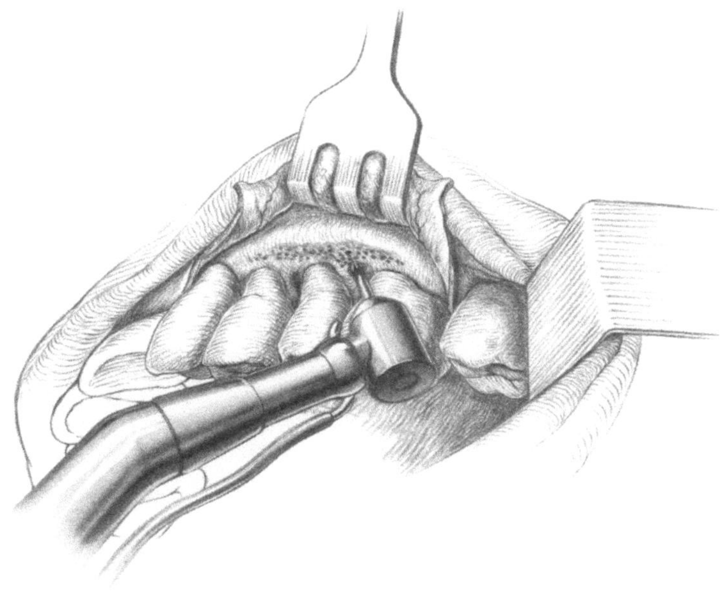

Contour the alveolar bone with the 70° angle
and friction-grip bur.

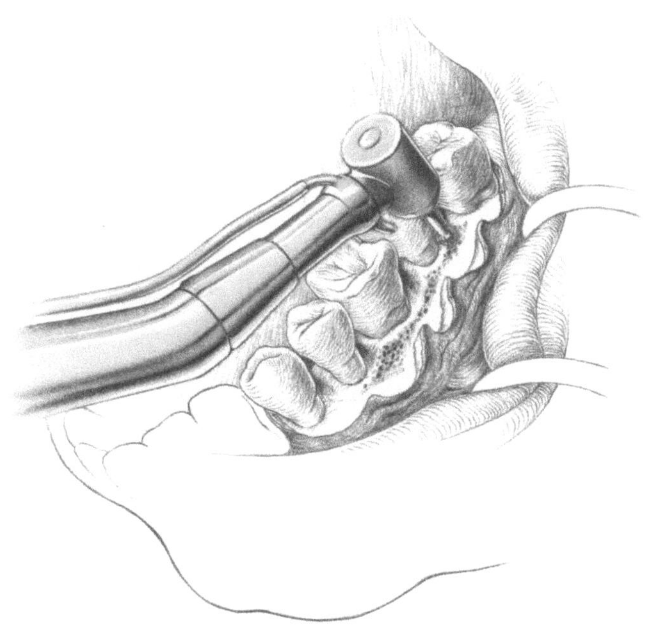

Operative Dentistry

The 70° angle and air drill are sterilizable and can therefore be used to perform dentistry in the operating room.

If a foot control is preferred it can be attached to the air drill. Assemble the air drill with foot control, push the safety lever forward on the drill and secure the throttle against the drill.

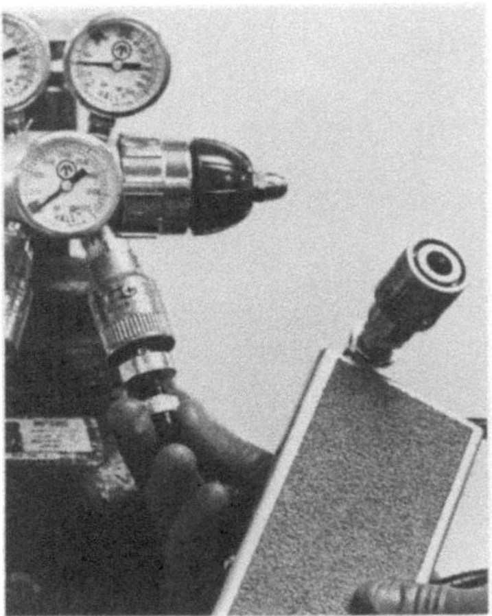

1. Plug the foot-control hose into the regulator.

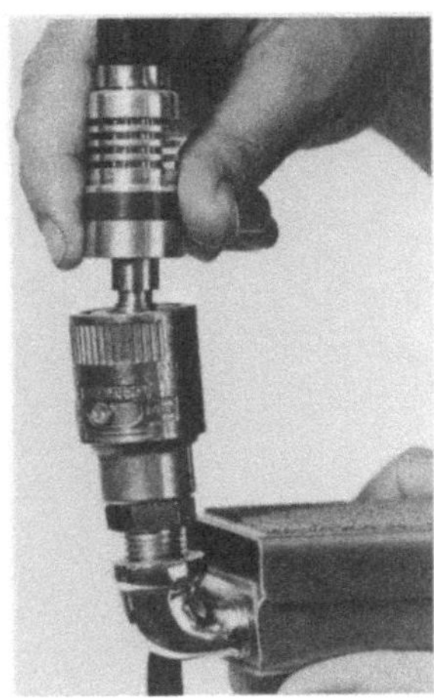

2. Connect the air-drill hose and foot control.

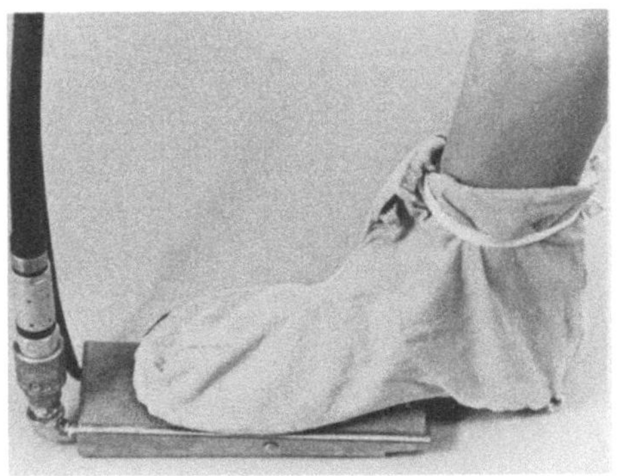

3. Place the foot control within easy reach of the surgeon's foot.

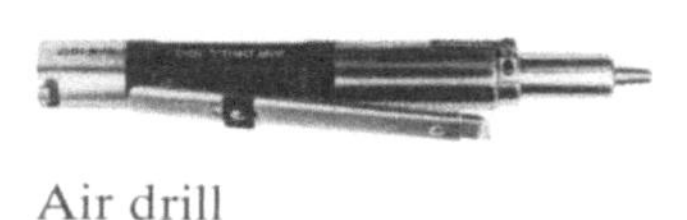

Air drill

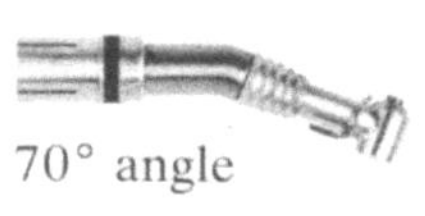

70° angle

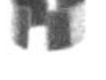

Throttle retainer

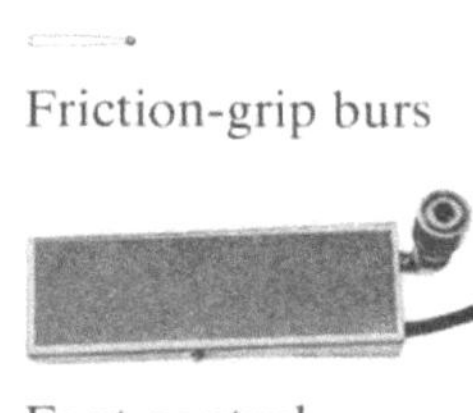

Friction-grip burs

Foot control

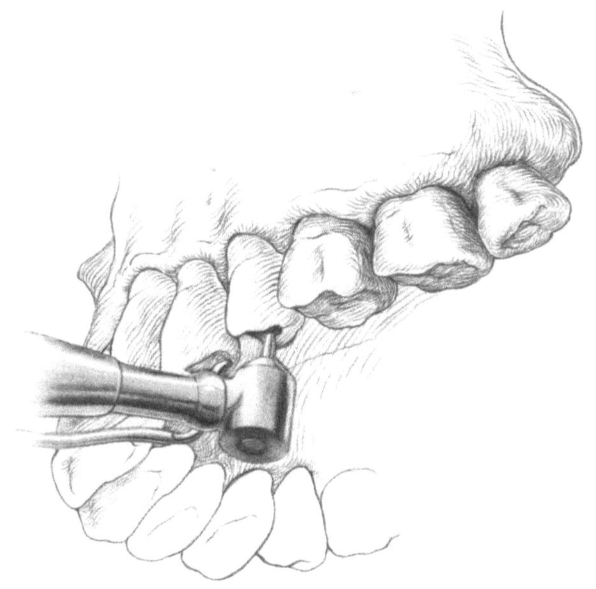

The air drill and 70° angle used for operative
dental procedures.

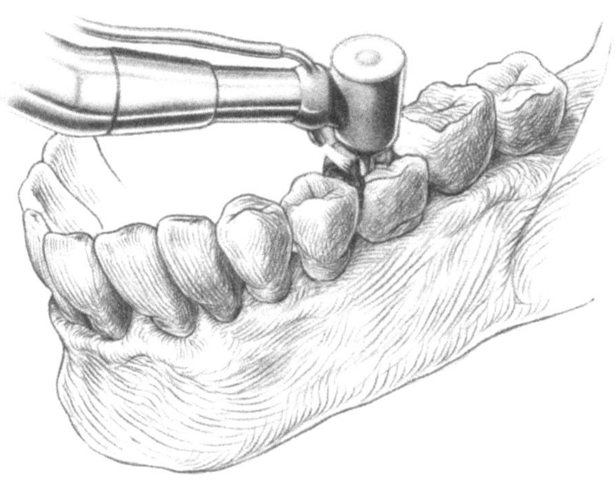

Technique Suggestions

Always wait until the drill stops before withdrawing the bur from the operative site. This will prevent accidental damage to adjacent tissue.

Substitute dissolving hemostatic foams for cottonoids or pledgets, as the former cannot be caught in the rotating drill.

Keep other equipment (e. g. suction tip) away from the drill point, which can burr a hole through metal.

Use a bur with a small tip in very restricted areas, as it is easier to control than a larger bur tip.

A combination of drilling, irrigation and suction will lubricate the bone and bur interface, clear the field and cool the bur tip.

Protect obscured or hidden soft tissue and bone with retractors before using the drill.

When unroofing a nerve or blood vessel, use a diamond bur that has a diameter equal to that of the nerve, etc. This bur will remove bone from a 180° circumference of the sheath and thereby preserve the nerve.

If extensive drilling is performed against or close to neural structures, a constant flow of irrigation fluid from an I. V. bottle and sterile tubing will help reduce heat and prevent neural damage.

For a slight increase in speed the pressure can be increased above 110 psi (7 atm); however, this is not recommended over long periods of time.

Lubricate the drill as indicated to keep the instrument in good condition.

The burs must always be sharp. Use a new bur for every operation.

Bibliography

Agren, E.: High-Speed or Conventional Dental Engines for the Removal of Bone in Oral Surgery. I. A Study of the Reactions Following Removal of Bilateral Impacted Lower Third Molars. **Acta. Odont. Scan.,** 21:585-625, December 1963.

Antoni, A. A.; Van de Mark, T. B. and Weinberg, S.; Surgical Treatment of Longstanding Malunited Horizontal Fracture of the Maxilla. **J. Canad. Dent. Ass.,** 31:22-25, January 1965.

Archer, W. H.: Oral Surgery, Fourth Edition. **W. B. Saunders Co.,** Philadelphia-London 1966.

Bell, W. H.: Surgical Correction of Mandibular Retrognathism. **Amer. J. Orthodont.,** 52:518-528, July 1966.

Bell, W. H.: Surgical Correction of Anterior Maxillary Retrusion. **J. Oral Surg.,** 26:58-60, January 1968.

Bell, W. H.: Surgical-Orthodontic Correction of Adult Bimaxillary Protrusion. **J. Oral Surg.,** 28:578-590, August 1970.

Bell, W. H.: Surgical-Orthodontic Treatment of Interincisal Diastemas. **(Personal Communication)** 1971.

Boyne, P. J.: Osseous Healing After Oblique Osteotomy of the Mandibular Ramus. **J. Oral Surg.,** 24: 125-133, March 1966.

Converse, J. M.: Horizontal Osteotomy of the Mandible. **Plast. and Reconstr. Surg.,** 34:464-471, November 1964.

Cunningham, M. P. and Slaughter, D. P.: A Face-Saving Procedure: Marginal Resection of the Mandible for Anterior Oral Cancer. **Illinois Med. J.,** 133: 166-169, February 1968.

Goldman, H. M. et al.: Current Therapy in Dentistry, Volume 3. **The C. V. Mosby Co.,** St. Louis, Missouri, USA 1968.

Gores, R. J.: Surgical Odontectomy for Unerupted Teeth. **Curr. Ther. in Dent.,** 3:510-526, 1968.

Hall, H. D. and O'Steen, A. N.: Free Grafts of Palatal Mucosa in Mandibular Vestibuloplasty. **J. Oral Surg.,** 28:565-574, August 1970.

Hall, R. M.: The Effect of High-Speed Bone Cutting Without the Use of a Water Coolant. **Oral Surg. Oral Med., Oral Pathol.,** 20:150: 153, August 1965.

Ham, J. W.; Patterson, S. S. and Healey, H. J.: An Evaluation of Handpiece Sterilization for Periapical Surgery. **J. Oral Surg.,** 28:353-355, May 1970.

Hinds, E. C. and Girotti, W. J.: Vertical Subcondylar Osteotomy: A Reappraisal. **Oral Surg. Oral Med., Oral Pathol.,** 24:164-170, August 1967.

Lipshutz, H.; Lerner, H. J. and Beckloff, G. L.: Hydroxyurea in the Management of Head and Neck Cancer. **Plast. and Reconstr. Surg.,** 40:240-242, September 1967.

Marlette, R. H.: Submucoperiosteal Wire Fixation of Mandibular Fractures. **J. Oral Surg., Anesth. & Hosp. D. Serv.,** 21:47-51, September 1963.

Bibliography *(continued)*

Meyer, I.: Alveoloplasty — The Oral Surgeon's Point of View. **Oral Surg.,** 22: 441-455, October 1966.

Moose, S. M.: Surgical Correction of Mandibular Prognathism by Intraoral Subcondylar Osteotomy. **J. Oral Surg.,** 22:197-202, May 1964.

Nicols, J. J.: Prognathism: Correction Using Sliding Osteotomy Technique. **Dent. Dig.,** 72:494-497, November 1966.

Pulec, J. L.: Facial Nerve Grafting. **Laryngoscope,** LXX1X:1562-1582, September 1969.

Robinson, M. and Shuken, R.: The L Splint for Immobilization of Iliac Bone Grafts to the Mandible. **J. Oral Surg.,** 24:10-14, January 1966.

Samuels, H. S. and Oatis, G. W.: The Use of Kirschner Wires in Facial Fractures: A Report of Cases. **J. Oral Surg.,** 28:382-385, 1970.

Singh, J. P.; Pinto Do Rosario, N. and Sangal, N. C.: Kirschner Wire Fixation of Fracture in an Edentulous Mandible. **J. Indian. Med. Ass.,** 49:557-560, December 1967.

Sowray, J. H. and Haskell, R.: Osteotomy at the Mandibular Symphysis. **Brit. J. Oral Surg.,** 6:97-102, November 1968.

Szmyd, L.: Combined Chisel-Air Turbine Technic for Impacted Mandibular Third Molar Surgery. **School of Aerospace Med.,** Brooks AF Base, Tex. SAM-TDR-62-78, June 1962.

Thoma, K. H.: Oral Surgery, Fifth Edition. **C. V. Mosby Co.,** St. Louis 1969.

Winstanley, R. P.: Subcondylar Osteotomy of the Mandible and the Intraoral Approach. **Brit. J. Oral Surg.,** 6:134-136, November 1968.

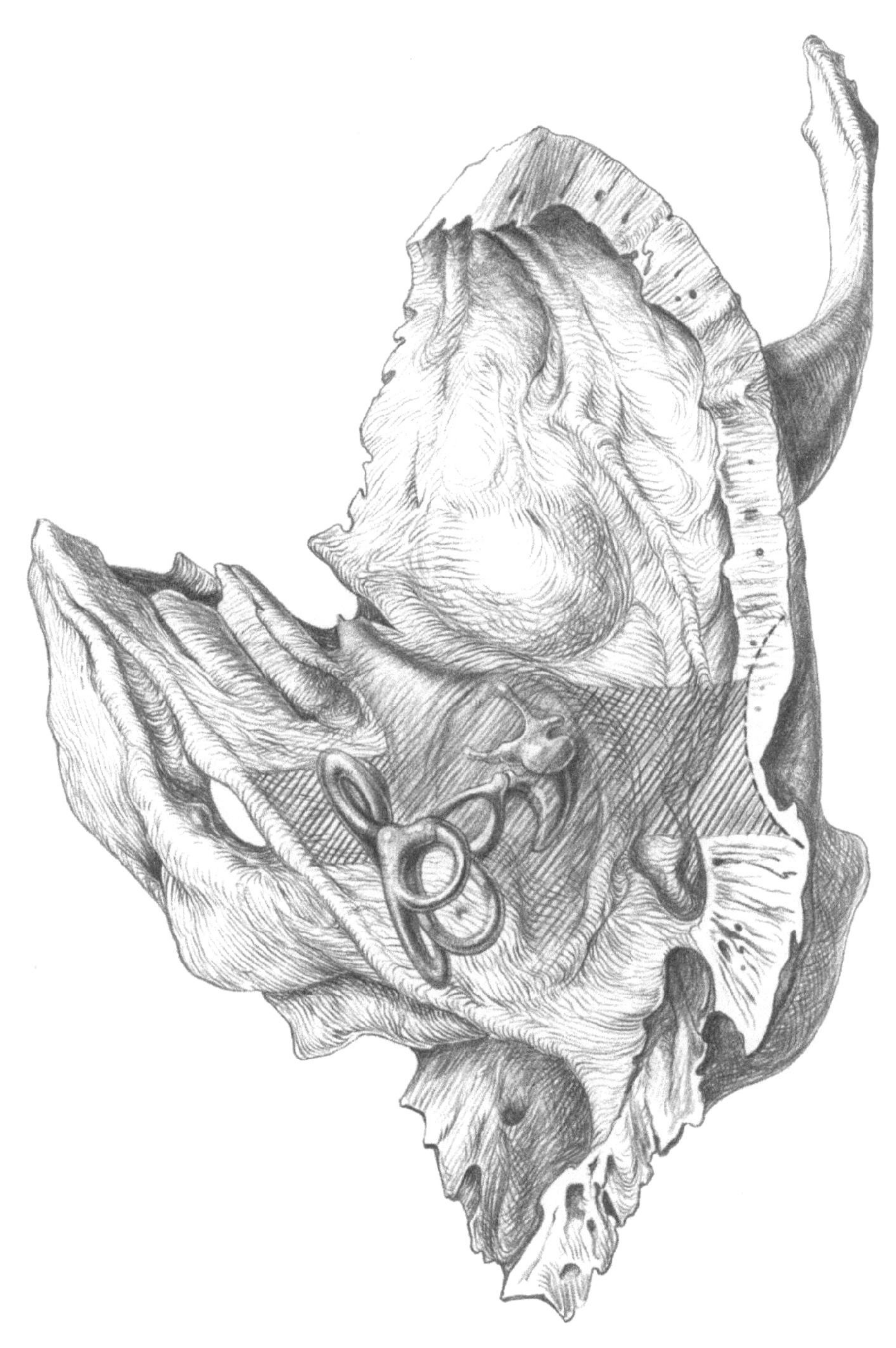

Introduction

Temporal bone surgery demands the most advanced and refined instrumentation. The advent of the surgical microscope makes new and anatomically exacting surgical procedures feasible.

The air drill can be used for many of these surgical techniques. A 20° angle attached to the air drill and controlled by the foot gives the surgeon full mastery over the bur tip.

The steel bur rotating at full speed quickly excises dense cortical bone. When approaching middle ear structures, a microsurgical bur, carbide-tipped or diamond, will effectively erase bone without harming surrounding soft tissue.

Most surgery requires irrigation and suction to clear and clean the operative site. Microsurgical techniques, however, require improved irrigation systems to protect neural structures from heat transmitted during bone drilling and also to lubricate the interface between bone and drill.

Contents

Excision of an Osteoma of the External Auditory Meatus

Assemble the air drill and 20° angle:

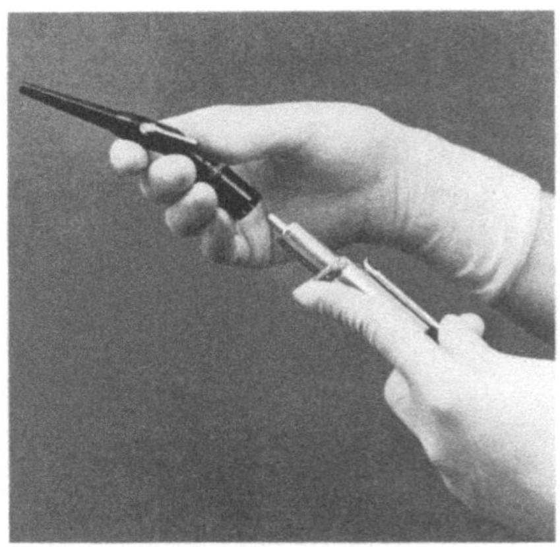

1. Slip 20° angle snugly over the shoulder of the air drill, while raising the lever 90°.

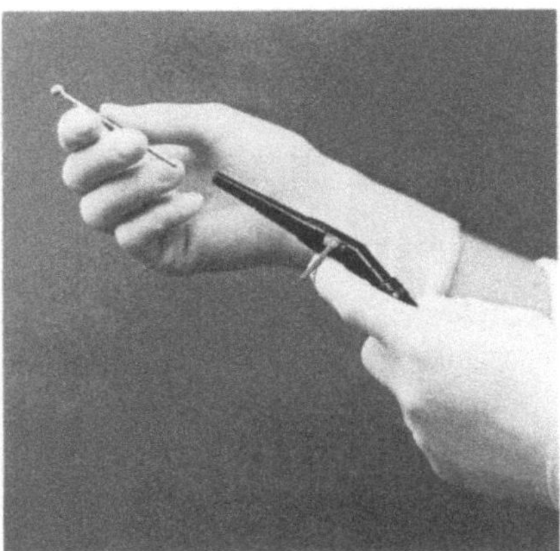

3. Push lever on angle forward; insert bur. Lock bur securely by returning lever flush against the instrument.

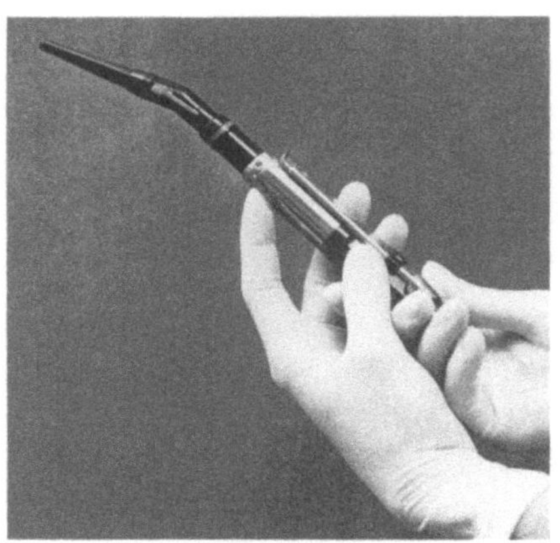

2. Return lever flush against the drill to lock 20° angle.

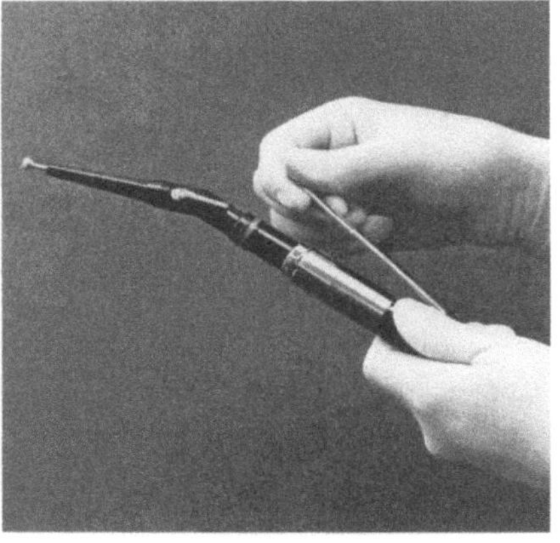

4. Use increased extension for finger-tip control.

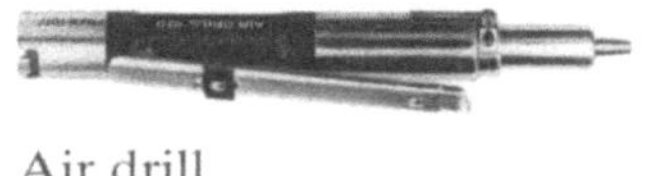

Air drill

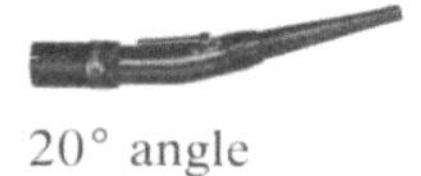

20° angle

23 long steel bur

5. Make a curved skin incision and elevate the tissue off the tumor.

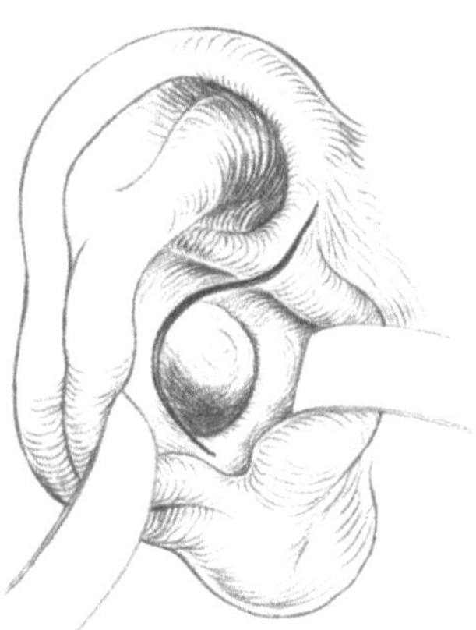

6. Excise the bone tumor with a steel bur. Intermittent irrigation clears the operative area of bone debris while reducing the heat generated by the rotating bur.

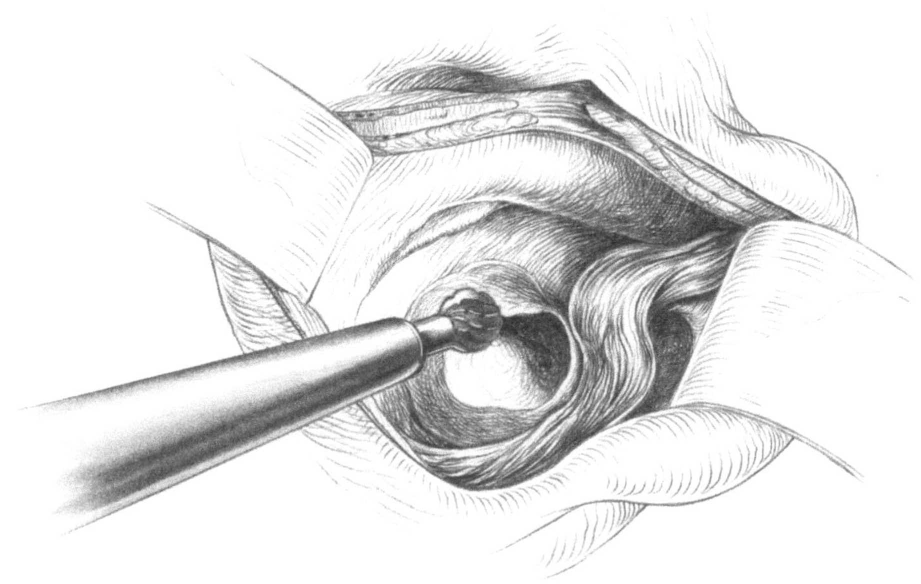

With a 23 steel bur excise the diseased cells of the mastoid bone. Do not apply pressure on the bur while drilling; a light constant movement of the bur over the bone surface will prove more effective for bone removal.

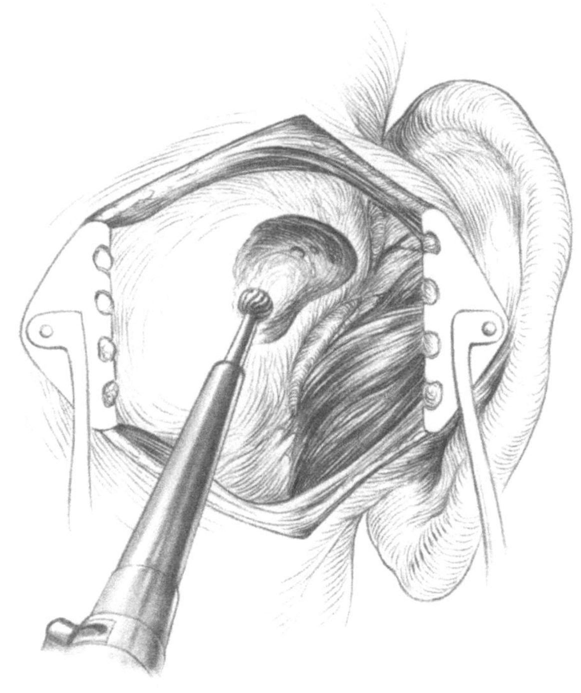

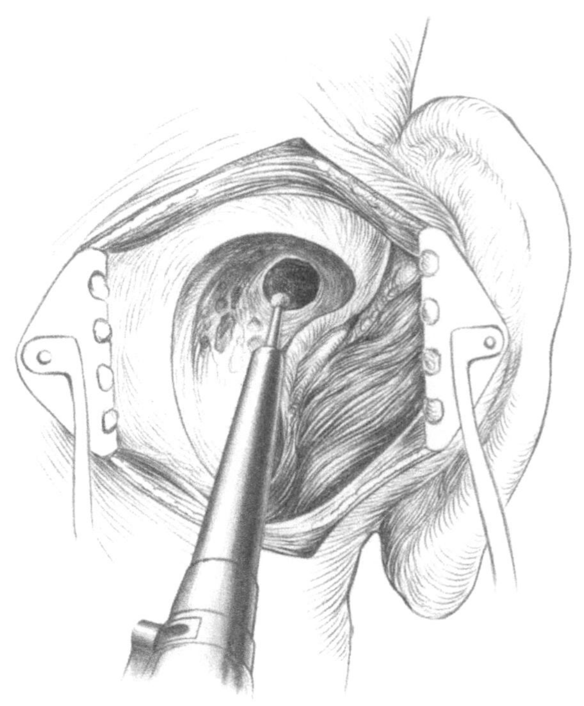

The edges on a steel bur are too severe for work close to soft tissue. The 23 diamond bur, being very abrasive, will cut bone, though more slowly, while causing no damage to soft tissue structures.

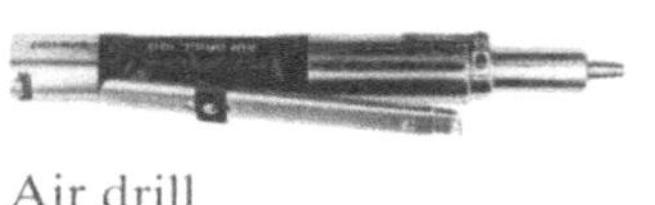

Air drill

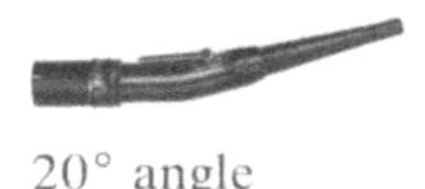

20° angle

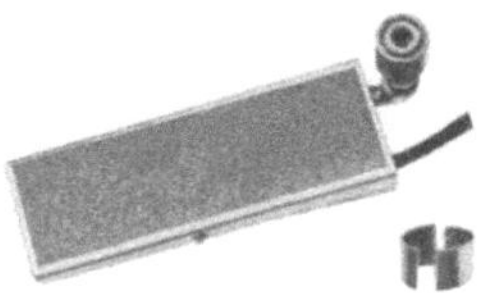

Foot control
Throttle retainer

23 long steel bur

23 long diamond bur

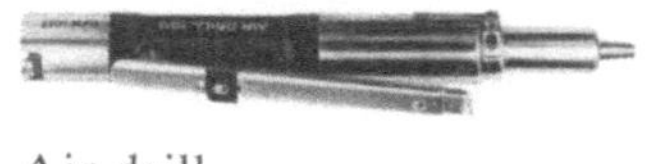

Air drill

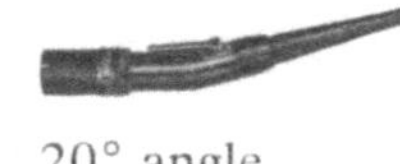

20° angle

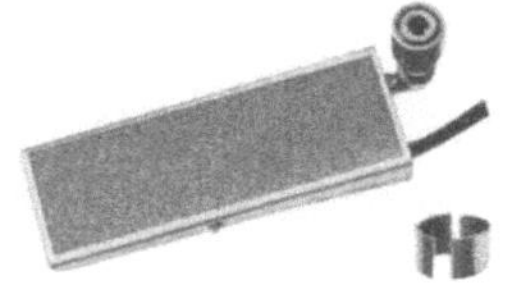

Foot control
Throttle retainer

23 long steel bur

23 long diamond bur

A Radical Mastoidectomy

A radical mastoidectomy requires a small round steel bur for removal of diseased bone cells. Make a connection between the middle ear and mastoid to form one large cavity. Burr away the posterior wall of the external auditory meatus and treat any further middle ear pathology. Middle ear bone removal should be completed with a diamond bur to avoid trauma to the facial nerve and other soft tissue structures.

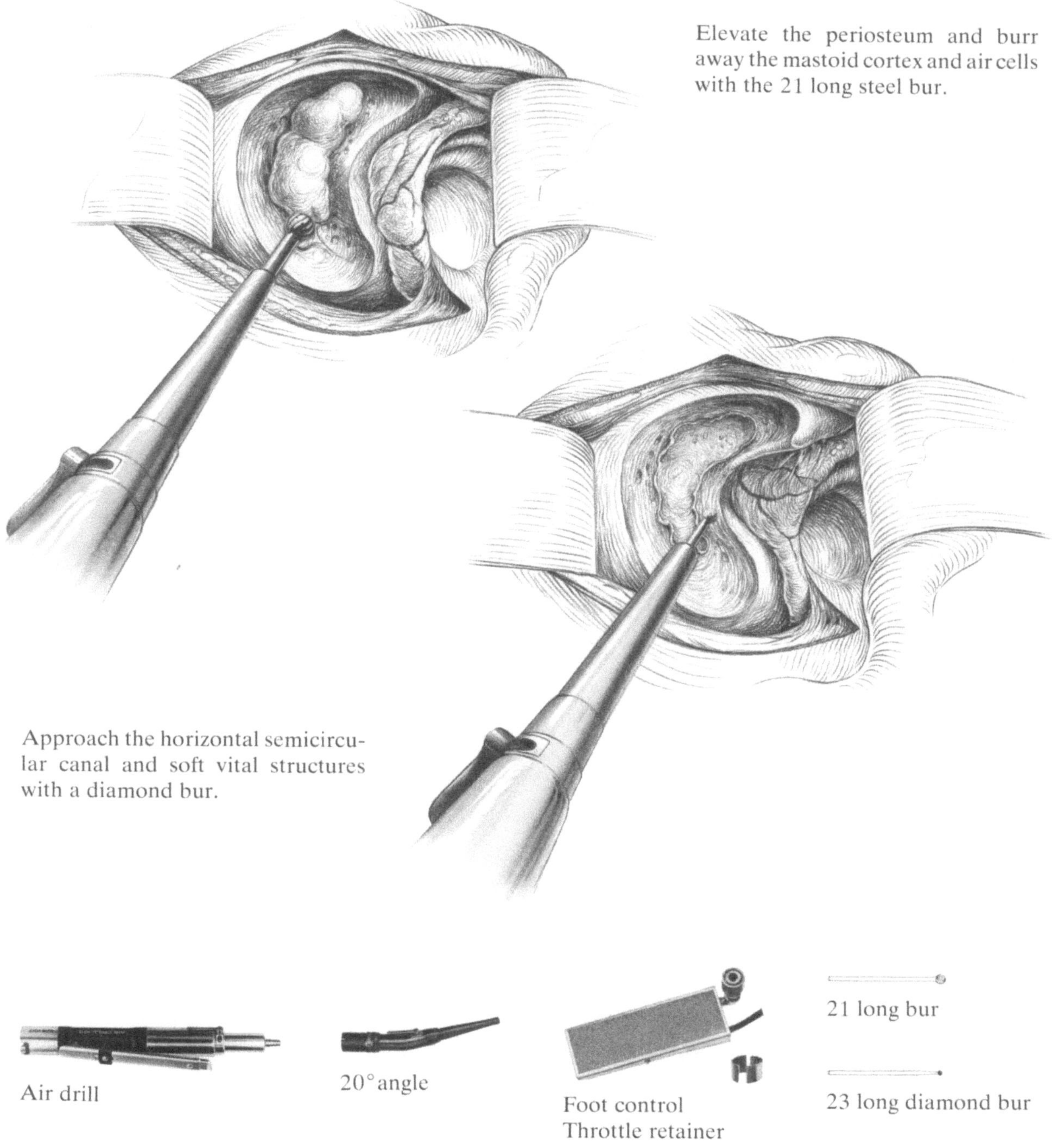

Elevate the periosteum and burr away the mastoid cortex and air cells with the 21 long steel bur.

Approach the horizontal semicircular canal and soft vital structures with a diamond bur.

Cryosurgical Treatment of Meniere's Disease

Make an endaural incision. Follow with a simple mastoidectomy to expose the horizontal semicircular canal.

Change to a diamond bur. Thin the posterior portion of the canal to allow maximum heat transfer between the interior of the canal and the tip of the freezing cannula. Abrade the bone until a grayish-blue line appears, while avoiding accidental cracking or puncturing of the bone.

1. Make the endaural incision.

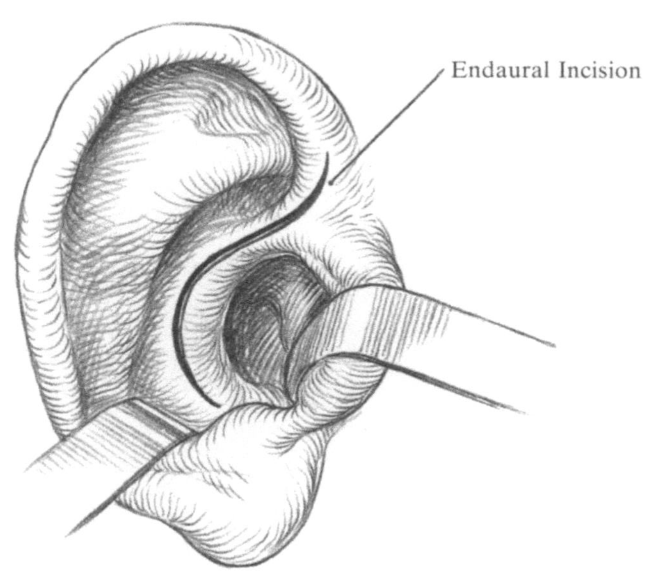

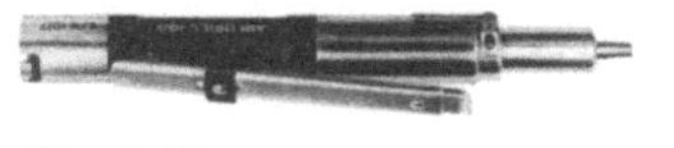

Air drill

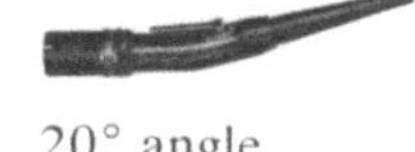

20° angle

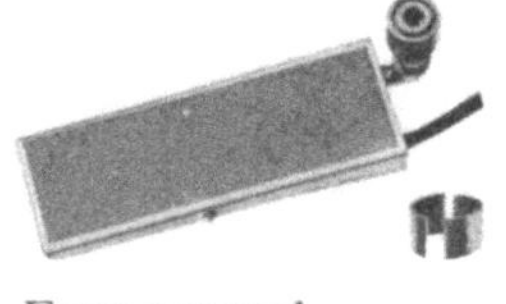

Foot control
Throttle retainer

22 long steel bur

28 long diamond bur

2. Use the 22 long steel bur to perform a simple mastoidectomy.

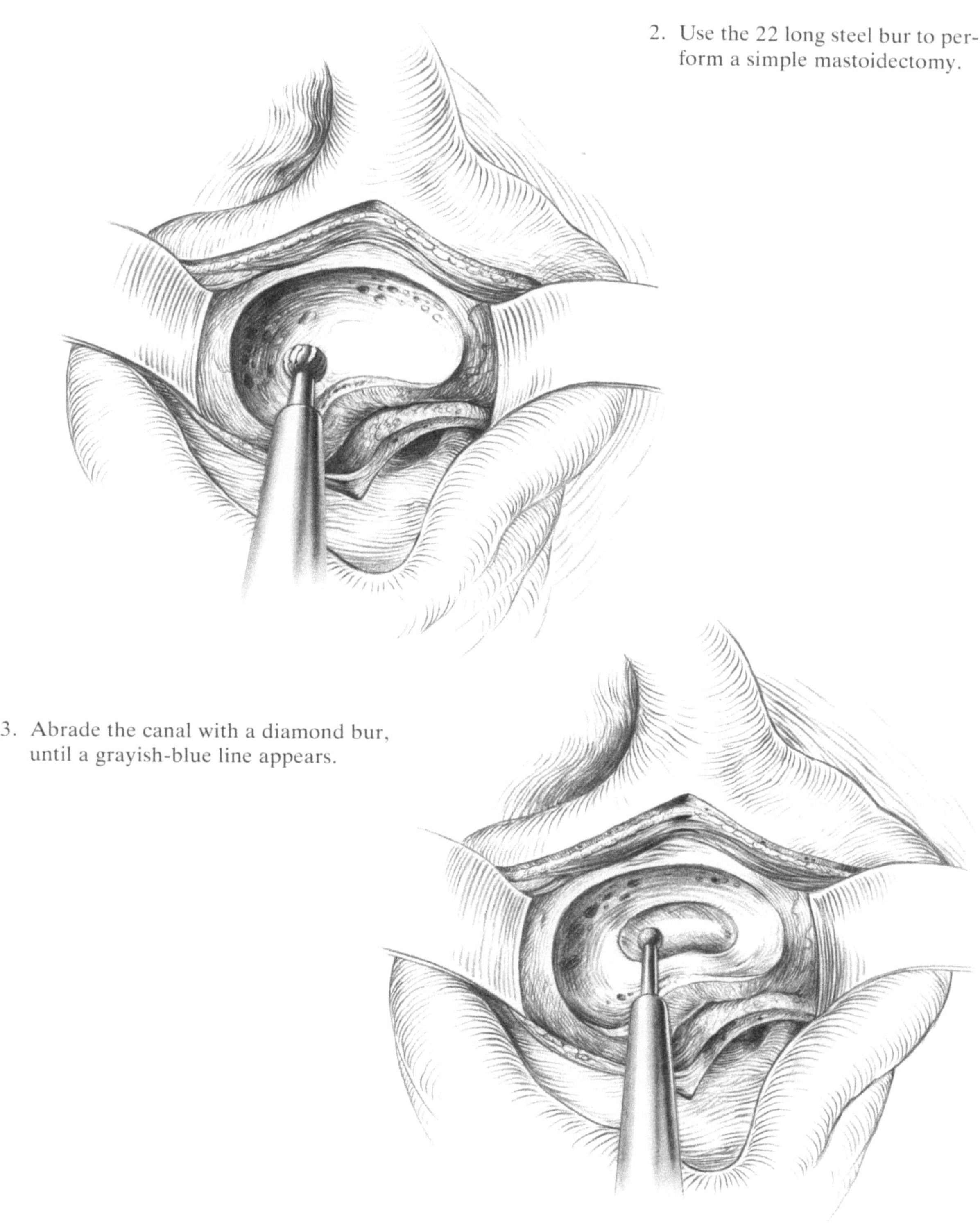

3. Abrade the canal with a diamond bur, until a grayish-blue line appears.

4. Apply a cryoprobe to the bone for several minutes. Warm the probe before removal to prevent adherence to the bone which may cause it to crack.

Exposure of the Middle Ear

To expose the inner ear and to carry out surgery there, extremely fine carbide and diamond burs are used with the projected micro air drill* with foot control. The drills will have a lower speed and more torque than any other drill presently available. The instrument will give the surgeon the desired balance. speed and comfort necessary to complete long and exacting procedures.

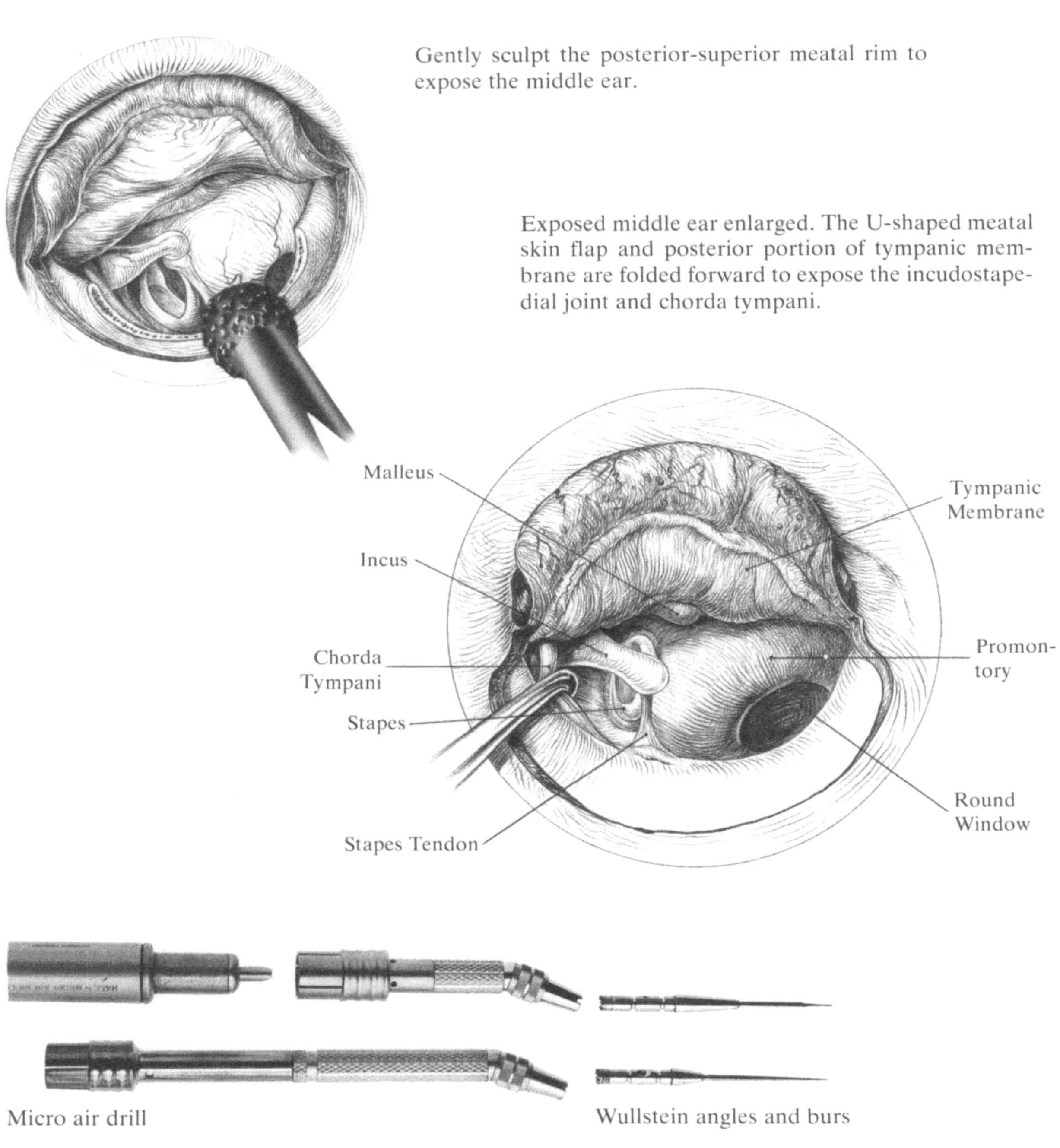

Gently sculpt the posterior-superior meatal rim to expose the middle ear.

Exposed middle ear enlarged. The U-shaped meatal skin flap and posterior portion of tympanic membrane are folded forward to expose the incudostapedial joint and chorda tympani.

Micro air drill

Wullstein angles and burs

---

* Under development.

Fenestration of the Solid Footplate

All the refinements of microneurosurgery come into play when surgery of the stapes footplate is necessary. The diamond bur is used to fenestrate, or drill out the solid footplate. A graft is placed over the oval window, and a prosthesis positioned to connect the incus and the graft.

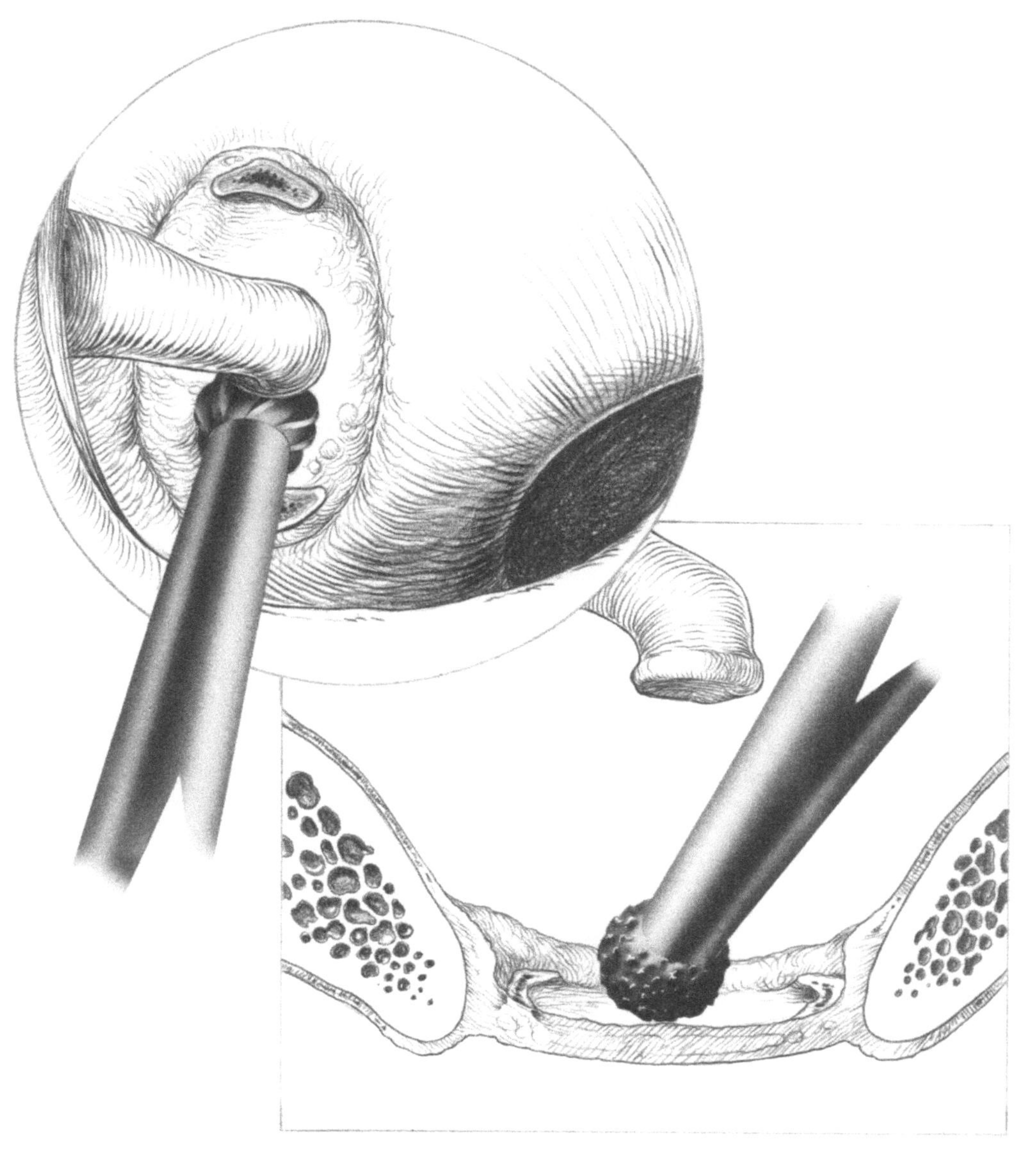

Gently fenestrate the stapes footplate with the diamond bur and micro air drill.

Transtemporal Translabyrinthine Approach to an Acoustic Neuroma*

With the 24 long steel bur perform a simple mastoidectomy. The exposure includes
the entire tegmen mastoidi, lateral sinus plate, sinodural angle, mastoid tip with
digastric ridge, horizontal semicircular canal, and short process of incus.

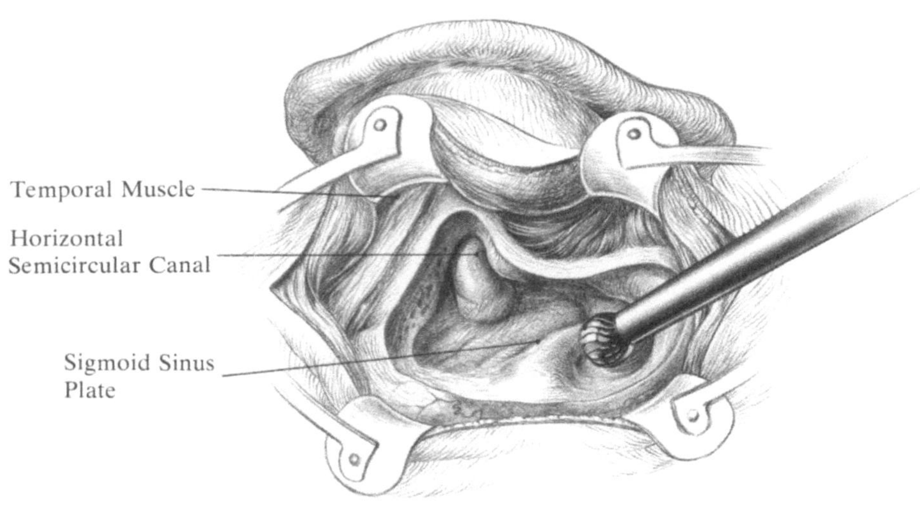

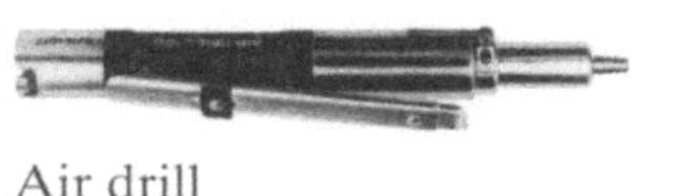

Air drill

Long bur guard

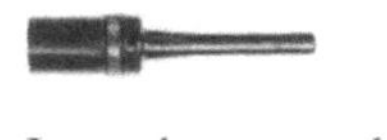

24 long steel bur

21 long diamond bur

---

* William W. Montgomery, M.D. (Personal Communication). Translabyrinthine Resection of the Small Acoustic Tumor.
  Arch Otolaryng Vol. 89, February 1969.

With a diamond bur make a small fenestra in the horizontal semicircular canal in order to obtain perilymph.

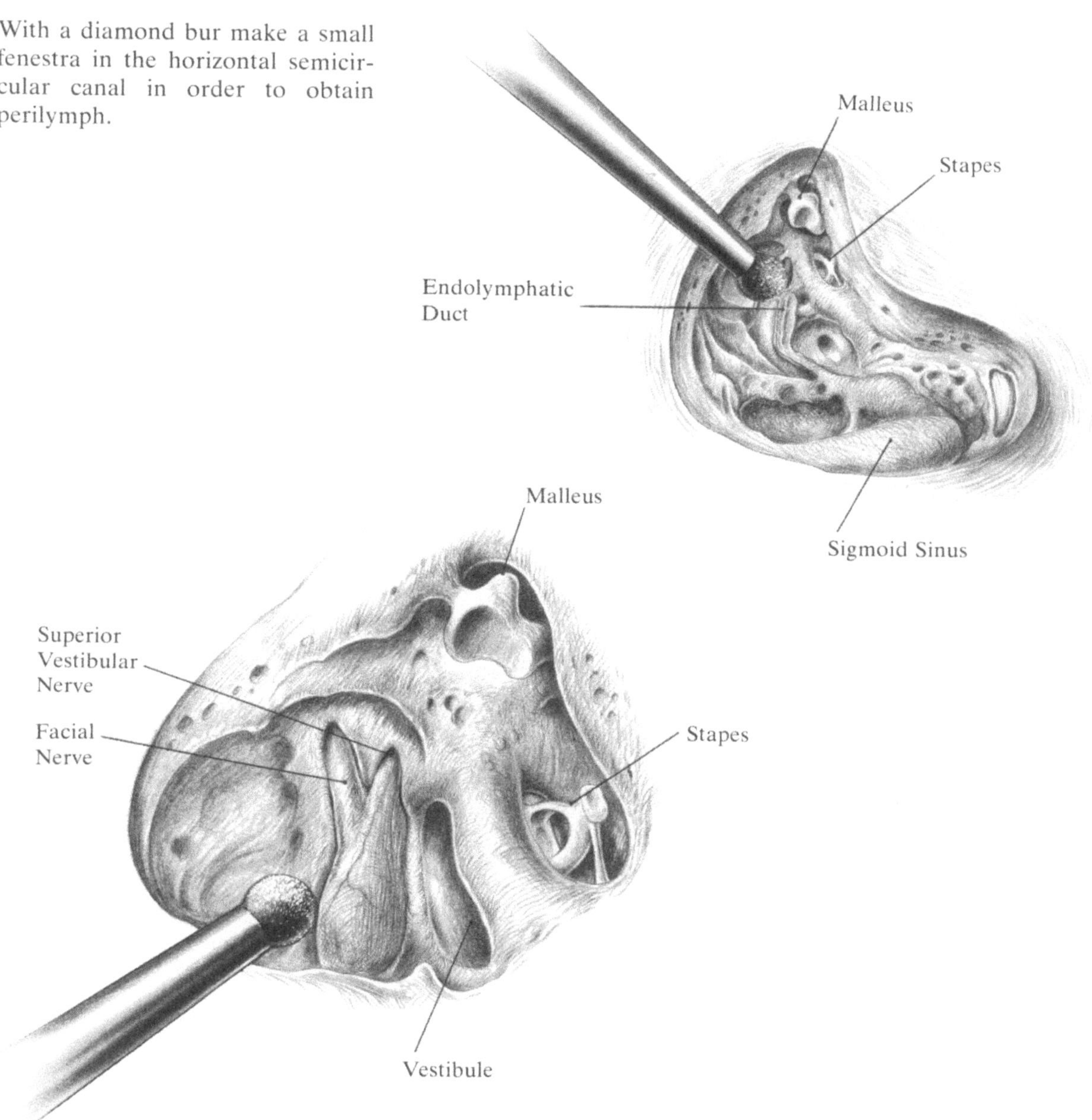

Using the same bur and a technique of drilling, irrigation and suction, unroof the petrous portion of the facial nerve and expose the dura covering the nerve tumor.

Preservation of the Posterior Canal Wall and Bridge in Surgery for Cholesteatoma*

1. Assemble the 20° angle and 19 long steel bur. Make a postauricular incision and using the steel bur perform a simple mastoidectomy-atticotomy. Thin the posterior canal wall to approximately 1.0 - 1.5 mm.

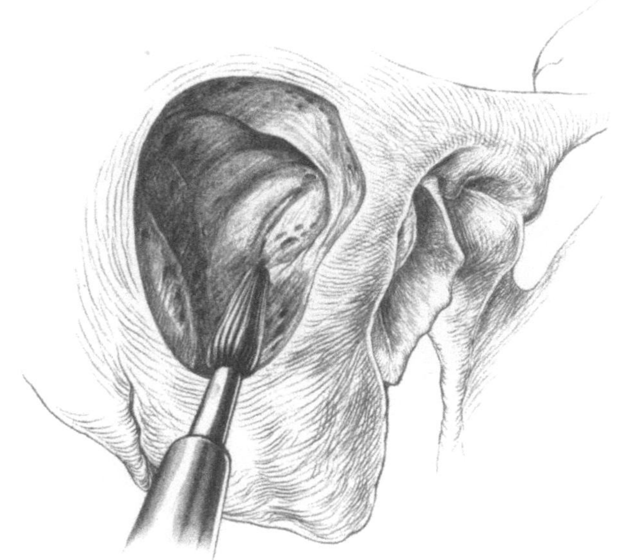

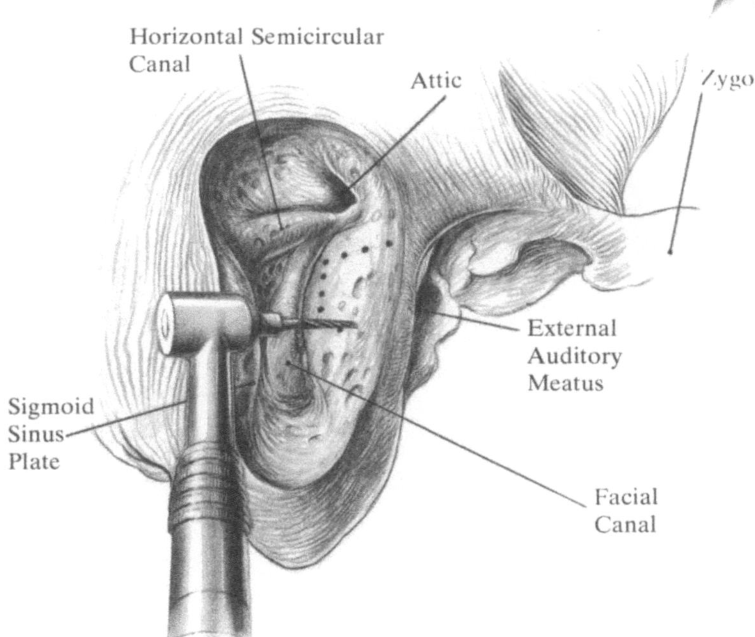

2. Make drill holes with the 90° angle and 10 short carbide-tip bur to outline a vertical osteotomy just below the level of the floor of the external canal. Outline a similar parallel osteotomy inferiorly at approximately the level of the floor of the external canal.

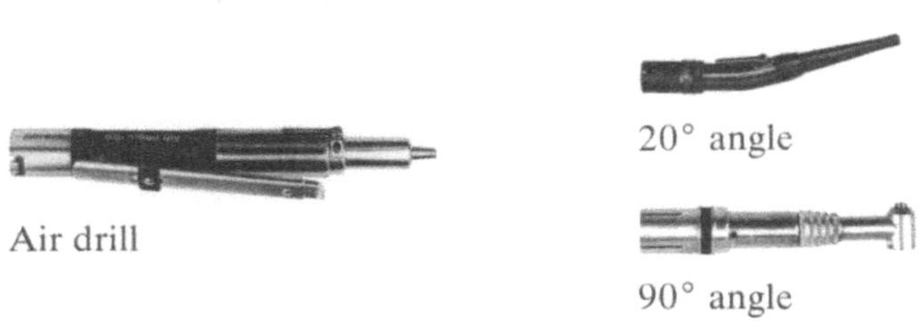

---

* A. Lapidot, M.D. and E. C. Brandow, M.D.: A Method for Preserving the Posterior Canal Wall and Bridge in the Surgery for Cholesteatoma. **Acta Oto-laryng** (Stockholm) 62 : 89 - 93, July 1966.

3. Connect the two osteotomies by a horizontal osteotomy approximately 1-2 mm above the facial ridge with the 04 short carbide-tip bur.

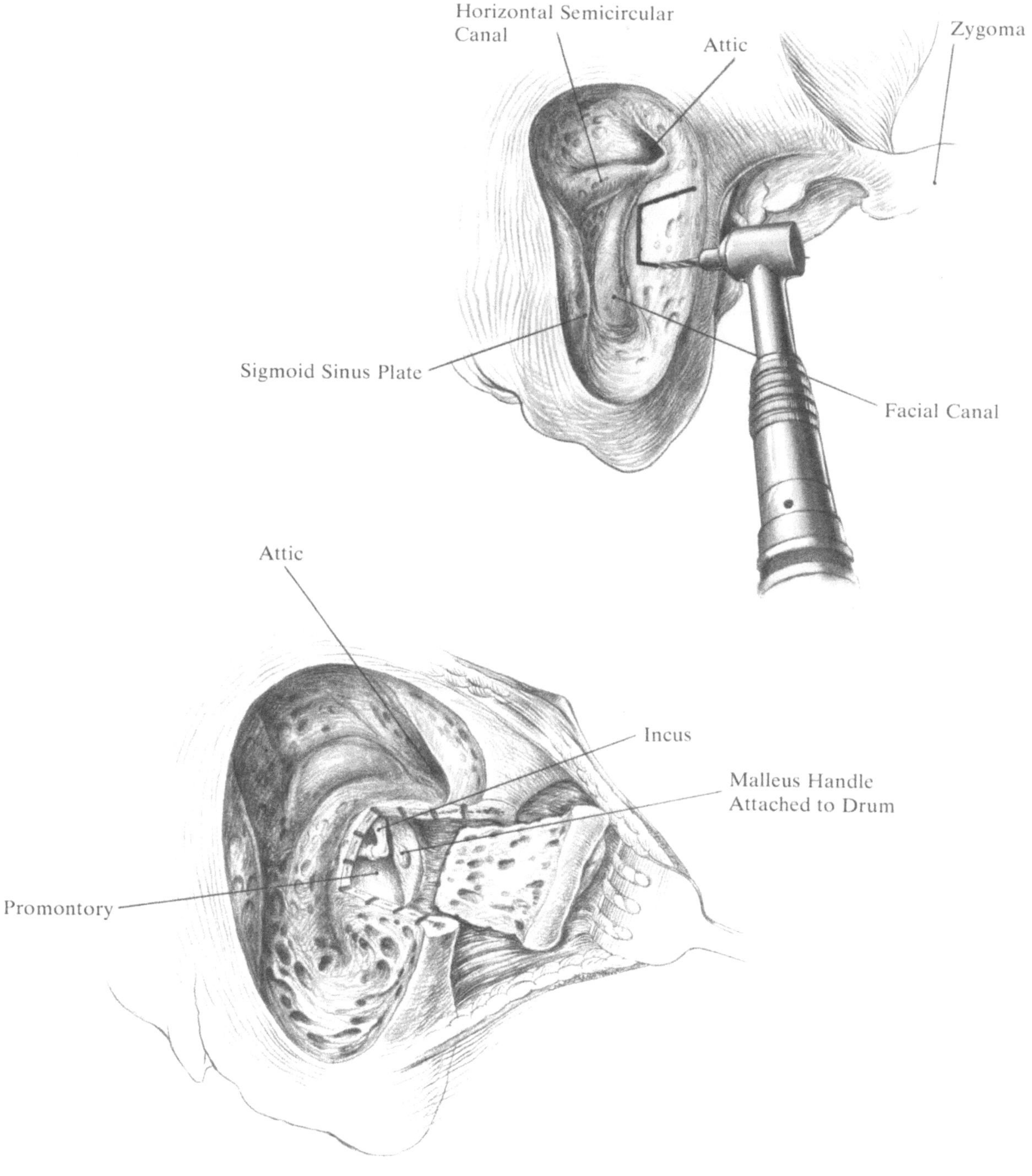

4. The isolated bone fragment can be elevated anteriorly and posteriorly for good visualization. Deliver the cholesteatoma sac posteriorly or anteriorly whichever is preferred to maintain continuity.

Technique Suggestions

Any high-speed drill used in microsurgical procedures should be tested first in the laboratory.

At first, there is a tendency to use a high-speed drill at too low a speed, thus requiring increased pressure against the bone. This can cause skidding of the bur. For best results, operate at maximum regulator pressure 100-110 psi (7-8 atm).

The air drill rotates only in a clockwise direction. Consequently, when pressure is applied to the bur the potential danger of skidding toward vulnerable brain structures should be recognized.

Irrigation fluid should be applied no faster than it can be suctioned away.

A drill in contact with bone produces some heat. This could be transferred to nearby neural structures, such as the optic nerve or facial and acoustic nerves. Reduce heat with irrigation.

Diamond burs, which are abrasive, must be used close to vital soft tissue structures. A steel bur could damage soft tissue if accidentally brought into contact with it.

When the drill is used under the microscope, a foot control is recommended. This allows the surgeon to control the movement of the bur with both hands and the speed of the drill with the foot.

Bibliography

Anonymous: Panel discussion on the problems of ear surgery. **J. Laryng.,** 81: 1212-4, November 1967.

Baron, S. H.: Modified radical mastoidectomy; preservation of the cholesteatoma matrix; a method of making a flap in the endaural technique. **Arch. Otolaryng.** 49:280, 1949.

Baron, S. H.: Management of aural cholesteatoma in children. **Otol. Clinics of N. A.,** February 1969.

Caparosa, R. J.: Bilateral acoustic neurinoma. Combined otoneurosurgical approach. **Laryngoscope,** 76:758-771, April 1966.

Caparosa, R. J.: Surgery of the internal auditory meatus. Development, surgical anatomy, and surgical techniques. **Laryngoscope,** 77:2077-102, Dec. 1967.

Coleman, C. C., Jr.: Removal of the temporal bone for cancer. **Amer. J. Surg.,** 112:583-90, October 1966.

Hanna, D. C. et al.: A suggested technic for resection of the temporal bone. **Amer. J. Surg.,** 114:553-8, October 1967.

Hilding, D. A. and Selker, R.: Total resection of the temporal bone for carcinoma. **Arch. Otolaryng.,** 89: April 1969.

Hitselberger, W. E. and House, W. F.: Acoustic tumor surgery. **Arch. Otalaryng.,** 84:255-265, September 1966.

House, W. F. and Crabtree, J. A.: Surgical exposure of petrous portion of seventh nerve. **Arch. Otolaryng.,** 81:506-507, May 1965.

House, H. P.: Surgery for otosclerosis. **Minn. Med.,** 50:817-822, June 1967.

House, W. F., Editor: **Arch. Otolaryng.,** 80: No. 6, December 1964.

House, W. F.: Cryosurgical treatment of Meniere's disease. **Arch. Otolaryng.,** 84:616-629, December 1966.

House, W. F. and Doyle, J.: Early diagnosis & removal of primary cholesteatoma causing pressure to the VIIIth nerve. **Laryngoscope,** LXXII, No. 8:1053-1063, August 1963.

House, W. F.: Middle cranial fossa approach to the petrous portion of the VIIth nerve. **Arch. Otolaryng.,** 78:406-469, October 1963.

House, W. F.: Surgical exposure of internal auditory canal and its contents through the middle cranial fossa. **Laryngoscope,** LXXI, No. 11:1363-1385, November 1961.

House, W. F.: Monograph. Transtemporal bone microsurgical removal of acoustic neuromas. **Arch. Otolaryng.,** 80:597-756, December 1964.

Jongkees, L. B. W.: Some remarks on the history of transtemporal bone acoustic neuroma surgery. **Arch. Otolaryng.,** 89: February 1969.

Ketcham, A. S.; Wilkins, R. H.; Van Buren, J. M., and Smith, R. R.: A combined intracranial facial approach to the paranasal sinuses. **Amer. J. Surg.,** 106:698, 1963.

Bibliography *(continued)*

Lapidot, A. and Brandow, E. C.: A method for preserving the posterior canal wall and bridge in the surgery for cholesteatoma. **Acta Otolaryng.** (Stockholm), 62:88-92, July 1966.

Lewis, J. S. and Page, R.: Radical surgery for malignancies of the ear. **Arch Otolaryng.,** 83:114, 1966.

Montgomery, W. W.: Translabyrinthine resection of the small acoustic neuroma. **Arch. Otolaryng.,** 89: February 1969.

Odon, G. L. et al.: Supratentorial skull flaps. **J. Neurosurg.,** 25:492-502, October 1966.

Portmann, M.: Stapedectomy problems. **J. Oto-Laryng. Society of Australia,** 2:82-5, March 1969.

Pulec, J. L.: Total facial nerve exposure. **Arch. Otolaryng.,** 89:179-183, January 1969.

Pulec, J. L.: Facial nerve grafting. **Laryngoscope,** LXXIX: No. 9, September 1969.

Rosenblut, B. et al.: Silicone implants in the mastoid portion of the temporal bone. **Ann. Otol.,** 75:889-902, September 1966.

Shambaugh, G. E., Jr.: Surgery of the ear. Second edition: pp. 518-582. W. B. Saunders Co., Philadelphia, Pa., 1967.

Sheehy, J. L.: Osteoma of the external auditory canal. **Laryngoscope,** LXVIII, No. 9: 1667-1673, Sept. 1958.

Sheehy, J. L.: Stapedectomy in the fenestrated ear. **Arch. Otolaryng.,** 78:574-577, October 1963.

Sheehy, J. L.: Stapes surgery in advanced otosclerosis. **Annals of Otology,** 3: September 1962.

Siirala, U.: Restoration of the air-containing middle ear in adhesive otitis. **Int. Surg.,** 49:205-11, March 1968.

Terz, J. J.; Alksne, J. F., and Lawrence, W., Jr.: En bloc resection of the pterygoid region in the management of advanced oropharyngeal carcinoma. **Surg., Gyn, & Ob.,** February 1970.

Wolfson, R. J. et al.: Clinical Symposia, 17: No. 4, October-November-December 1965.

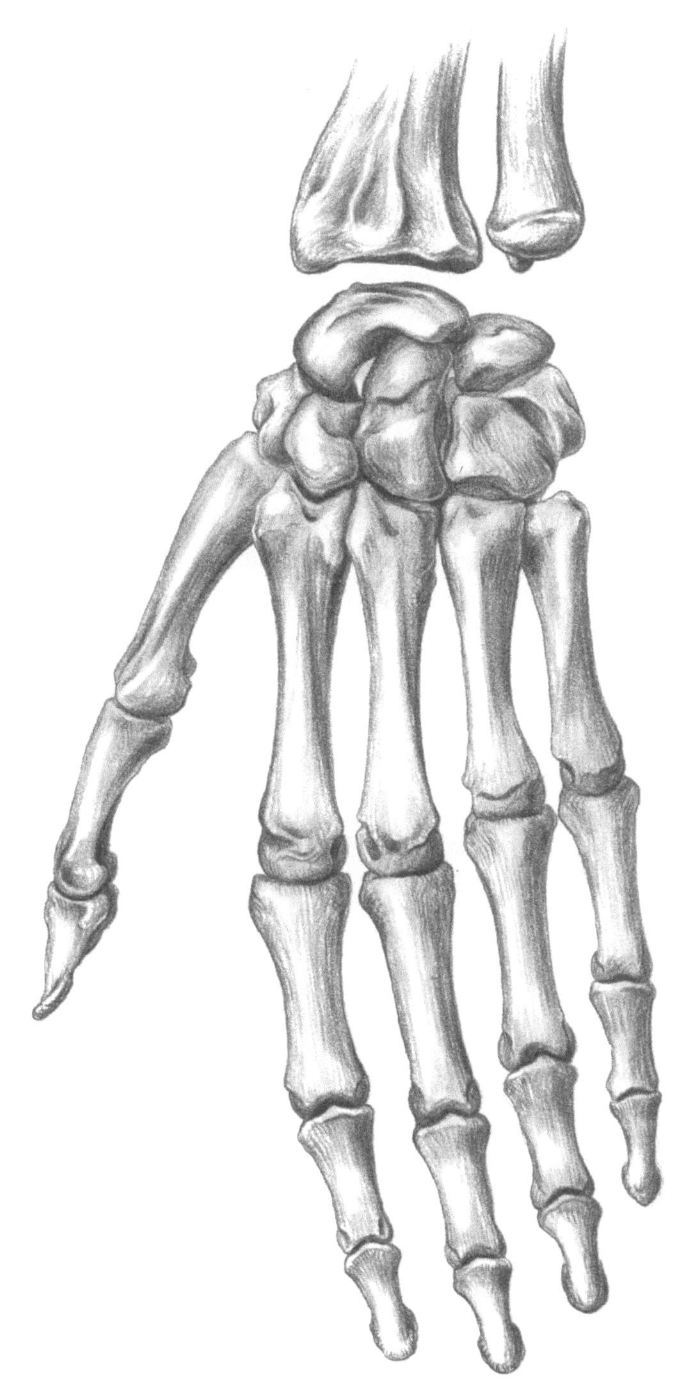

Introduction

Advances in Hand Surgery, as in surgery of trauma, have historically centered around the medical accomplishments of wartime. World War II saw the development of this field into an organized method, led by the great Sterling Bunnell. In the past thirty years, the knowledge of functional and surgical anatomy and the development of new operative techniques have made this field one of the most dynamic in surgery. The industrial development of synthetic materials that can be tolerated in human tissues has given the surgeon new tools for human engineering. The use of implants in reconstructive surgery has become an established method of treatment.

Simultaneously, the development of powered surgical instrumentation has facilitated more sophisticated procedures. The use of the air drill in surgery has begun a new era in surgical instrumentation. The precision possible with this procedure makes bone carpentry simple. Operating time can be significantly shortened because of the speed. Certain hand operations are now made possible because they can be done within the limited period of time a tourniquet can be used – a problem with the older methods.

The safety, versatility, efficiency and simplicity of the air drill method makes it an important instrument system which every hand surgeon should have available.

An atlas of these surgical techniques should prove useful to those who have this specialized interest.

Alfred B. Swanson, M.D., F.A.C.S.

Contents

Insertion of a Silastic® Carpal Scaphoid Implant*

The development of inert silicon rubber as an implant material has made possible the many reconstructive techniques developed by Dr. Alfred B. Swanson. These techniques require instruments that can sculpt, resect and ream bone with the delicacy necessary in hand surgery. The air drill runs at 100,000 rpm and has a low stall torque, often an advantage when working close to vital nerves and tendons.

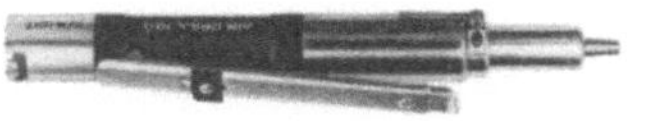

Air drill

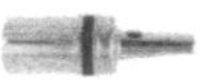

Medium bur guard

06 carbide-tip bur

---

* Alfred B. Swanson, M. D.: Silicone Rubber Implants for the Replacement of the Carpal Scaphoid and Lunate Bones. **Orthop Clin N Amer** 1 : 299-309, November 1970.

® Registered trademark of the Dow-Corning Corporation.

To assemble the burs:

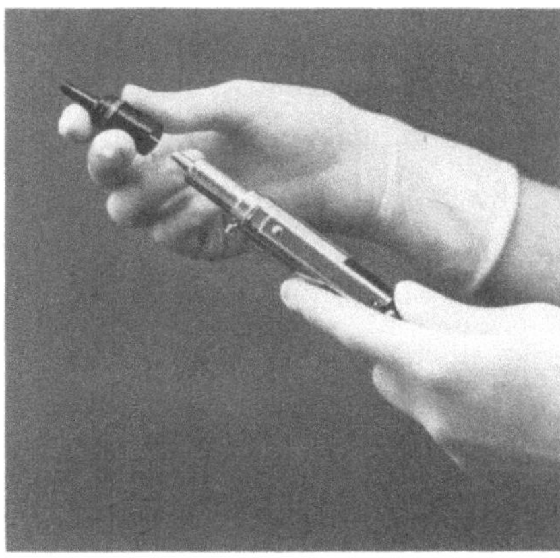

1. With safety lock off, place the medium bur guard over the drill shoulder.

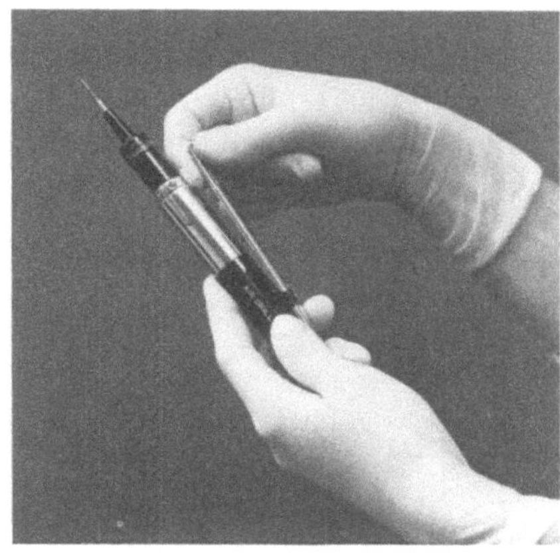

3. Return lever flush against drill to lock bur. Use extension lever for additional speed control.

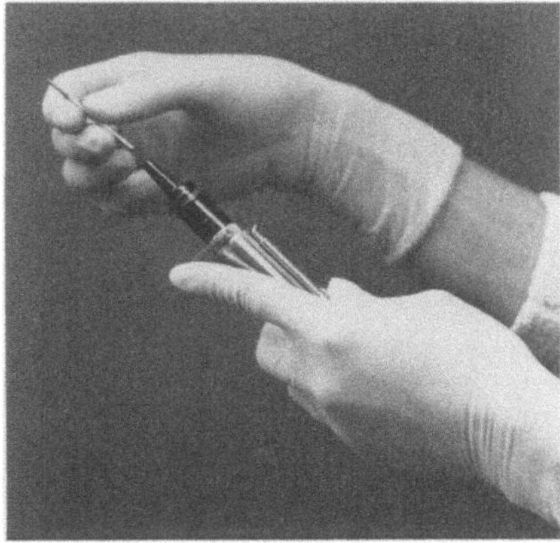

2. Push release lever to 90°. Insert bur deep into collet.

Insertion of a Silastic® Carpal Scaphoid Implant *(continued)*

4. Make a skin incision longitudinally over the anatomical snuffbox. Carefully protect the radial nerve branches and radial artery. Expose the scaphoid bone between the tendons of the extensor pollicis brevis and extensor carpi radialis longus. Incise and carefully preserve the capsule and ligaments.

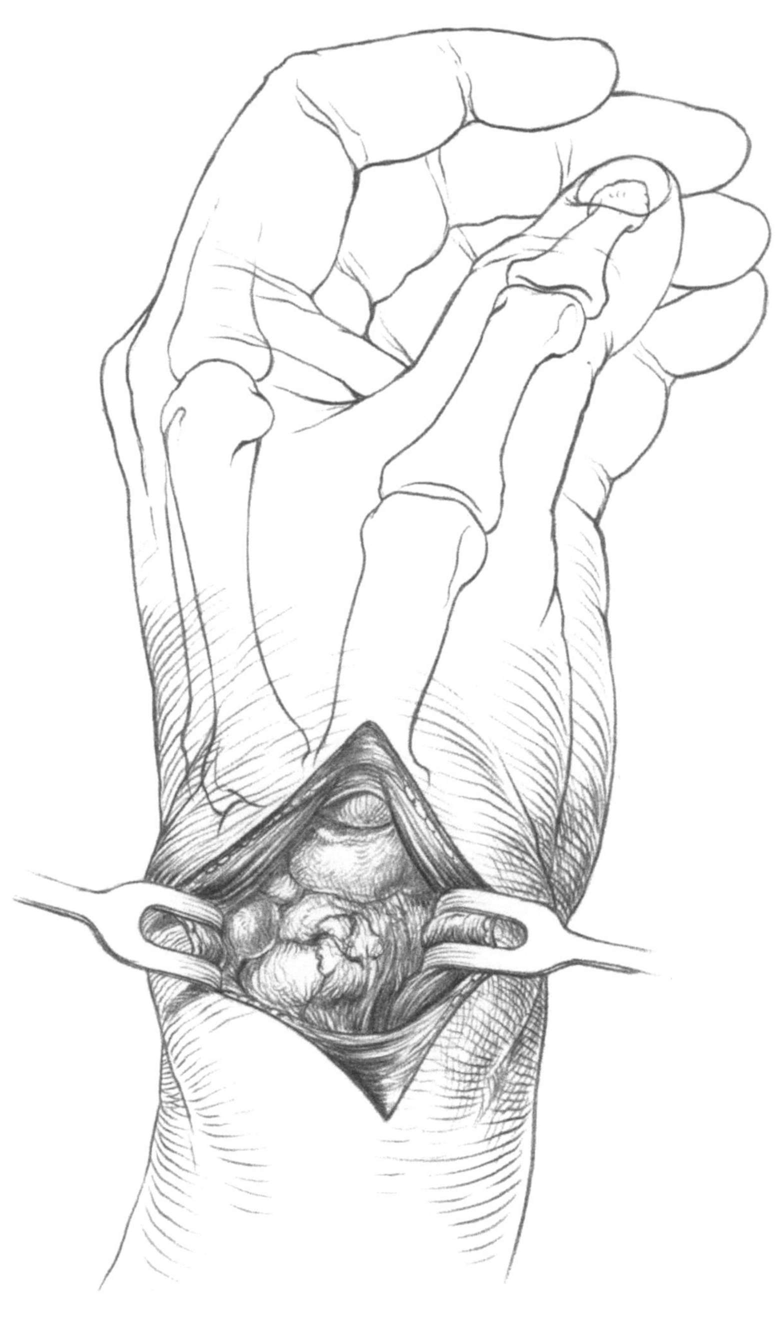

5. Identify the scaphoid, by roentgenogram if necessary. Remove the entire bone en bloc or piecemeal. The implant* is available in three sizes, designed for the left and right wrist. It should be approximately the same size as the removed scaphoid, and fit easily in the space left.

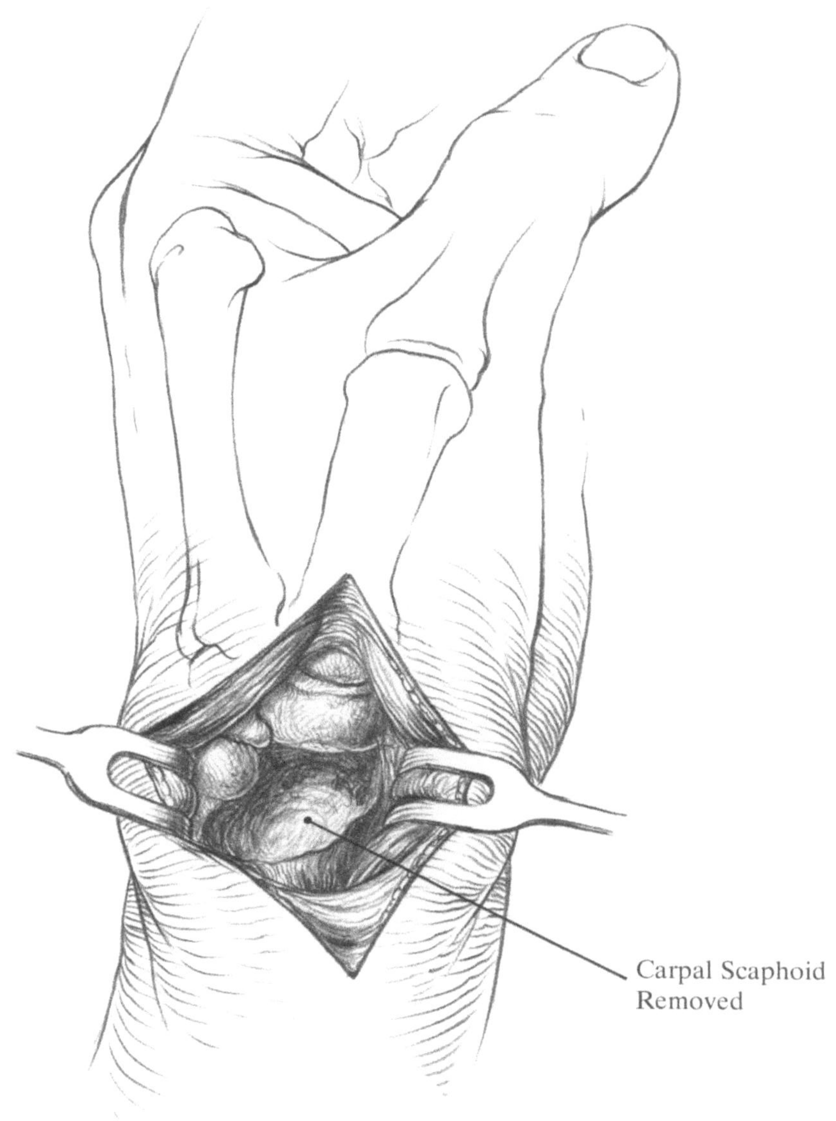

---

* Available from Dow-Corning Corporation, Midland, Michigan/USA.

Insertion of a Silastic® Carpal Scaphoid Implant *(continued)*

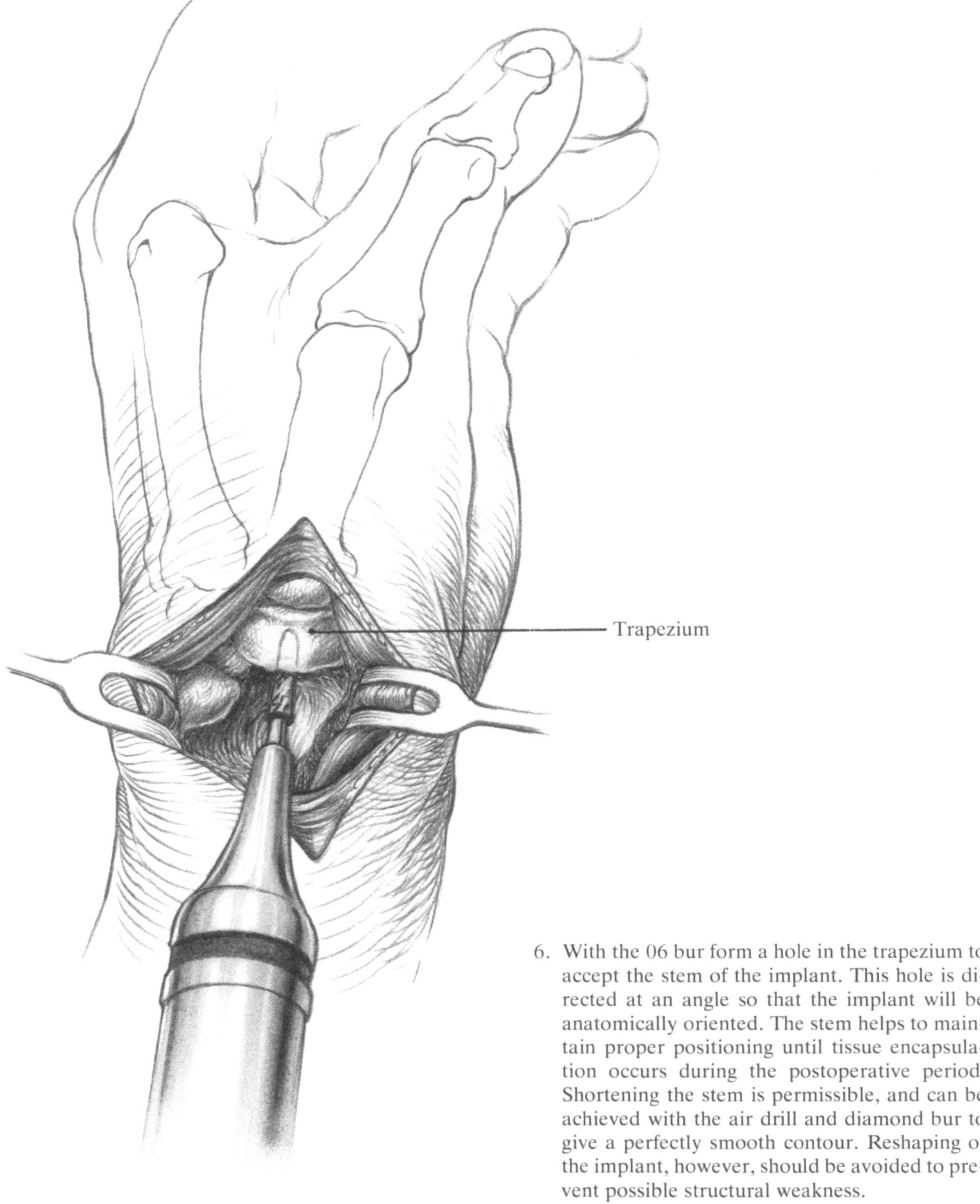

6. With the 06 bur form a hole in the trapezium to accept the stem of the implant. This hole is directed at an angle so that the implant will be anatomically oriented. The stem helps to maintain proper positioning until tissue encapsulation occurs during the postoperative period. Shortening the stem is permissible, and can be achieved with the air drill and diamond bur to give a perfectly smooth contour. Reshaping of the implant, however, should be avoided to prevent possible structural weakness.

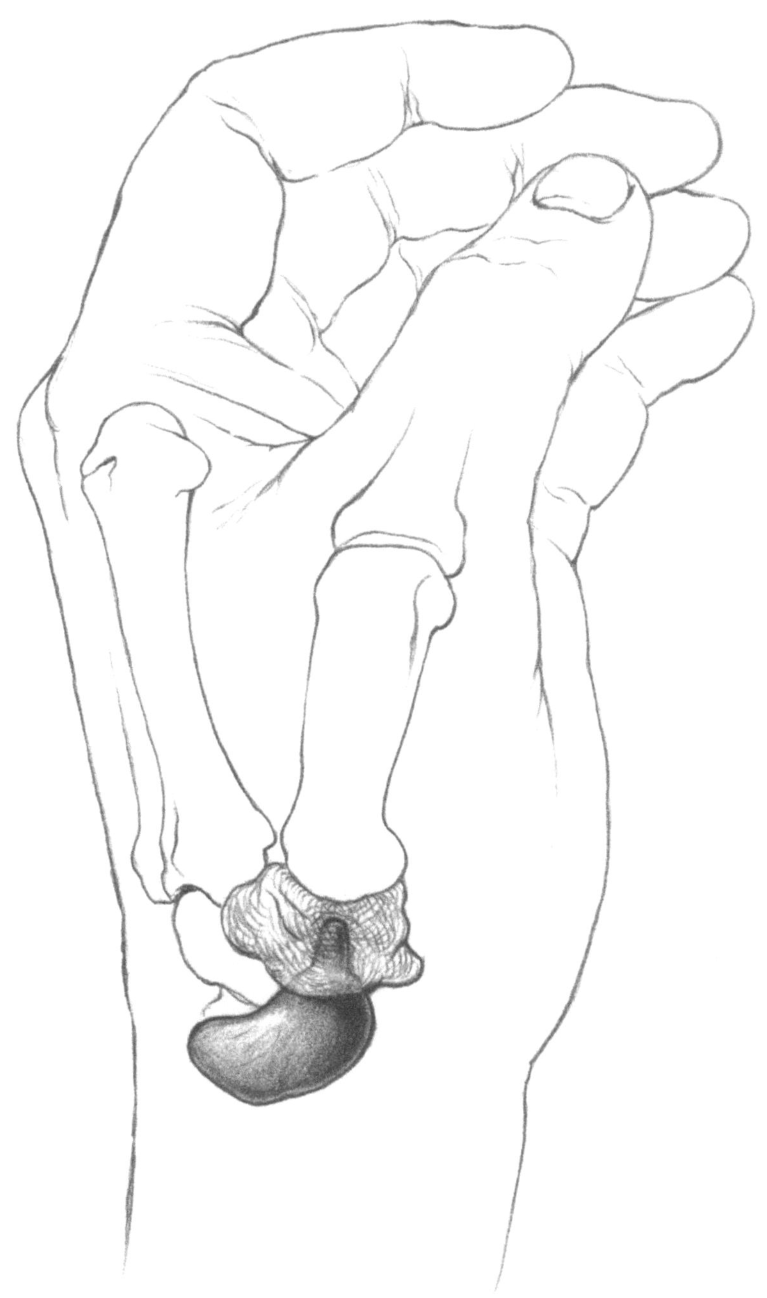

7. Insert the implant and suture the capsule securely with
   Dacron 4-0, using a buried knot technique. Leave a small
   drain in the wound. Apply a voluminous conforming dressing and posterior molded plaster splint. **Post-operative care:**
   After the postoperative swelling has decreased, usually three
   to four days, apply a short arm cast, including the thumb.
   This is worn from four to six weeks. Allow full activity at
   twelve weeks.

Insertion of a Silastic® Trapezium Implant in Trapeziometacarpal Arthroplasty*

Make a two-to three-inch incision parallel to the extensor pollicis brevis tendon centered over the trapezium. Carefully dissect down to the trapezio-scaphoid joint, avoiding injury to the branches of the superficial radial nerve. Retract the overlying branches of the radial artery off the trapezium with an elevator. The capsule is incised longitudinally and reflected by sharp dissection. Dissect out the trapezium, working close to the bone to avoid damage to the deep-lying radial artery and flexor carpi radialis longus tendon. Incise the capsule longitudinally and reflect by sharp dissection.

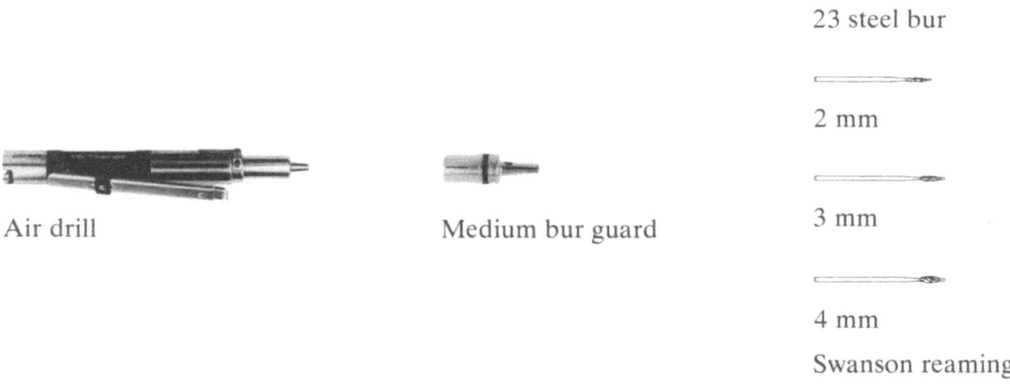

---

* Alfred B. Swanson, M. D. Silicone Rubber Implants for Replacement of Arthritic and Destroyed Joints in the Hand. **Surg Clin N Amer** 48:1113-1127, October 1968.

Arthroplasty in Traumatic Arthritis of Joints of the Hand. **Orthop Clin N Amer** 1:285-298, November 1970.

1. Remove the entire trapezium in a piecemeal method, including its medial portion, by sectioning it into two or three pieces with an osteotome and making, the final excision with a biting rongeur. Avoid injury to capsular ligaments. If they are torn, they should be sutured. If there is any evidence of osteophytes or irregularity of the scaphoid, trim them with the 23 steel bur.

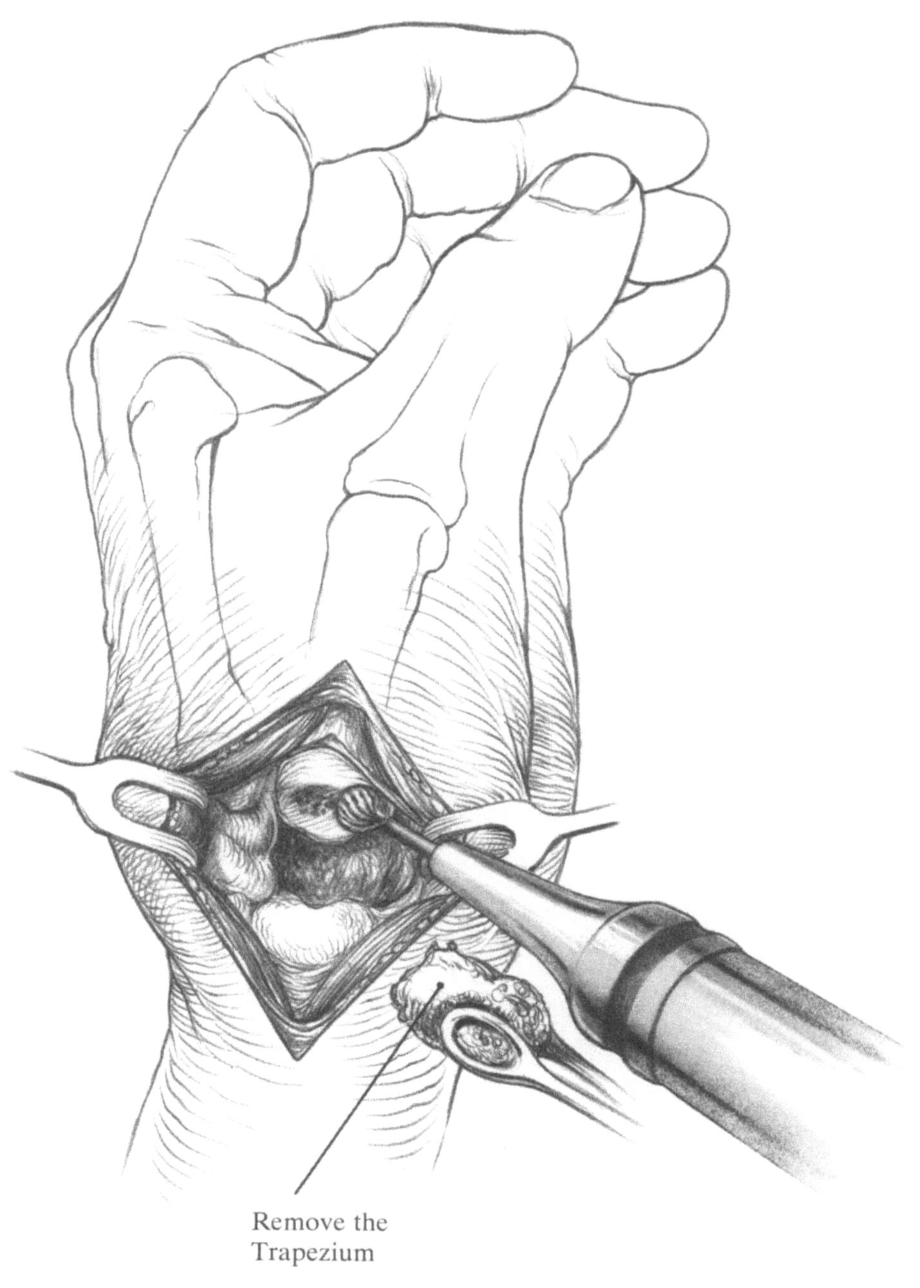

Remove the
Trapezium

Insertion of a Silastic® Trapezium Implant in Trapeziometacarpal Arthroplasty (*continued*)

2. Square off the base of the metacarpal leaving most of the cortical bone intact. Make a hole in the base of the metacarpal to open up the intramedullary canal. Drill the hole with the appropriate reaming bur. The hole should not be reamed too much, only enough for easy insertion of the stem of the implant. Before inserting the implant, carefully inspect the anterior capsule in the depth of the wound for inadvertent tears. A firm capsular support is essential for a good result.

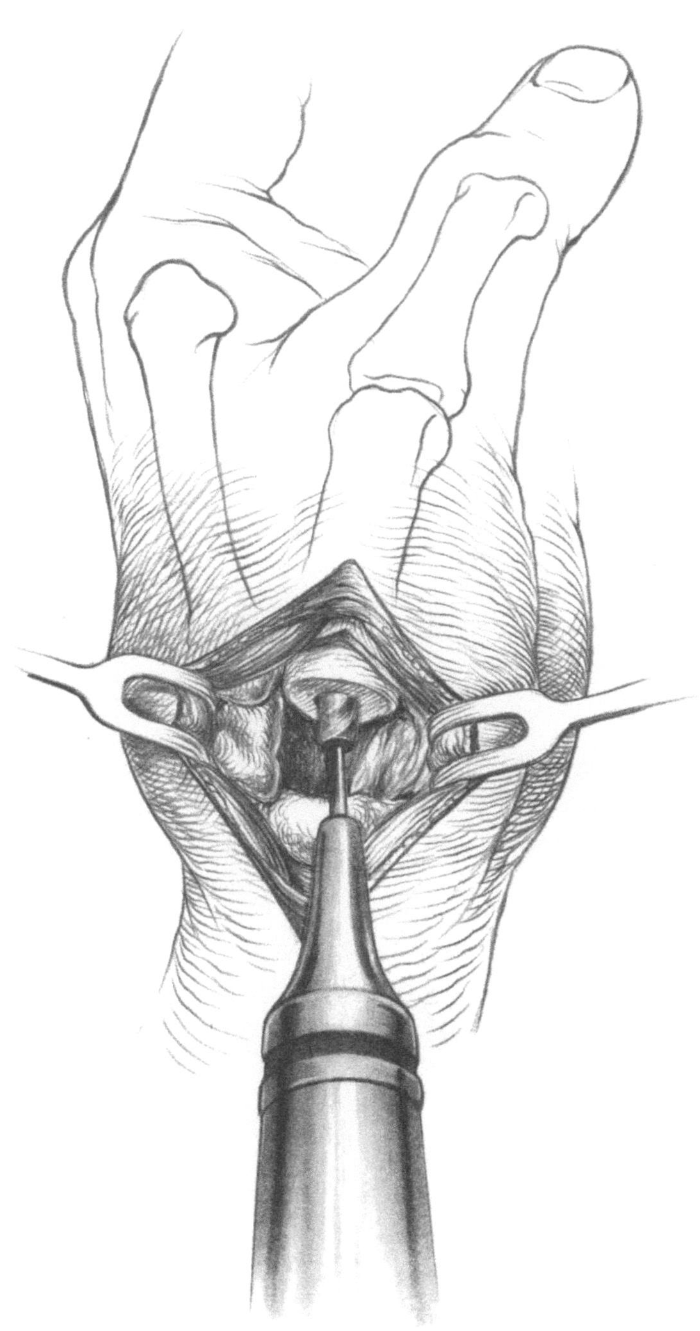

3. Using instruments, insert the stem of the implant into the intramedullary canal of the metacarpal. It is important to have the collar of the implant in intimate contact with the base of the metacarpal to avoid wobbling. Hold the thumb in abduction; this will place the implant well into the recess left by the trapezium. Carefully suture the preserved capsule over the implant using three to four non-absorbable sutures with an inverted knot technique.

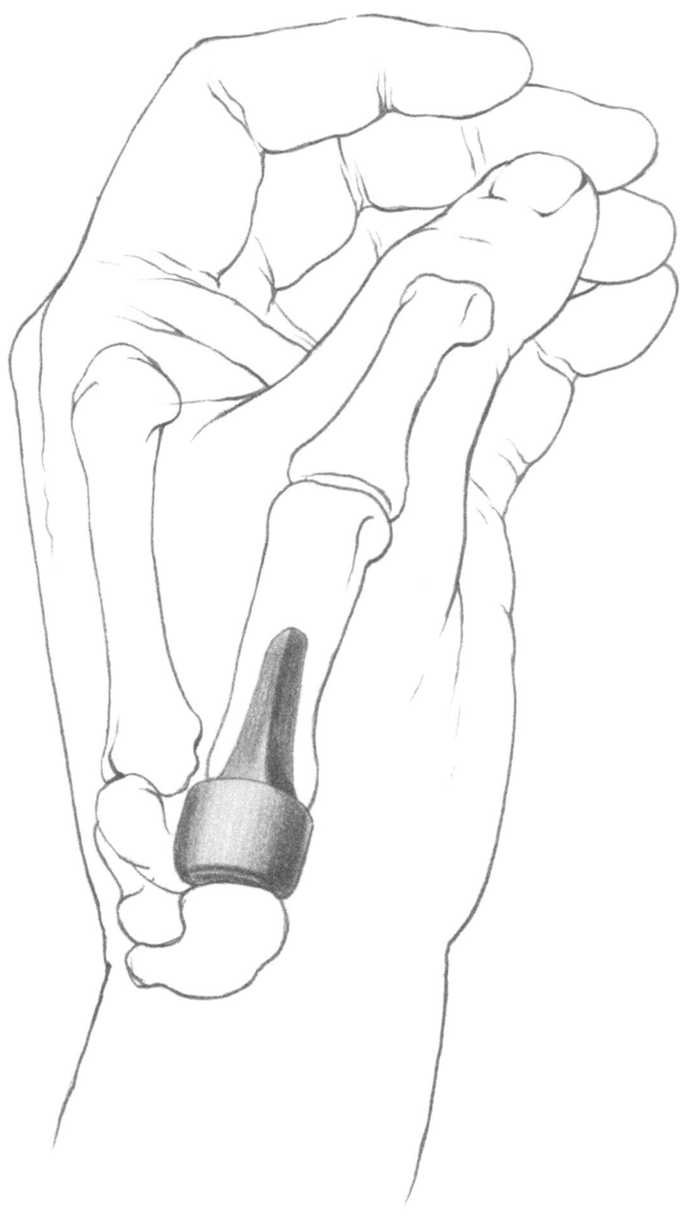

Insertion of a Silastic® Trapezium Implant in Trapeziometacarpal Arthroplasty (*continued*)

4. If loose, the capsule should be imbricated. If the capsule is thin or inadequate it can be reinforced with a slip of the abductor pollicis longus tendon. The tendon slip is cut two inches proximal from its insertion to the base of the first metacarpal and dissected distally to its metacarpal attachment.

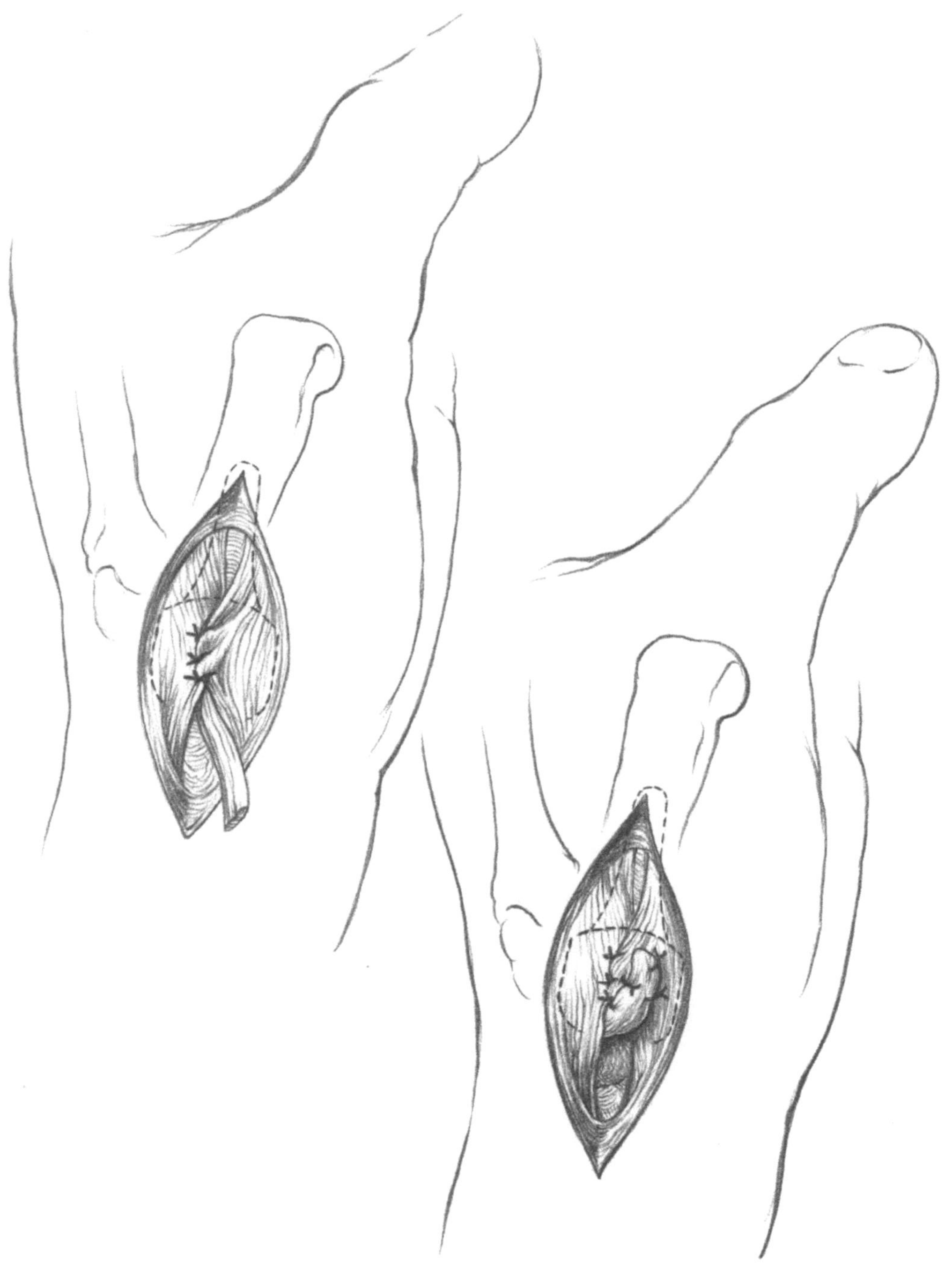

5. It is then placed under the capsule and folded over the capsule during its closure. This reinforcement provides a firmer radial capsular support for the implant when the capsule is thinned out. The wound is closed, leaving a small drain for three to four days. Apply a voluminous conforming dressing, placing a roll of cotton or Dacron batting between the first and second metacarpals to maintain 40 to 60 degrees of palmar abduction. A plaster splint is then applied to the pressure dressing.

6. Special Considerations

Adduction contracture of the first metacarpal, if severe and untreated, will seriously affect the result. If 45 degrees abduction between the first and second metacarpals cannot be achieved, proximal release of the origin of the adductor pollicis muscle from the third metacarpal must be done through a separate incision.

Hyperextension deformity of the metacarpophalangeal joint further contributes to the imbalance of the thumb forces:

a. If the MP joint hyperextends less than 10 degrees usually no other treatment is necessary than care in applying the cast so that the metacarpal is in abduction and not the proximal phalanx.

b. If the MP joint hyperextends from 10 to 20 degrees, insert a Kirschner wire obliquely across the joint with 10 degrees flexion.

c. If hyperextension of the MP joint is greater than 20 degrees, stabilization of the joint is essential, either by capsulorrhaphy or by fusion. Place the MP joint in 10 degrees flexion with 15 degrees abduction and slight supination. Insert a longitudinal wire in retrograde fashion across both the IP and MP joints and leave 5 to 10 mm extruding from the tip of the thumb. Insert a second wire obliquely across the MP joint to fix the position desired. Firmly compress the fusion area to assure good contact between the raw bony surfaces. Small cancellous bone grafts from the excised trapezium may be applied.

After three to four days apply a scaphoid-type cast. This is worn for four to six weeks. A good stable capsule is usually formed by this time.

Insertion of a Silastic® Carpal Lunate Implant*

1. Use the dorsal approach and make a longitudinal or S-shaped incision. A volar approach is suggested when the lunate bone is dislocated. Transversely incise the wrist capsule between the third and fourth dorsal compartments. Carefully preserve the capsule. Exposure is made between the tendons of the extensor pollicis longus and extensor digitorum communis. Make a positive identification of the lunate bone using roentgenograms if necessary, and remove it completely either en bloc or piecemeal. Care should be taken to avoid cutting the capsular ligaments on the palmar aspect. If injured, they should be sutured together to give a firm palmar support.

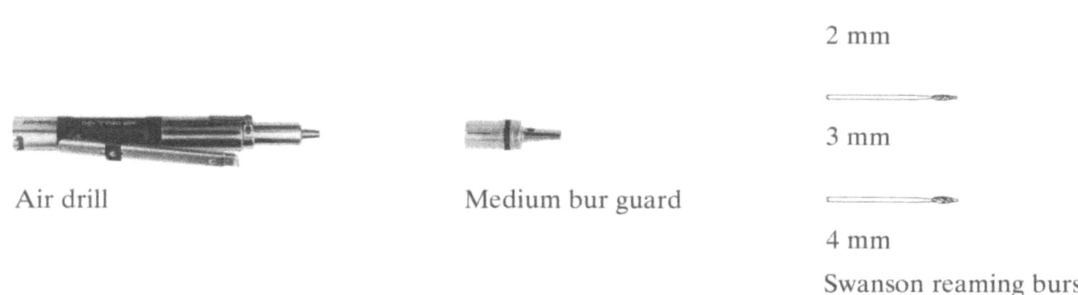

---

* Alfred B. Swanson, M. D.: Silicone Rubber Implants for the Replacement of the Carpal Scaphoid and Lunate Bones. **Orthop Clin N Amer** I: 299-309, November 1970.

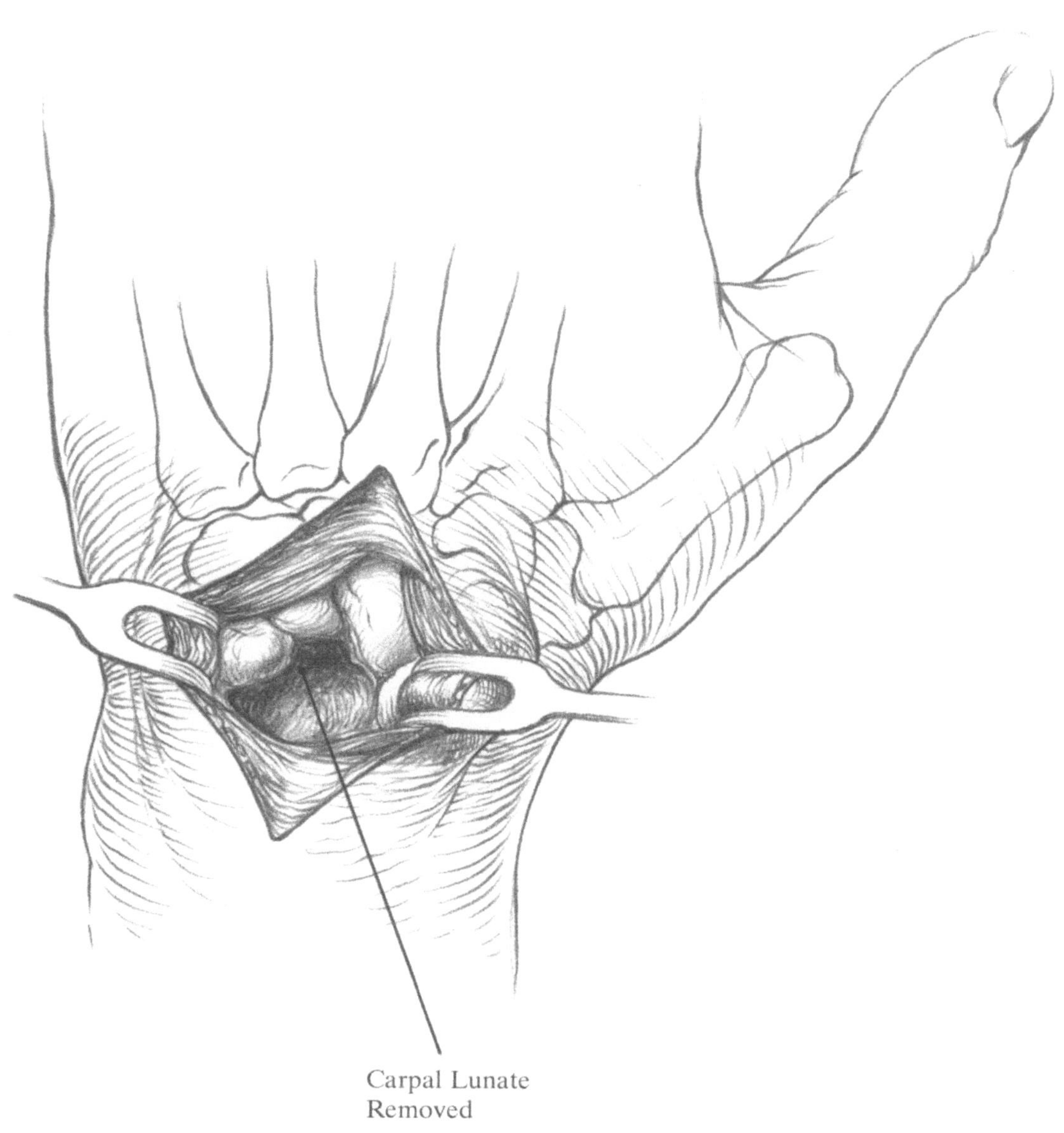

Carpal Lunate
Removed

Insertion of a Silastic® Carpal Lunate Implant *(continued)*

2. With the air drill, drill a small hole in the triquetrum to accept the implant stem snugly. The stem helps to maintain proper positioning until tissue encapsulation occurs during the postoperative period. Three implant sizes are available, and an implant approximately the same size as the excised lunate should be inserted.

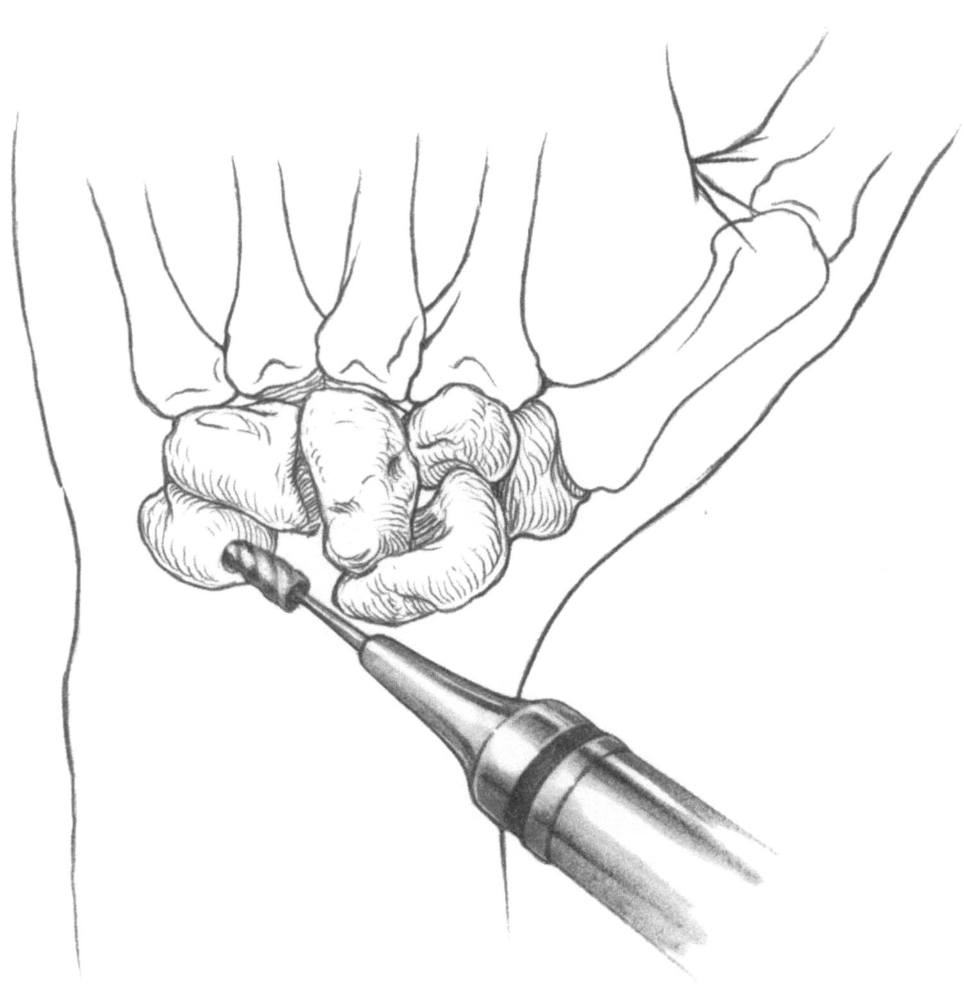

3. Insert the carpal lunate prosthesis. Tightly suture the preserved capsule with non-absorbable sutures and insert a small wound drain. Apply a voluminous conforming dressing and molded plaster splint. After three to four days apply a short arm cast with the wrist in neutral position; this is worn from four to six weeks. Allow full activity at twelve weeks.

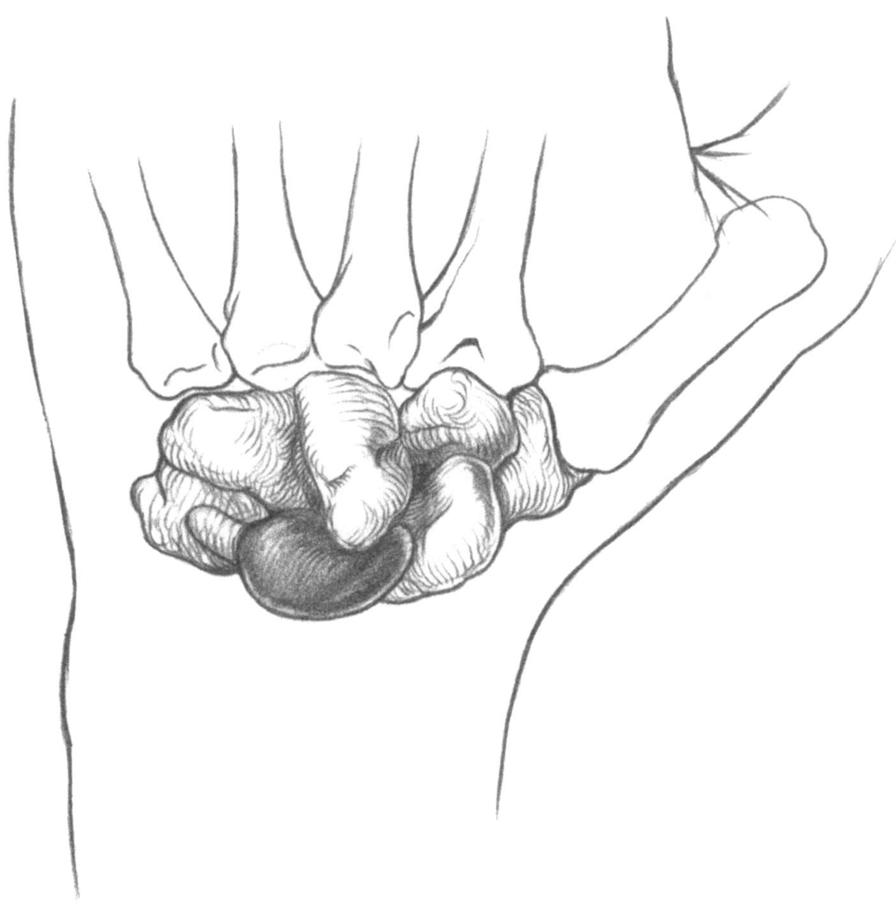

Silastic® Implants for Replacement of Arthritic or Destroyed Joints of the Hand*

Make a long transverse incision on the dorsum of the hand over the necks of the metacarpals. Dissect down through the subcutaneous tissue to expose the extensor tendons. Carefully release the dorsal veins which lie between the metacarpals by longitudinal dissection and retract them laterally. Expose the extensor hood to the base of the proximal phalanx. Incise the extensor hood fibers parallel to the extensor tendon on its ulnar aspect.

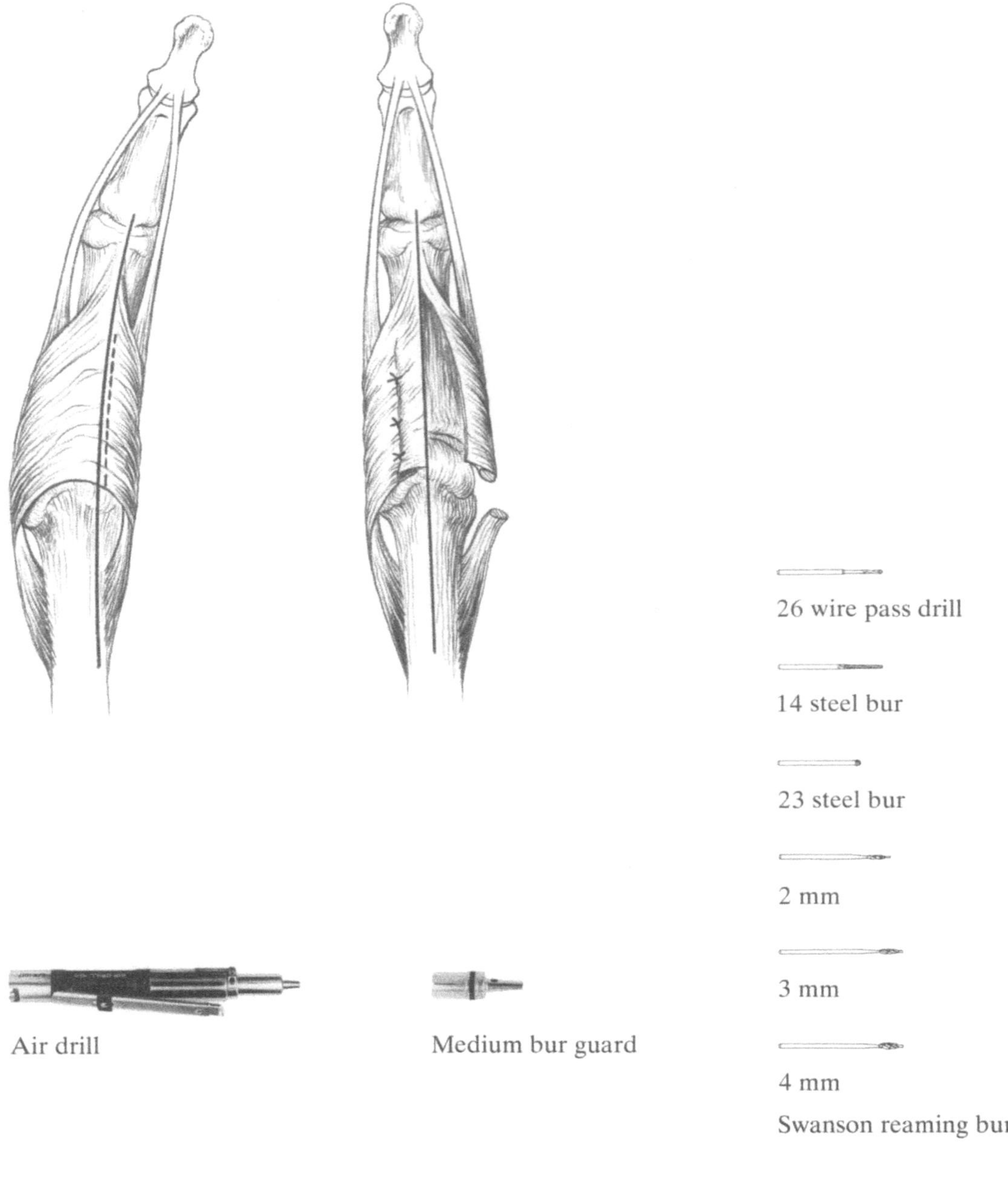

---

* Alfred B. Swanson, M. D.: Silicone Rubber Implants for Replacement of Arthritic and Destroyed Joints in the Hand. **Surg Clin N Amer** 48:1113-1127, October 1968.
Arthroplasty in Traumatic Arthritis of the Joints of the Hand. **Orthop Clin N Amer** 1:285-298, November 1970.

1. With clear exposure of the metacarpal head, dissect the neck of the metacarpal subperiosteally and transsect with the air drill and 14 steel bur. The air drill will minimize the danger of splintering the bone. Remove the head of the metacarpal while preserving the collateral ligaments and capsule attachments. Remove all involved synovia from the joint capsule and surrounding tissue. A pituitary rongeur is useful for this purpose.

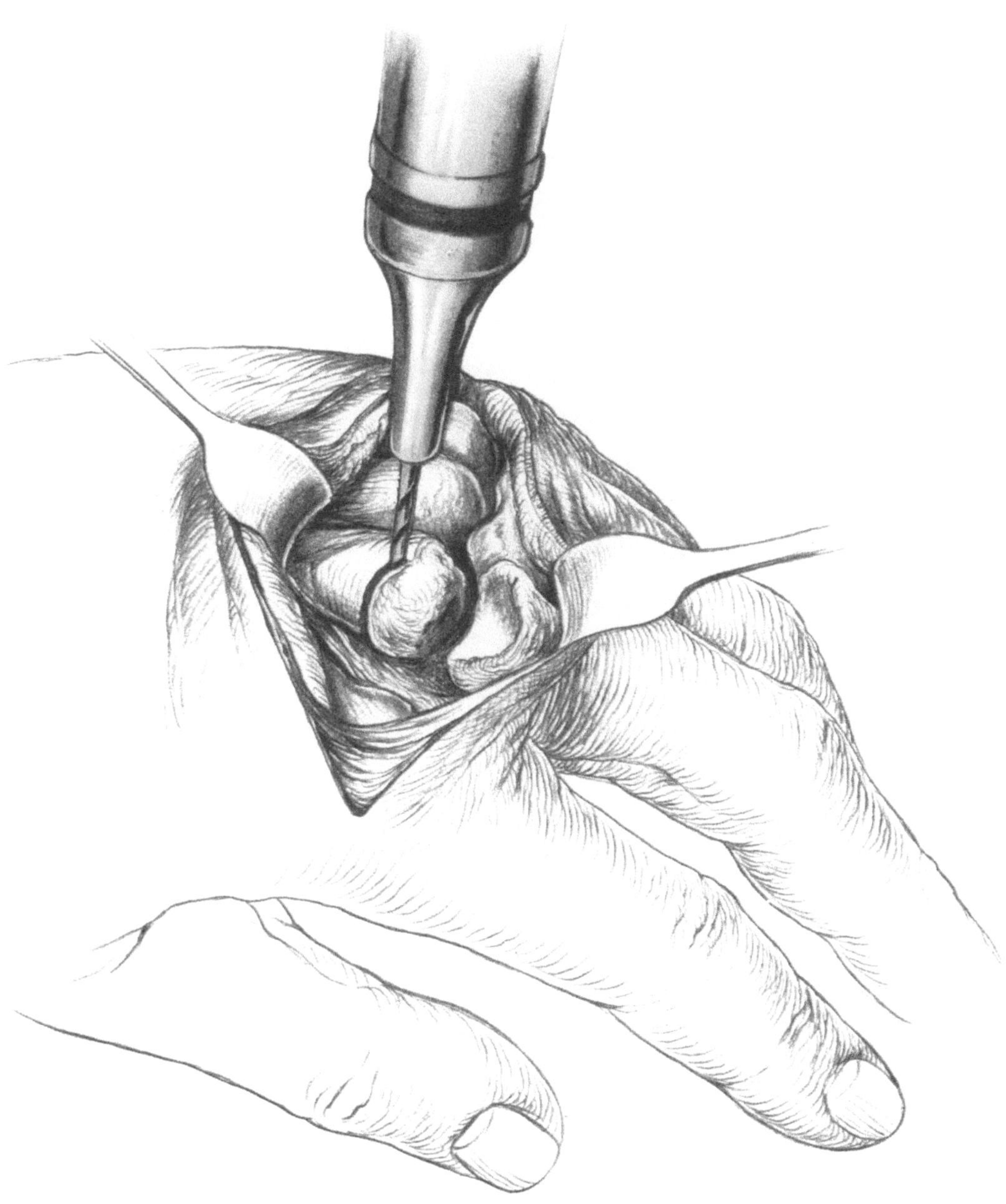

Silastic® Implants for Replacement of Destroyed Joints *(continued)*

2. Perform a comprehensive soft tissue release so that the base of the proximal phalanx can be displaced dorsally above the metacarpal. This is done symmetrically and may require incision of the palmar plate and collateral ligament attachments from the proximal phalanx. Identify the ulnar intrinsic tendon. If it is tight it is sectioned at the myotendinous junction. With a blunt hook pull up the tendons of the abductor digiti minimi and the flexor digiti minimi into the wound and section them avoiding injury to the ulnar digital nerve.

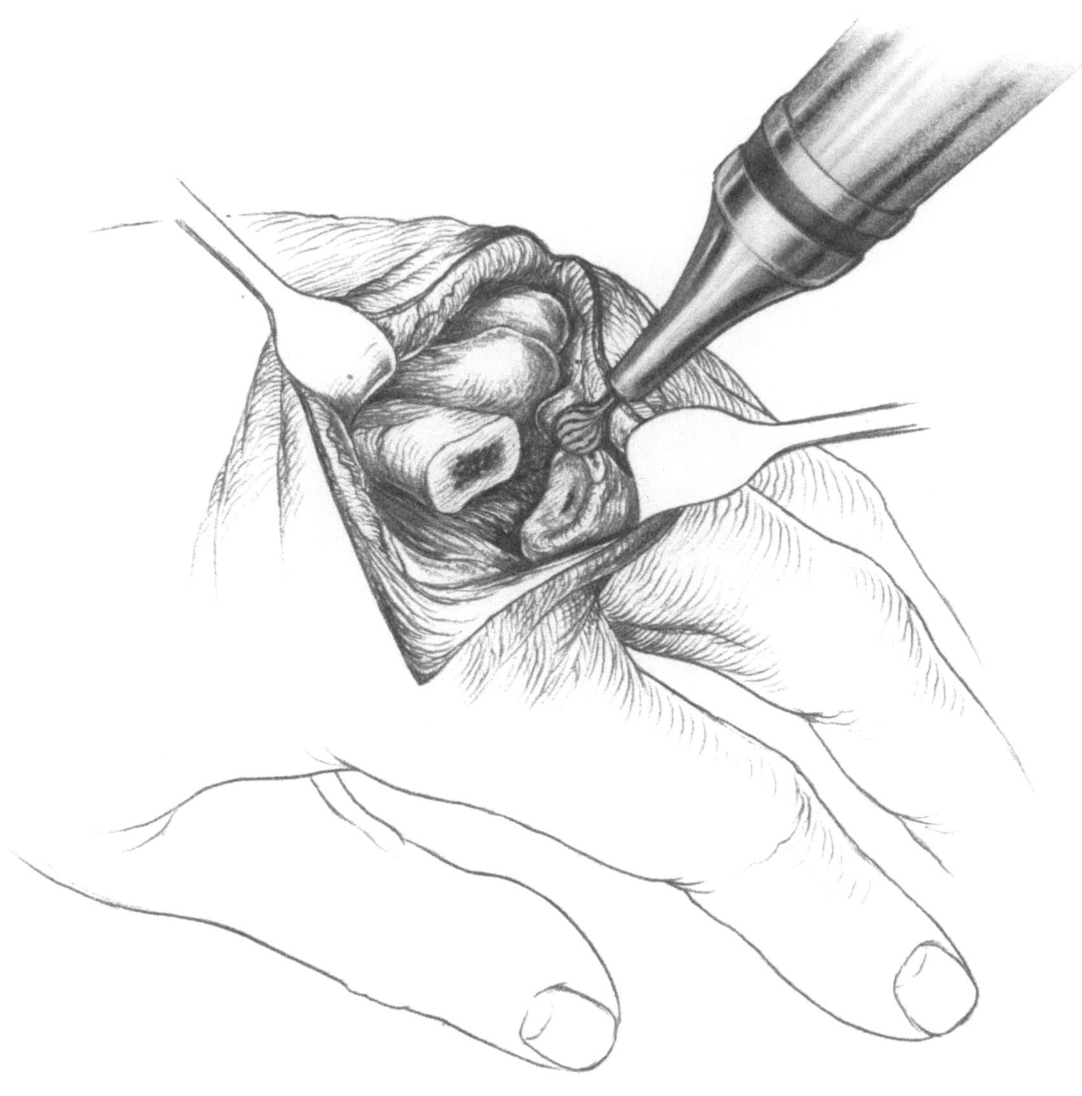

3. It is not usual to perform a bony resection at the base of the proximal phalanx. Remove any marginal osteophytes which might interfere with the implant with a 23 steel bur. Occasionally the deformity of the proximal phalanx may be severe and reshaping of the base of the phalanx may be necessary.

4. Use a broach or 14 steel bur to penetrate the medullary canal. With a Swanson bur ream the metacarpal canal. The burs are available in three sizes, 2 mm, 3 mm and 4 mm diameter, to accommodate all sizes of metacarpal phalange intramedullary canals. The pilot tip on the bur is non-cutting and prevents penetration of the lateral cortex. The reverse cutting threads back out the cancellous bone as the bur moves forward, preventing damming-up of bone at the bur tip. The intramedullary canal of the ring metacarpal is often quite small and requires careful preparation.

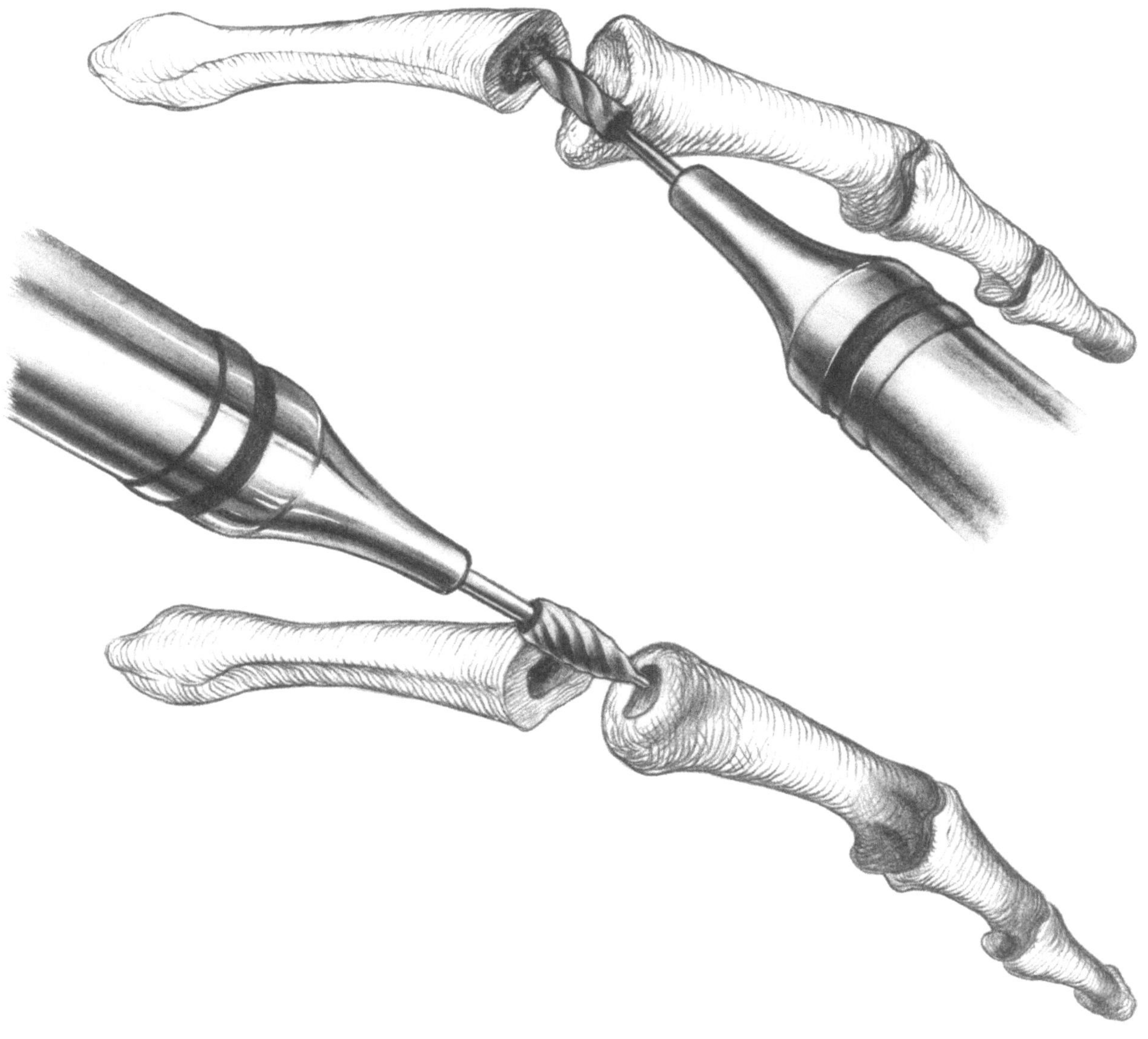

5. Ream the canal of the proximal phalanx with the same bur. The limited torque of the air drill may cause the bur to stall which, in this delicate technique, is an additional safety factor.

Silastic® Implants for Replacement of Destroyed Joints *(continued)*

6. The implants are available in nine sizes to meet most surgical requirements. Select the largest implant size that the bones can accommodate. Use a test implant to determine the correct implant size. The implant stems should fit well down into the canal so that the transverse mid section of the implant abuts against the bone end. Thoroughly irrigate the joints with saline to remove all debris. Use a "no-touch technique" to insert the implants. Handle with a blunt instrument to avoid traumatization and contamination.

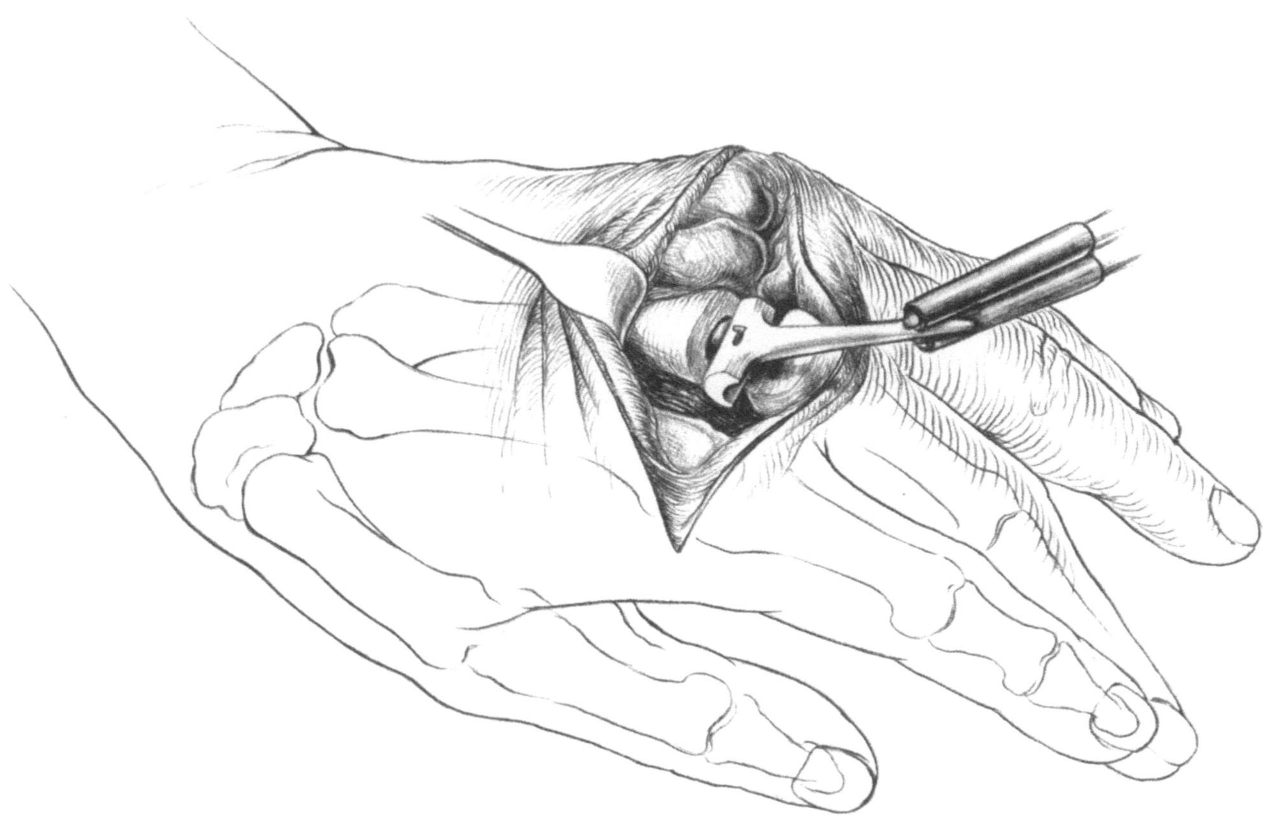

7. After inserting the stem into the proximal metacarpal, distract the joint, flex the implant and insert the distal stem into the proximal phalanx. With 4-0 Dacron sutures, using a buried knot technique, reef in an overlapping fashion the radial portion of the sagittal fibers of each extensor hood mechanism so that the extensor tendon is brought slightly to the radial side of the center of the joint.

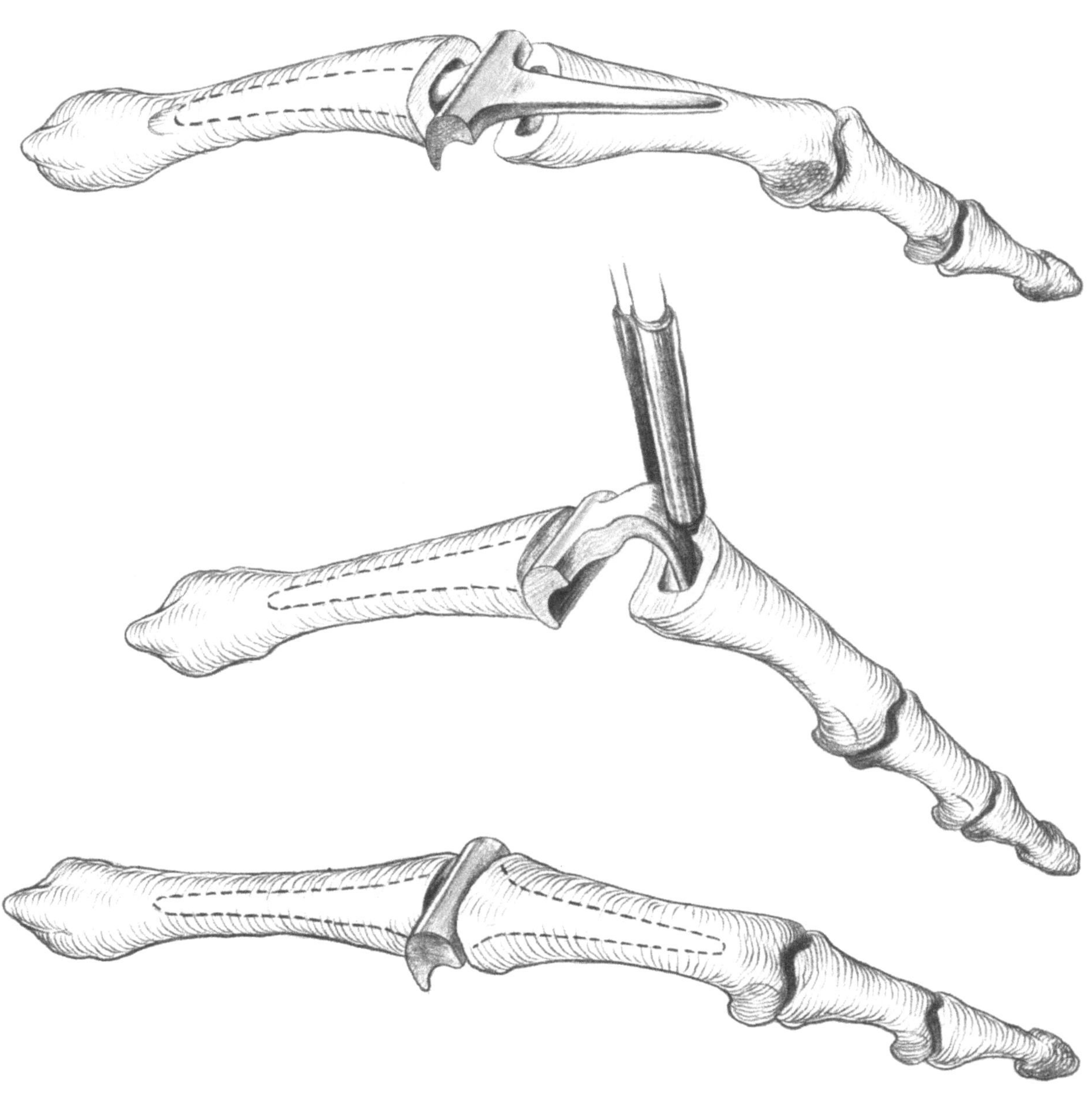

8. The implant pistons to a small degree within the medullary canal as the digit flexes and extends. This movement provides a greater range of motion and increases the flex life of the implant. Fixing the stems of the implant does not allow the device to act as a dynamic spacer for the new-formed joint.

Silastic® Implants for Replacement of Destroyed Joints *(continued)*

9. Reconstruction of the radial collateral ligaments is done in patients who have an inadequate first dorsal interosseous muscle or a tendency for pronation deformity of the index finger. Make a distally based flap of the radial portion of the palmar plate and separate the collateral ligament from the underlying intrinsic muscles and tendon. Attach this 1.5 to 2 cm flap around the radial aspect of the neck of the metacarpal to a hole in the dorsal radial portion of the neck of the bone. This procedure slightly decreases flexion of the index metacarpophalangeal joint, but seems to improve rotational deformities and may be important in certain cases.

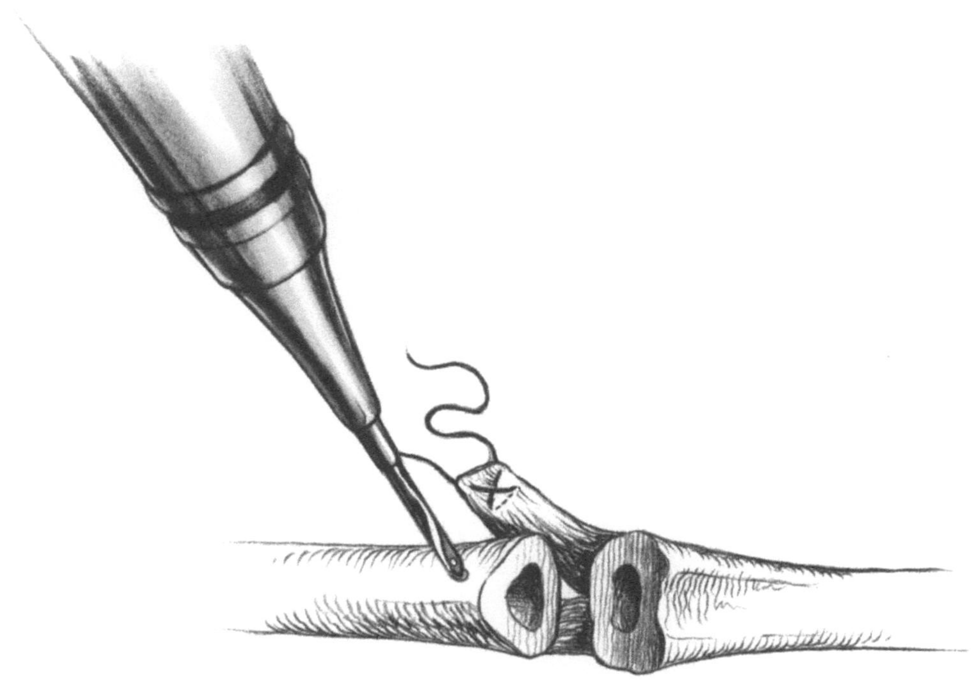

10. Close the incision with interrupted sutures, inserting two small drains under the skin. Apply a non-adherent dressing over the wound and shape a voluminous conforming dressing over the hand and forearm. Include a narrow palmar plaster splint. Between the third and fifth postoperative day change the voluminous dressing to a light one and start using the dynamic brace*. Adjust the brace to allow a range of motion from zero degrees of extension to 90 degrees of flexion. Use the flexion cuff device if the patient has difficulty in maintaining 70 degrees of flexion. The extension part of the brace is usually worn day and night for three weeks, and sometimes longer in patients who show a tendency to extensor lag or recurrent deformity. A careful postoperative program and follow-up are essential to a good final result.

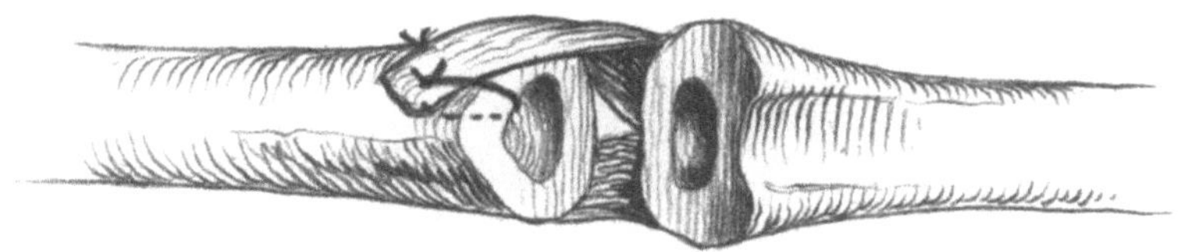

---

* Pope Brace Foundation, Kankakee, Illinois/USA.
  Alfred B. Swanson, M. D.: A Dynamic Brace for Finger-Joint Reconstruction in Arthritis. **Inter-Clinic Information Bull,** New York University, New York, 10:1-7, May 1971.

Silastic® Implants for Replacement of Destroyed Joints *(continued)*

11. When the thumb metacarpophalangeal joint is involved, fusion of the joint is recommended. Make chips from the metacarpal head and stabilize the joint with two wires.

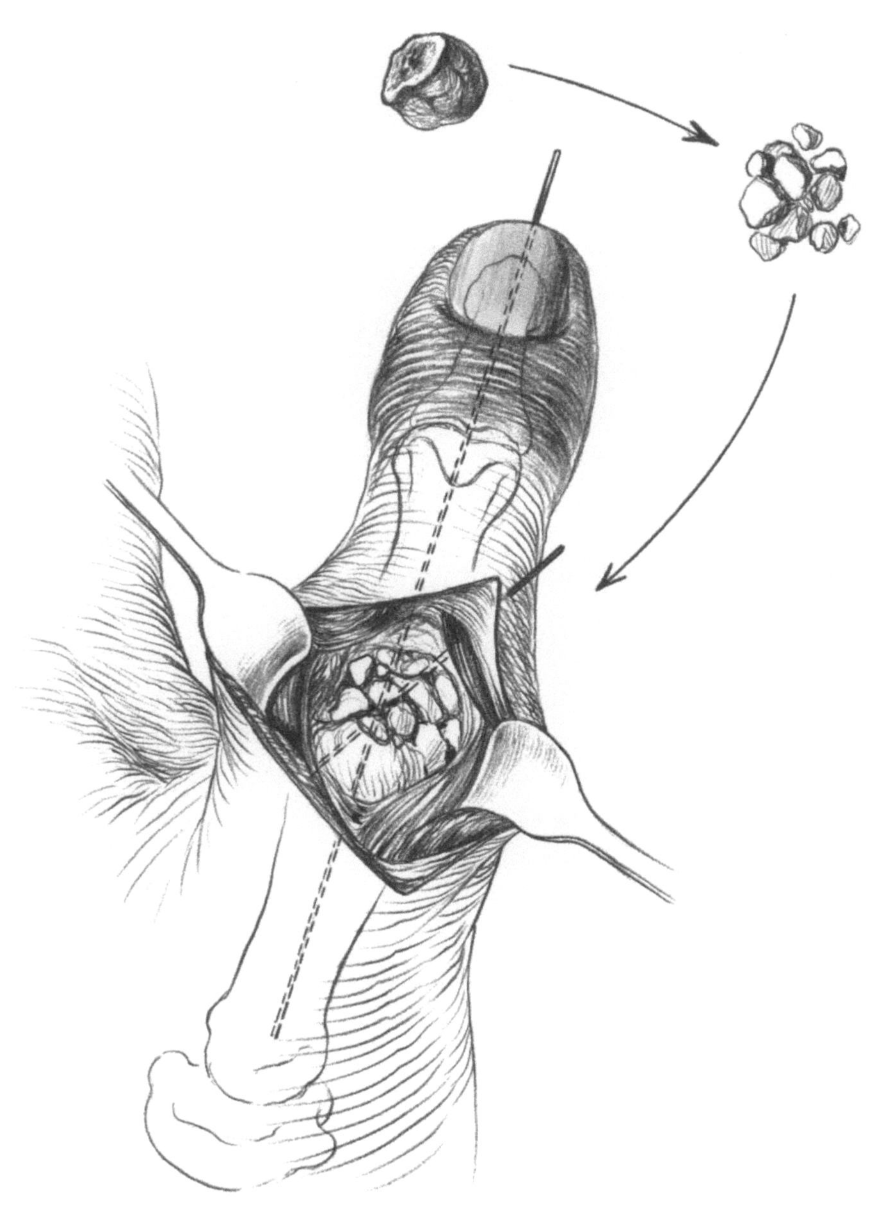

Technique Suggestions

All soft tissue and vital structures should be retracted and protected prior to application of air equipment.

Incise or elevate the periosteum before using the equipment. Burs and blades do not work well close to soft tissue.

Score a line with the bur to mark a line of incision and resection.

A thin cut is achieved with the thinnest bur.

Do not apply pressure against the bur tip. This will cause the bur to slow down and the increase in friction and heat may damage the bone.

Excessive pressure may cause the bur to stall.

Move the bur constantly across the area of resection for a faster, cooler, cleaner cut.

Use intermittent physiologic saline irrigation with the air instruments. The liquid cools the bone and clears the operative site of bone debris.

Use only sharp burs and blades.

Set the pressure of the regulator with the instrument running.

Burs must be assembled with the appropriate bur guards.

Running burs without a bur guard or with a bur guard of incorrect length may cause the bur to whip or break.

Bibliography

Agner, O.: Treatment of Non-United Navicular Fractures by Total Excision of the Bone and the Insertion of Acrylic Prostheses. **Acta. Orthop. Scandinav.**, 33:235-245, 1963.

Brannon, E. W. and Klein, G.: Experiences with a Finger-Joint Prosthesis. **J. Bone and Joint Surg.**, 41-A:87-102, January 1959.

Dawkins, A. L.: The Fractured Scaphoid: A Modern View. **Med. J. Aust.**, 1:332-333, February 1967.

Swanson, A. B.: Silicone Rubber Implants for the Replacement of the Carpal Scaphoid and Lunate Bone. **Orthop. Clin. N. Amer.**, 1:299-309, November 1970.

Swanson, A. B.: Silicone Rubber Implants for Replacement of Arthritic and Destroyed Joints in the Hand. **Surg. Clin. N. Amer.**, 48:1113-1127, October 1968.

Swanson, A. B.: Arthroplasty in Traumatic Arthritis of Joints of the Hand. **Orthop. Clin. N. Amer.**, 1:285-298, November 1970.

Swanson, A. B.: A Dynamic Brace for Finger-Joint Reconstruction in Arthritis. **Inter-Clinic Information Bull.**, New York University, New York. 10:1-7, May 1971.

Urbaniak, J. R.: McCollum, D. E. and Goldner, J. L.: Metacarpophalangeal and Interphalangeal Joint Reconstruction. **South. Med. J**, 63:1281-1290, November 1970.

Verdan, C. and Narakas, A.: Fractures and Pseudarthrosis of the Scaphoid. **Surg. Clin. N. Amer.**, 48:1083-1095, October 1968.

Wallace, P. F.: Fractures of the Carpal (Wrist) Navicular Bone. **Med. Trial. Techn. Quart.**, 10:79-82, September 1963.

Weinman, D. T. and Lipscomb, P. R.: Degenerative Arthritis of the Trapeziometacarpal Joint: Arthrodesis or Excision. **Mayo Clin. Proc.**, 42:276-287, May 1967.

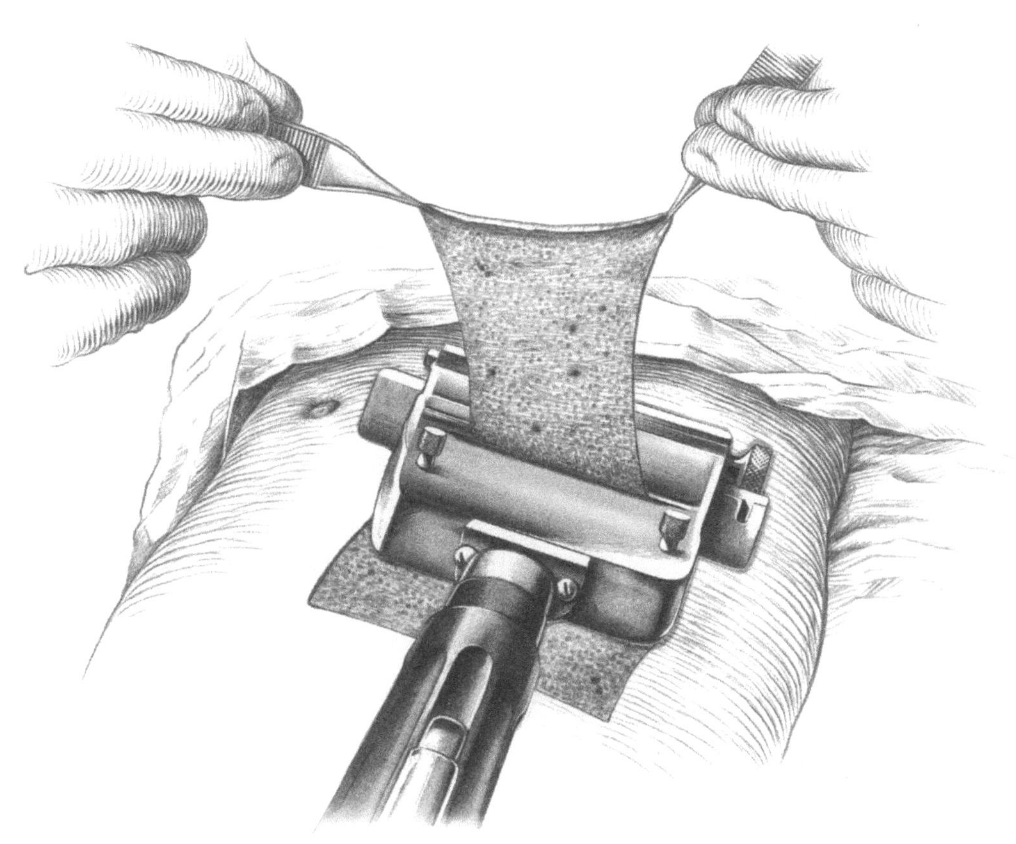

Introduction

The surgical application of any type of air drill in soft tissue surgery is limited. The techniques described demonstrate specifically how the drill aids the surgeon in his work.

The skin grafting instrument is probably most familiar to all surgical personnel, and has been described in detail. Techniques of liver biopsy and aortic valve surgery etc. are, however, not so well known and are fully illustrated.

People are becoming ever more critical of their own appearance, and so the plastic surgeon is developing techniques for improving disfiguring skin conditions. Several such operations are included in this section. All require considerable familiarity with the instruments to develop skill in controlled and even application of the burs. In addition the technique suggestions should be read and understood before beginning to use the instruments in surgery.

New operations are slowly being perfected for cosmetic surgery. Alongside these operations instruments are designed to meet the new demands of the surgeon. The omission of any techniques or instruments from this chapter is probably due to their recent addition to the surgeon's skill or instrumentarium.

Contents

Dermabrasion

A diamond dermabrader rotating at 100,000 rpm will remove minor skin deformities with a light surgical touch. Heavy pressure applied to the skin will cause the drill to stop, and this prevents deeper planing or cutting of the skin.* It is helpful to use magnification, and dot with methylene blue the high points of a scar ridge or fullness. These are removed selectively and in a very limited field down to an even surface, and only then is a generalized planing of the area done. To try and cover a wide area as with the whole length of the cylinder will not give as good a result as smoothing a preliminary of marks or ridges alongside of the scar.

Following assembly of the equipment**, it is advisable to begin with a reduced pressure from the nitrogen tank; with repeated use and practice, it can be turned up to maximum pressure, 110 psi (7 atm), to obtain peak efficiency.

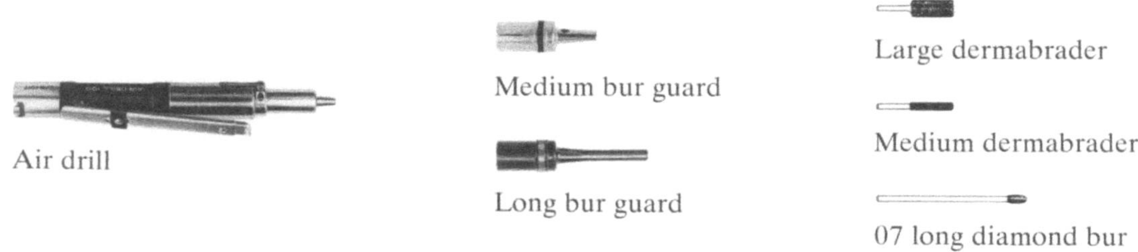

---

 * William H. Frackleton, M.D. (Personal Communication, November 1969).
** H. Lipshutz, M.D.: The Air Drill with Diamond Abrader, a New Useful Adjunct for Dermabrasion. *Plastic and Recon Surg.* 39:521-522, 1967.

1. With the slim medium dermabrader, dermabrade the small crevassed areas of the nasolabial folds.

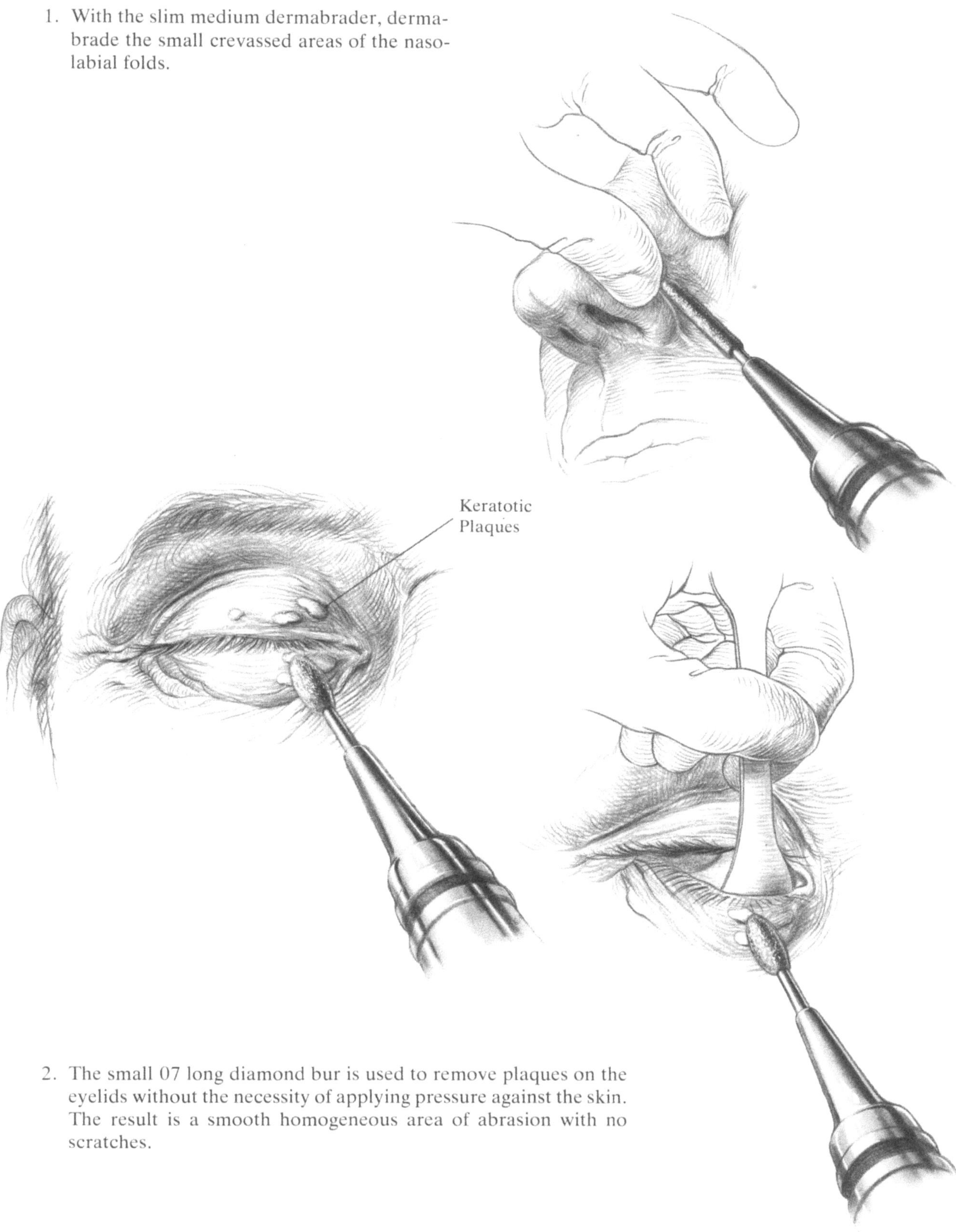

2. The small 07 long diamond bur is used to remove plaques on the eyelids without the necessity of applying pressure against the skin. The result is a smooth homogeneous area of abrasion with no scratches.

Dermabrasion *(continued)*

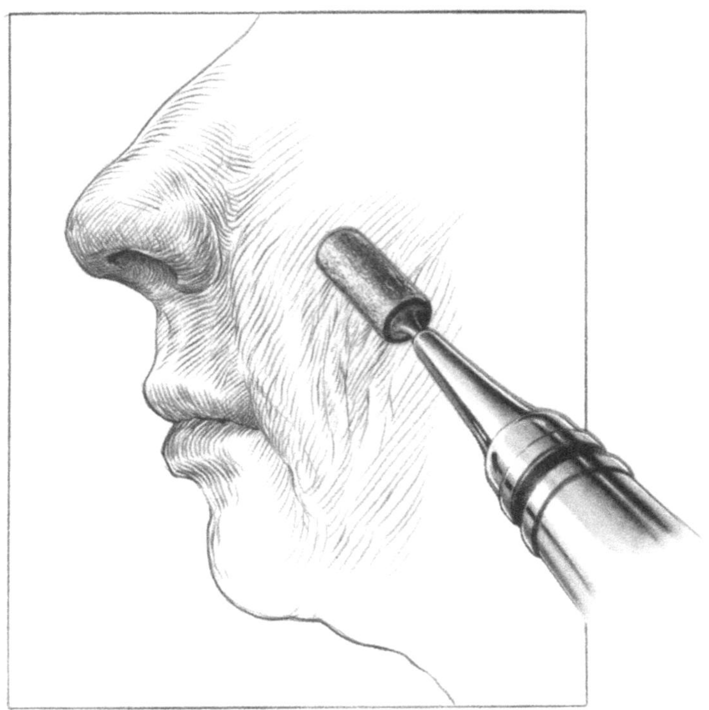

3. Treat flat areas of the face, cheeks and forehead with the large dermabrader.

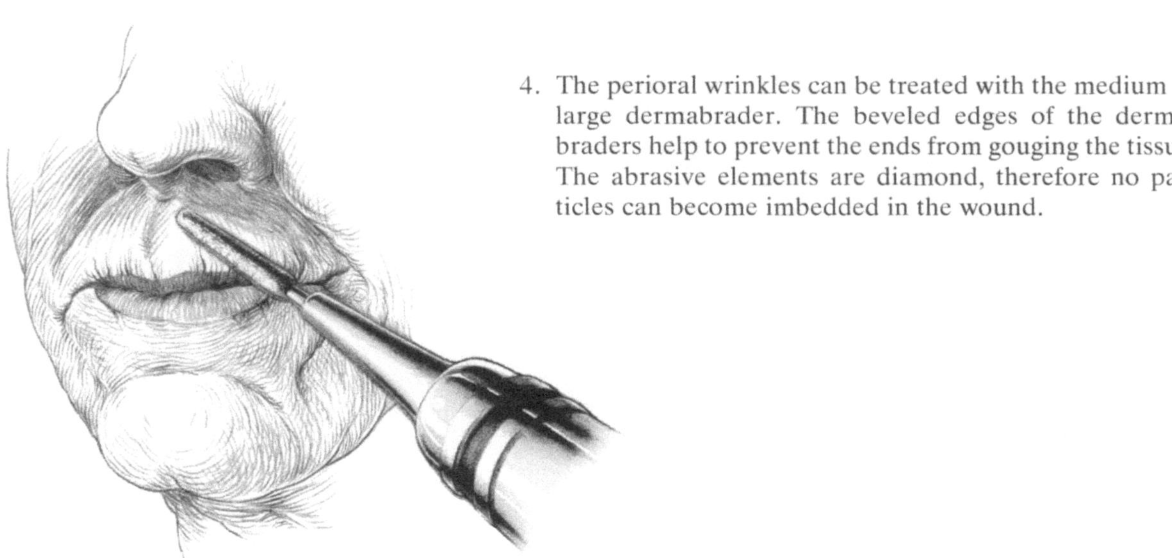

4. The perioral wrinkles can be treated with the medium or large dermabrader. The beveled edges of the dermabraders help to prevent the ends from gouging the tissue. The abrasive elements are diamond, therefore no particles can become imbedded in the wound.

Discussion of Methods of Management of Lower Extremity Soft Tissue Trauma in Arteriosclerotic Patients*

Sloughs:

Skin sloughs secondary to the extravasation of intravenously administered vaso-constrictors are not uncommon and can be disastrous, sometimes causing a far greater problem in management and resultant morbidity than the patient's original condition. In the event of skin necrosis, treatment is conservative. Wet dressings are instituted early to macerate the eschar and to facilitate bedside debridement. Necrosis down to and including bone can further complicate the picture.

It is possible with the air drill and wire-pass bur to drill multiple holes through the cortex of the tibial bone to promote ingress of granulation tissue. The formation of granulation tissue over decorticated bone will permit the application of split-thickness skin grafts.

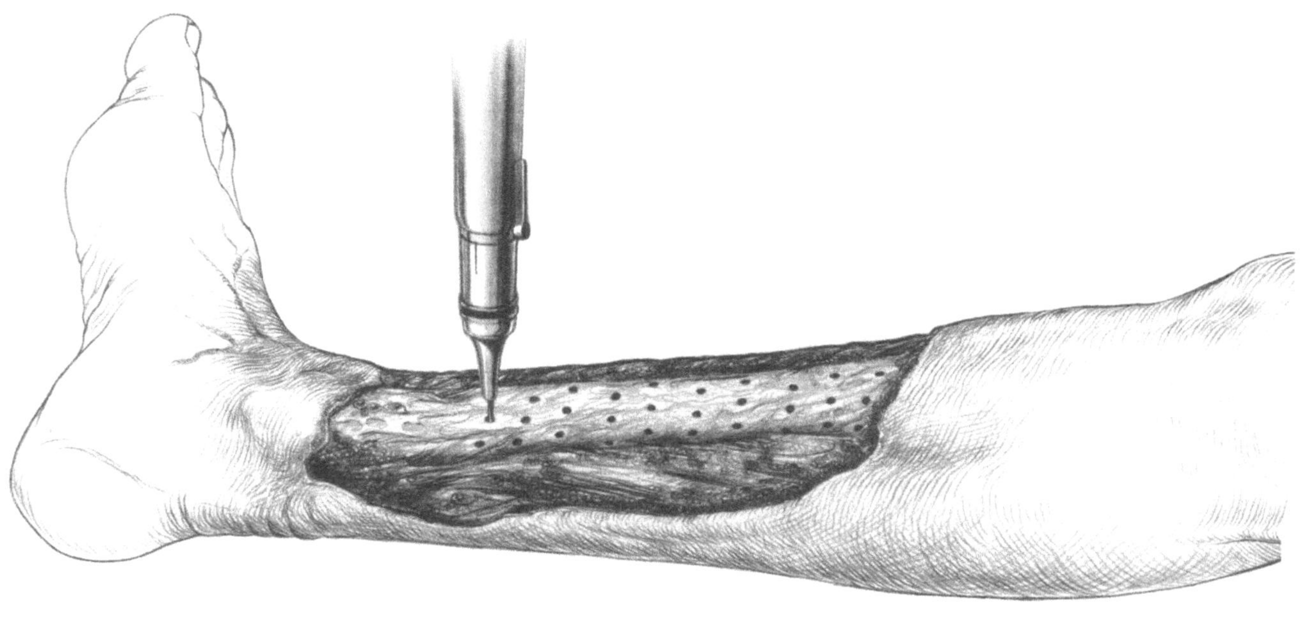

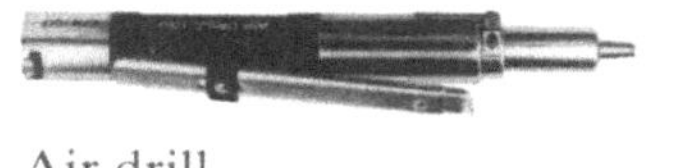

Air drill

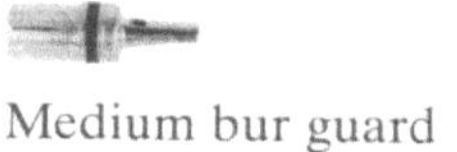

Medium bur guard

27 wire-pass bur

---

* Melvin Spira, M.D., D.D.S. et al.: Discussion and Methods of Management of Lower Extremity Soft Tissue Trauma in Arteriosclerotic Patients. **J of Trauma.** 9:874-886, 1969.

Permanent Camouflage of Capillary Hemangiomas*

Microscopically, the nevus flammeus is composed of thin-walled capillaries. These capillaries vary in their position and depth in the dermis. Take a biopsy to determine the type of lesion present. The deep dermal or subdermal lesions respond most favorably to the deposition of insoluble pigments. There must be a layer of uninvolved dermis overlying the vascular dilations if the pigment is to be effective.

Deposit the inert white pigment deep into the skin to the stratum granulosum but superficial to the pathologic capillaries. Only the pigment deposited in the dermis (overlay) will be permanent; as this is below the level of the vessels of the subepidermal hemangioma, the masking effect in such cases is not apparent.

The instrument** is designed to allow the needles to penetrate the dermis at controlled depths and operates through an air-driven flexible shaft.

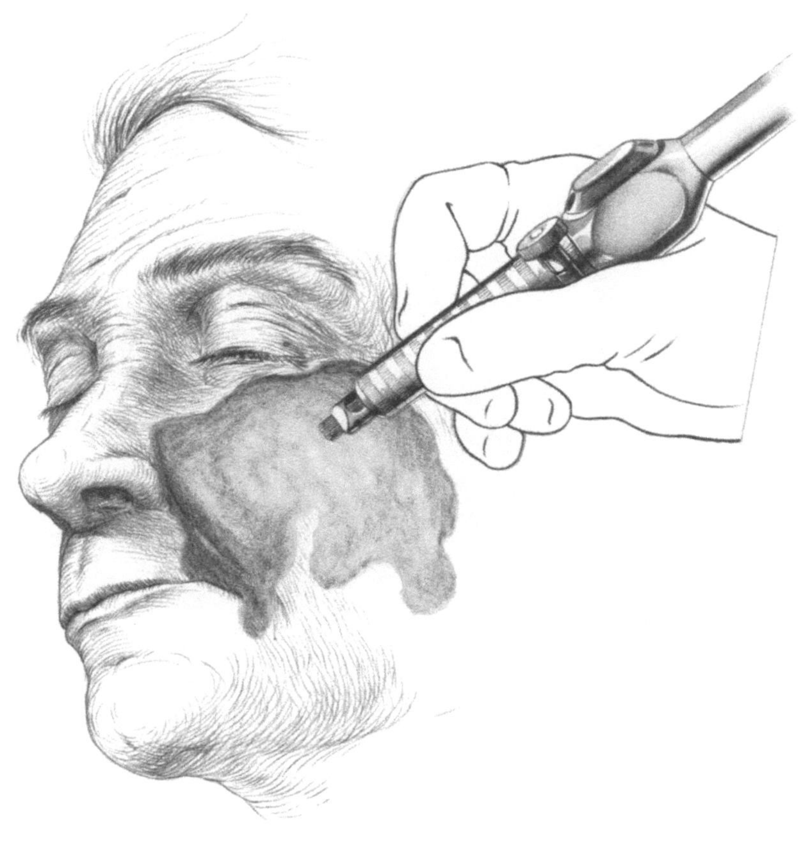

---

  * H. Conway, M. D., F. A. C.S. and R. E. Montroy, M. D.: Permanent Camouflage of Capillary Hemangiomas of the Face by Intradermal Injection of Insoluble Pigments (Tattooing): Indications for Surgery. **New York State J of Med** 65:875-885, April 1965.
 ** Available from Stryker Corporation, Kalamazoo, Michigan, USA.

The rate of injection is controlled with the foot and the depth of penetration by a set-screw attachment. It is not necessary to shave the hair. Outline the margins of the lesion with methylene blue and anesthetize the area. With the pigment applied to the dermatattoo, hold the instrument like a pen so that the needles penetrate the skin at an angle of 60°. This makes for even and uniform distribution of the pigment. Following treatment, apply impregnated gauze and sterile dressings.

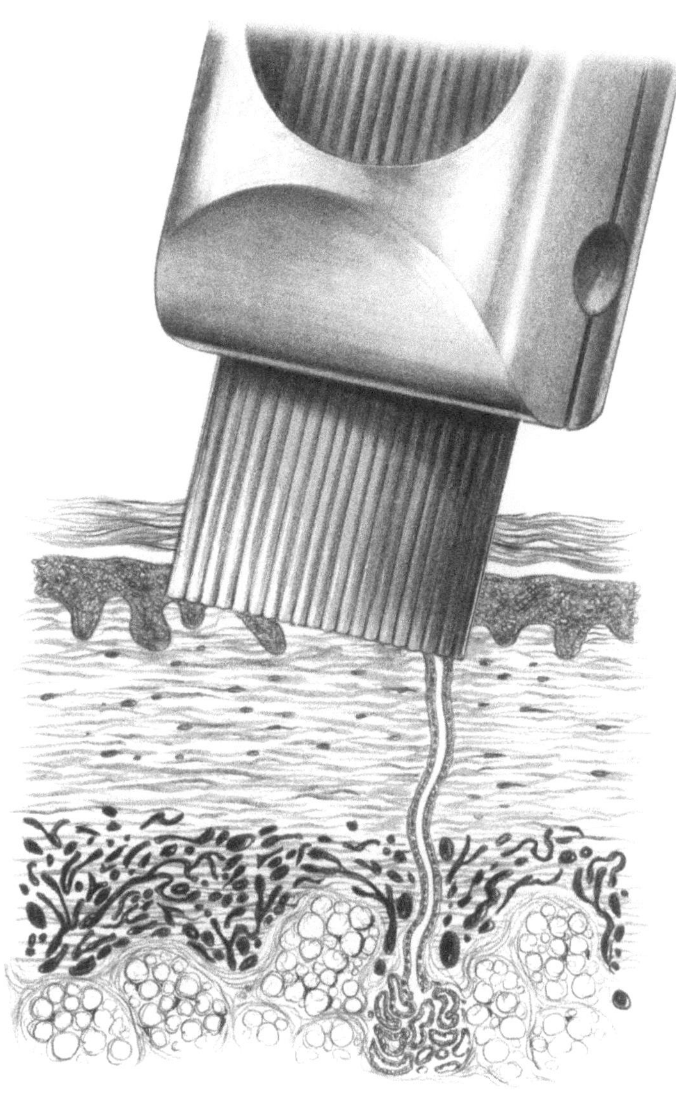

Tissue Biopsy

A tissue biopsy can be taken at a 90° angle or with the straight medium bur guard, from any area of the surface tissue. Burs have an inside diameter ranging between 4.4 mm and 1.2 mm. The depth of all biopsy burs is reduced in one millimeter increments from 13 mm to a depth of 10 mm. Biopsies can be rapidly excised. The high-speed circular knife minimizes tissue trauma and postoperative edema. The specimen is a clean intact segmental core, excellent for pathological examination.

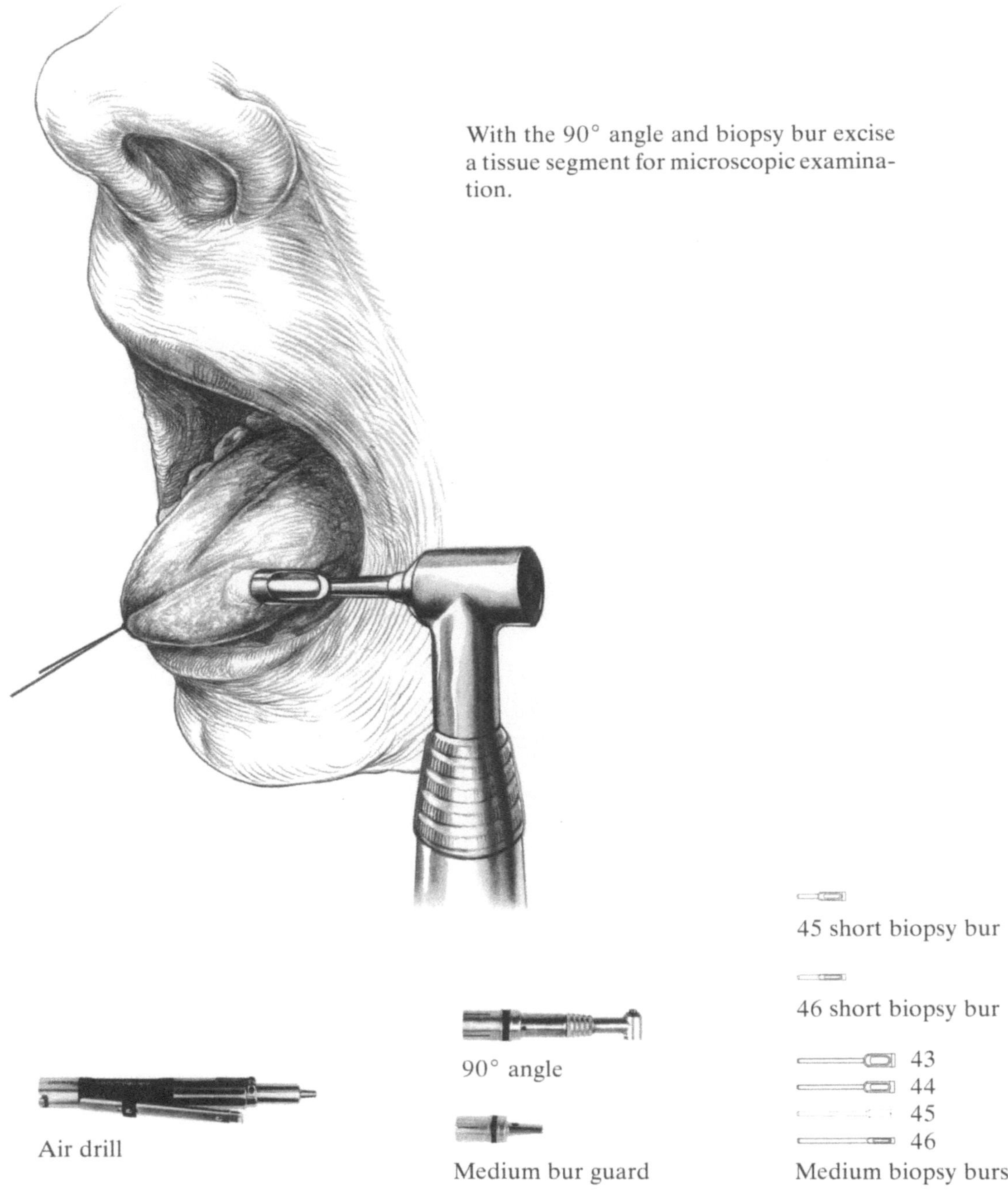

Excision of a Fibroma

Small intraoral tumors can be rapidly excised with a tissue or bone biopsy bur.
The circular knife action reduces hemorrhage and postoperative edema. When both
tissue and bone are required for biopsy, as for examination of a fibroma, the bone
biopsy burs can excise a continuous segmental core as a specimen.

Bone-biopsy burs with an inside diameter of 6.0 mm, 5.0 mm and 4.0 mm are
available for the medium and long bur guards. The depth of biopsy burs is reduced
in one millimeter increments from 13 mm to 10 mm.

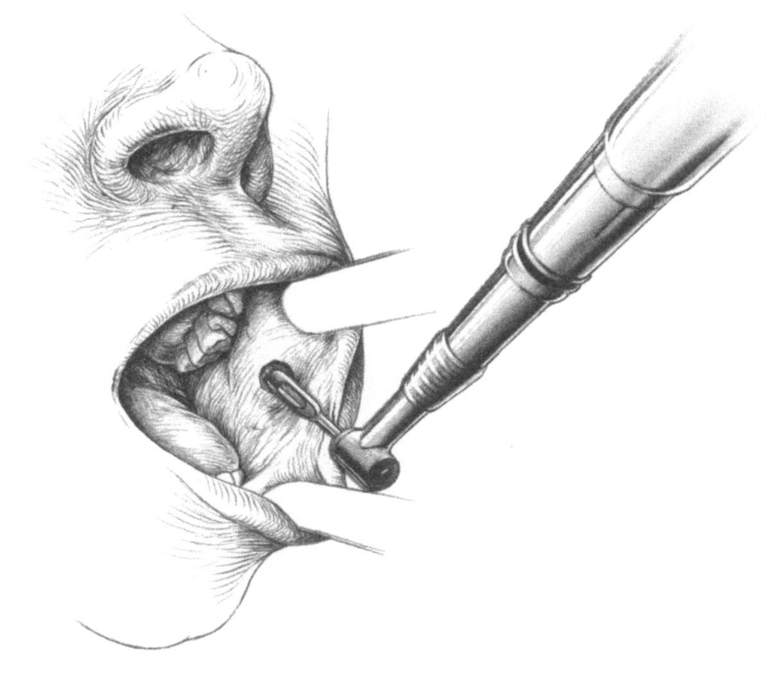

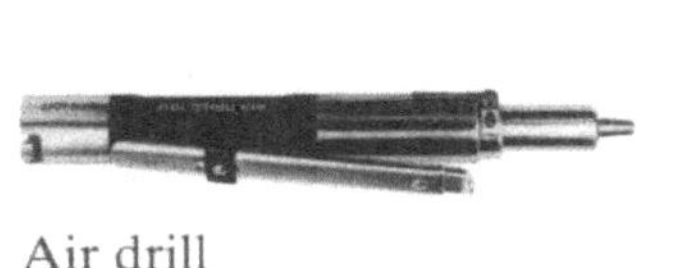

Air drill

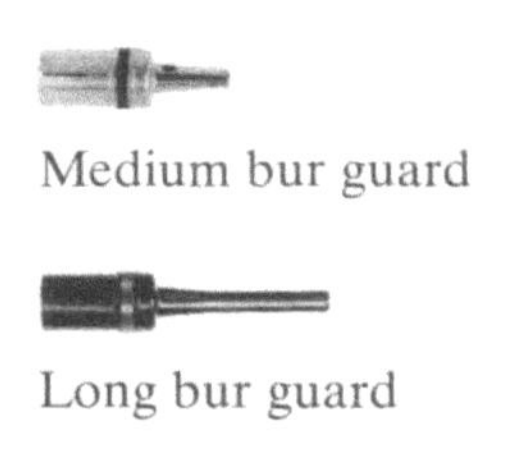

Medium bur guard

Long bur guard

51 medium bone-biopsy

52 medium bone-biopsy

53 medium bone-biopsy

51 long bone-biopsy

52 long bone-biopsy

53 long bone-biopsy

Liver Biopsy*

Almost any tissue lends itself to drill biopsy, which obviates the need for a more formal surgical procedure.
The high-speed drill minimizes trauma to both host tissues and biopsy specimen and thereby reduces the possible hazard of malignant cell dissemination.

Assemble the biopsy-needle adapter and biopsy needle:

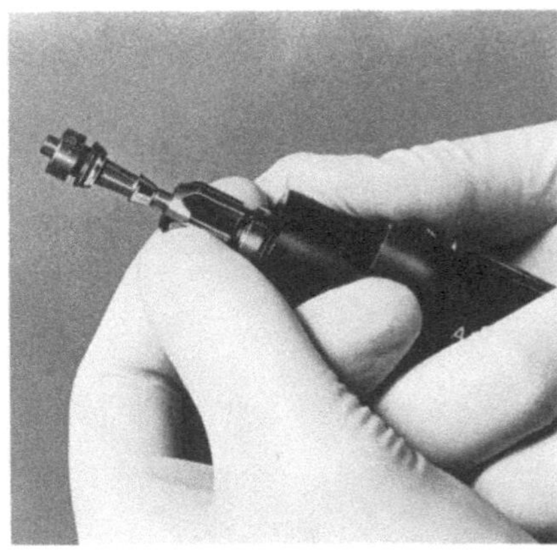

1. Insert biopsy-needle adapter into air driver collet. Maintain hold on button and turn collet to lock adaptor.

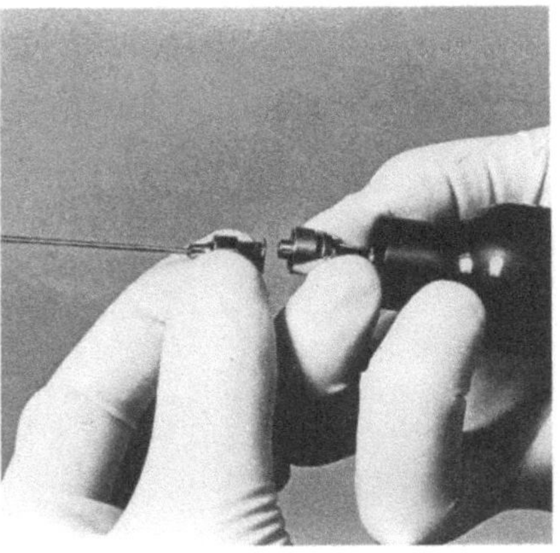

3. Remove center trocar point from the biopsy needle and engage needle and adapter.

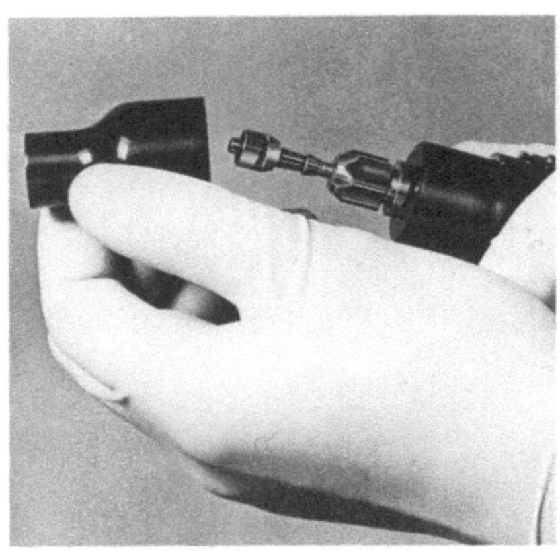

2. Place wire-pass guard over the adapter and air driver shoulder, and seat firmly.

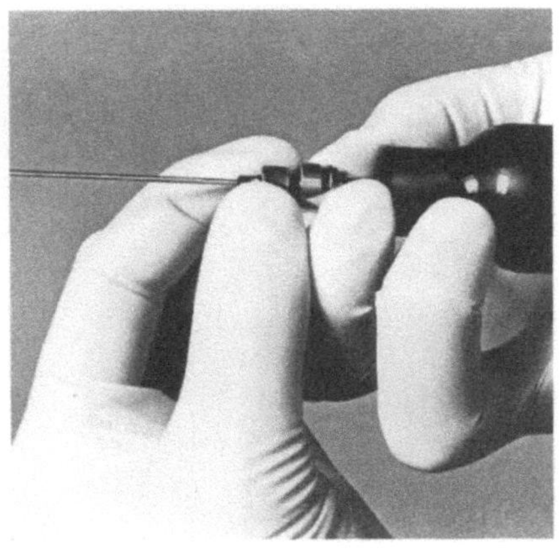

4. Turn needle within the biopsy-needle adapter.

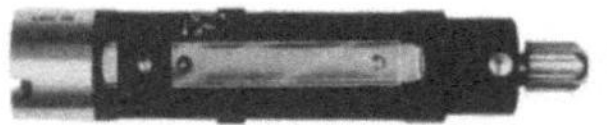
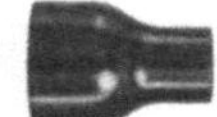
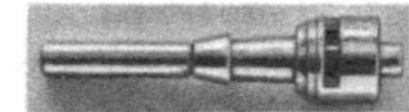
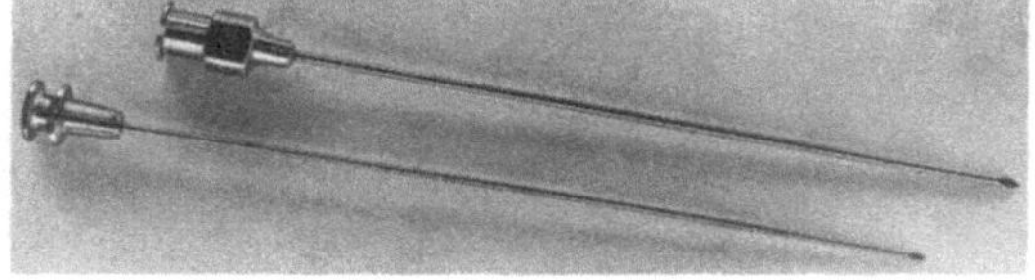

Air driver   Wire-pass guard   Biopsy-needle adapter   Biopsy needles

---

* B. R. Meyerwitz, M. D. et al.: Pneumatic Drill for Tissue Biopsy. **Amer J Surg** 109:536-538, April 1965.

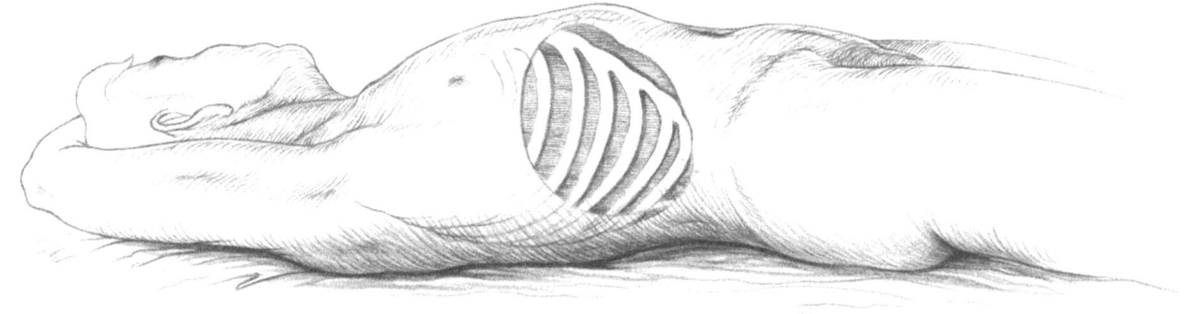

5. Perform the biopsy under aseptic conditions. Locally anesthetize the biopsy site, and make a small skin incision.

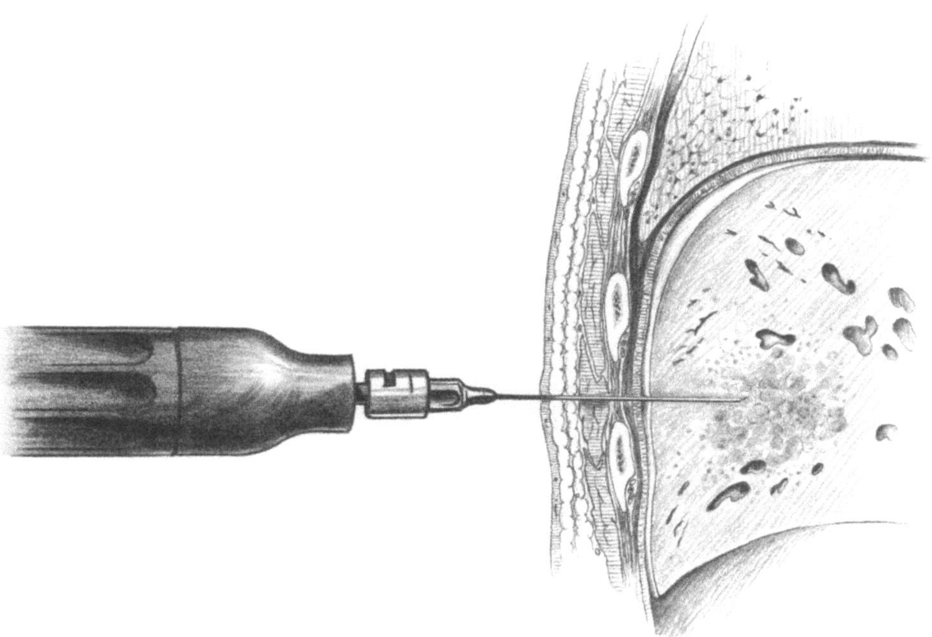

6. Fit the needle into the biopsy-needle adapter and drill and insert it into the stab wound. Stabilize the area of entry with one hand and guide the direction of the drill with the other. Completely depress the throttle. Apply no force. A brisk "in and out" application of the needle will ensure a satisfactory specimen. If the needle becomes detached as the drill is withdrawn, attach a syringe to remove the needle while maintaining suction with the syringe. The biopsy section when examined shows no fragmentation and is free of crushing artifacts. Intact biopsies are ideal for frozen section processing.

7. The drill and attachments can also be used for lung biopsy**.

** Anonymous: Drill Biopsy: Not for the inexperienced. **J Amer Med Ass** 223: 1094-1095, March 1973.

Operative Management of Heavily Calcified Aortic Valve*

Calcific embolization, especially to a coronary or cerebral artery, is a serious and frequently fatal complication in operations for replacing a heavily calcified aortic valve. Early in the course of the development of our operative technique for valve replacement, several such episodes of calcific embolization occurred. Specific techniques were then devised or adopted to prevent this complication. One of these techniques, described here, is excision of the valve with a high-speed air drill. When valve replacement is indicated, take the 02 carbide-tip bur and air drill and begin excision of the densely calcified valve at the central orifice. Once a portion of the valve is removed, fill the ventricular cavity with loosely packed gauze. Avoid contact between the drill and gauze packing. Any loose fragments of valve or debris are enmeshed in this gauze.

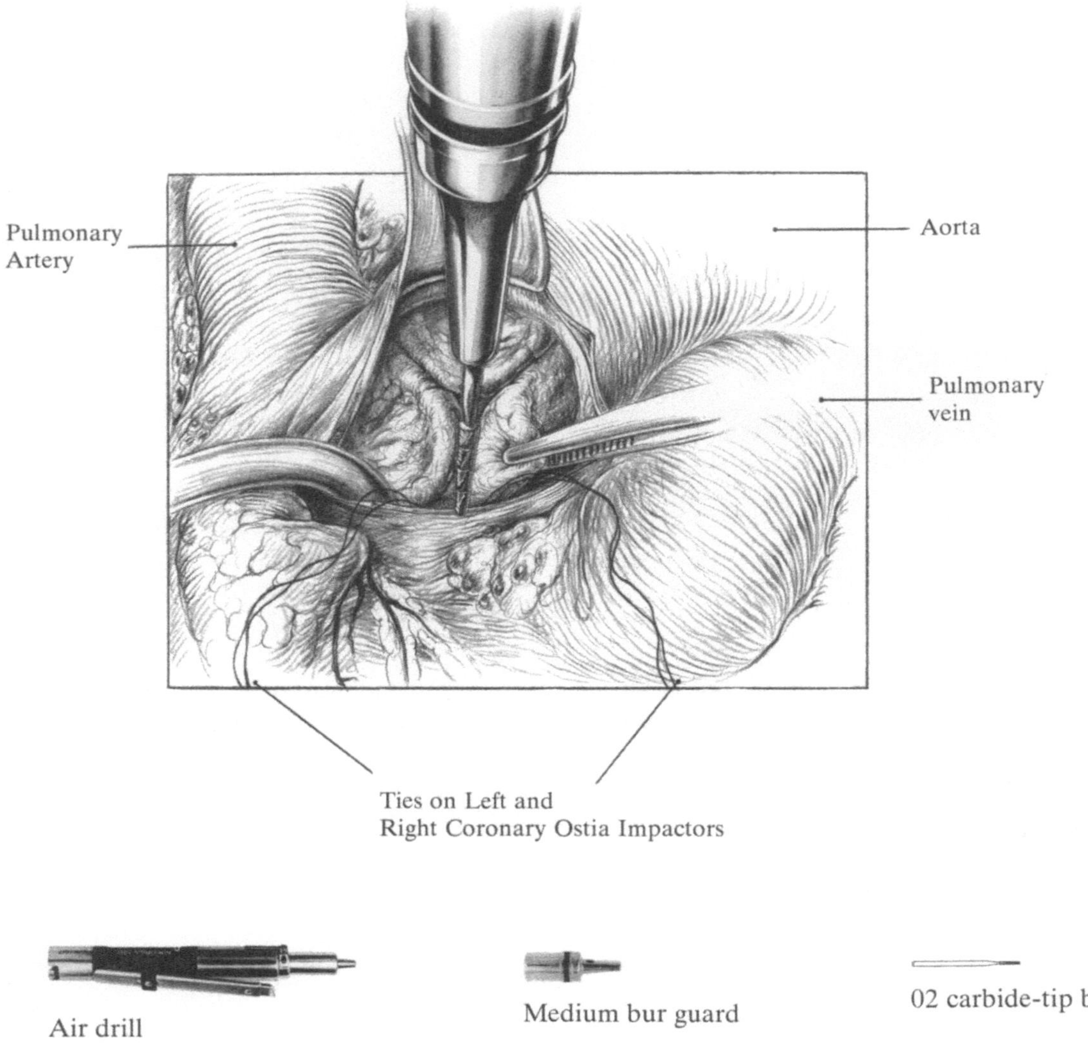

---

* G. J. Haupt, M.D., et al.: Operative Management of the Heavily Calcified Aortic Valve. **J of Thor and Cardiovas Surg** 51:656-659, May 1966.

The drill is capable of cutting soft tissue as well as densely calcified material. It is possible to scribe a very fine precise line of excision around the entire circumference of the valve. Excise the noncoronary cusp at the annulus. Carefully remove the ventricular packing and freely irrigate the cavity with several liters of cold saline. For insertion of the prosthesis follow the commonly used techniques for the Starr-Edwards or Magovern valve. After aortic closure, make careful efforts to assure complete displacement of air from the ventricular cavity prior to defibrillation. When the heart is beating effectively, the left ventricular vent is removed and cardiac bypass is discontinued.

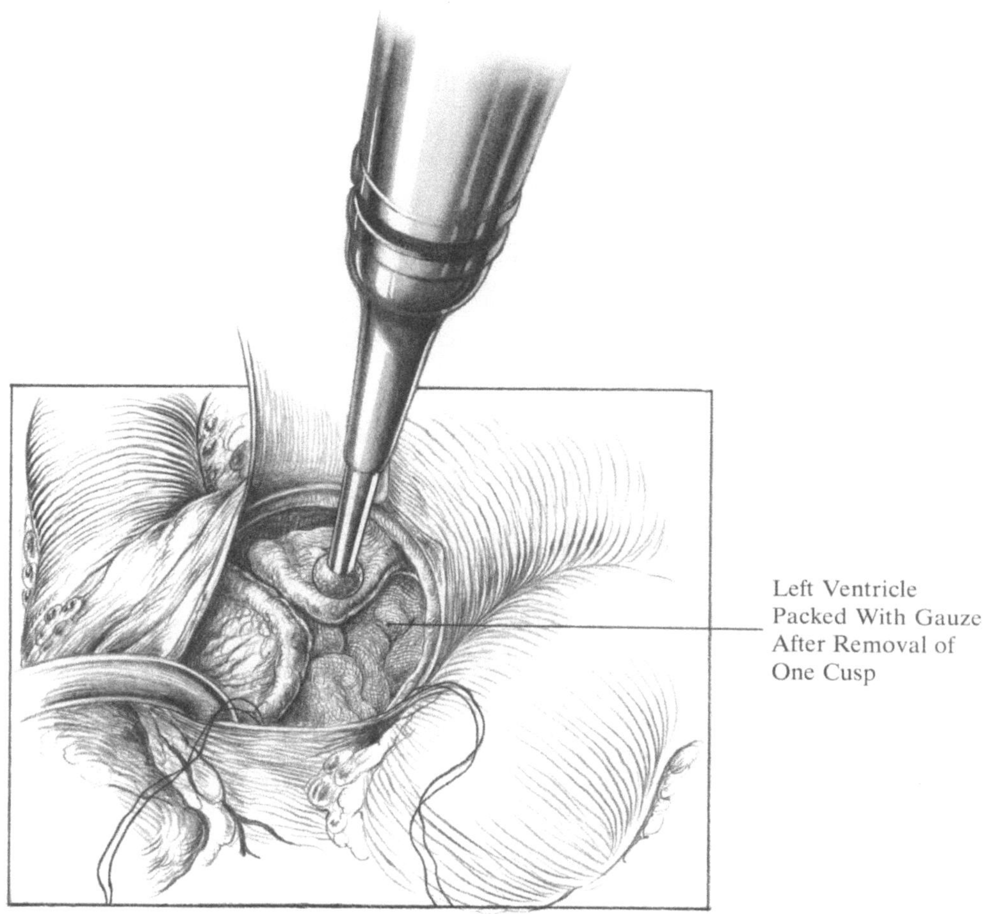

Intimectomy*

Dissect the occluded arterial segment in both directions as far as necessary to attain a soft and patent vessel. Isolate the branches and for hemostatic control apply double loops of 00 Mersilene. Secure clamps distally and proximally. Open the distal clamp and inject a diluted heparin solution into the vessel distal to the occlusion. Perform the same procedure proximal to the occlusion.
With the aid of fine dissectors remove clot and intraluminal atheromatous material. Resect protruding intimal swellings with care, using a sharp scalpel. Scrape ulcers with sharp scoops and smooth the borders. Resect any calcified plaques present in the edge of the arteriotomy to facilitate later suture of the patch graft.
With the drill and 07 steel bur treat the intima to remove all irregularities. A smooth finish can be attained with final application of a diamond bur.

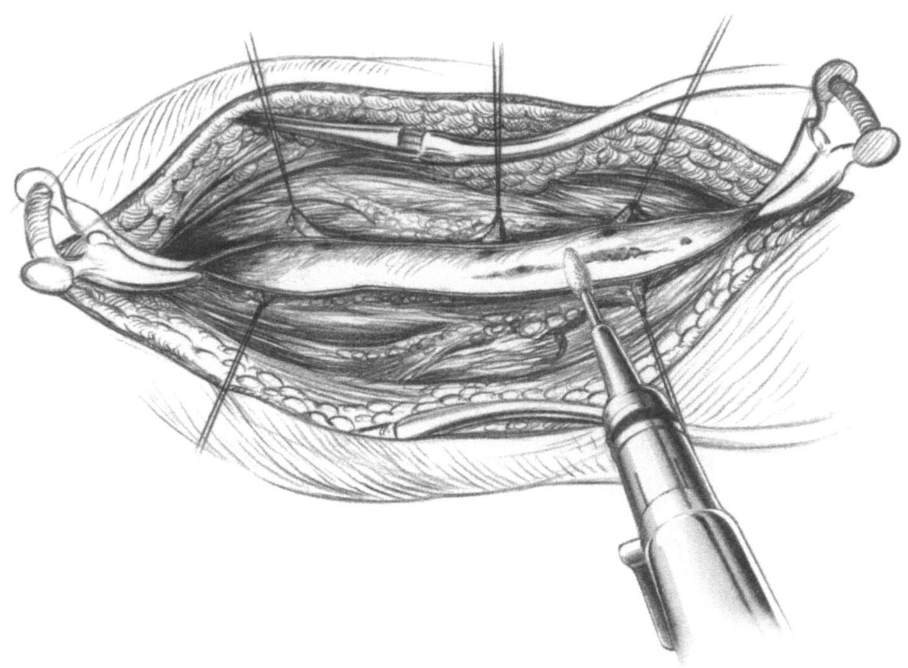

Excise and prepare a graft for suturing to the vessel. After the patch has been sutured in, remove the clamps. Exert careful pressure on the graft with dry gauze. Hemostasis is soon complete. Sometimes it is necessary to apply an additional mattress suture to arrest a hemorrhage between two stitches. For this purpose use 6-0 Mersilene.

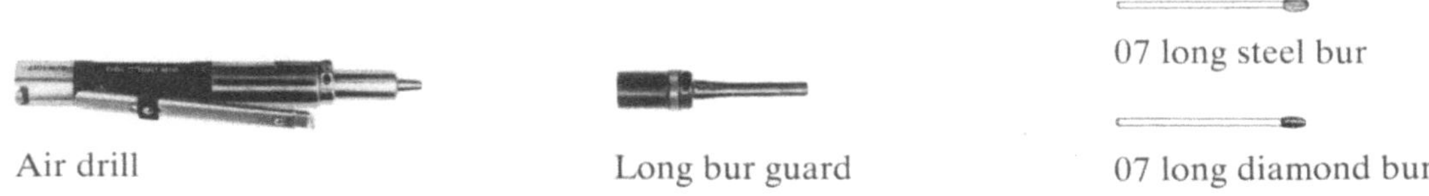

---

* van Dangen, R. J. A. M.: Photographic Atlas of Reconstructive Arterial Surgery. **Springer-Verlag, H. E. Stenfert Kroese N. V.** 1970.

Technique Suggestions

Do not apply pressure on dermabraders, as this may cause too deep planing of the skin. Use the drill at full speed with a light delicate touch.

Although special burs have been designed for dermabrasion, any of the diamond burs can be used in the smaller, less acessible areas of the soft tissue.

A foot control is available if preferred to the finger-tip operation.

Adhere carefully to the recommended lubrication instructions for the air drill and air driver found at the end of this book.

Diamond burs maintain their cutting qualities indefinitely but steel burs will dull after use. The drill is only as effective as the sharpness of the bur. Change the burs regularly.

Never use a bur without the appropriate bur guard. An unprotected bur may snap off and cause an accident.

Gauze in close contact with the drill may become tangled in the bur. Use Gelfoam wherever possible, as this eliminates the danger of bur entanglement.

Use intermittent irrigation and suction to clear the operative site and reduce heat between bur and tissue.

Never place air motors in liquids, especially saline solution. The salt will damage the smooth running parts.

All instruments can be gas or steam sterilized. Ultrasonic cleaning of the equipment, with the exception of the burs, is not recommended.

Bibliography

Anonymous.: Drill Biopsy: Nor for the Inexperienced. **J. Amer. Med. Assoc.** 223:1094-1095, March 1973.

Conway, H. and Montroy, R. E.: Permanent Camouflage of Capillary Hemangiomas of the Face by Intradermal Injection of Insoluble Pigments (Tattooing). Indications for Surgery. **New York State J. Med.,** 65:875-885, April 1965.

Deeley, T. J.: Drill Biopsy Results with a High Speed Pneumatic Drill. **Acta. Union Interna.,** 16:338-340, 1960.

van Dongen, R. J. A. M.: Photographic Atlas of Reconstructive Arterial Surgery (Intimectomy). **Springer-Verlag** New York Inc., **H. E. Stenfert Kroese N. V./** The Netherlands, 1970.

Haupt, G. J.: Operative Management of the Heavily Calcified Aortic Valve. **J. Thor. and Cardiovas. Surg.,** 51:656-659, May 1966.

Lipshutz, H.: The Air Drill with Diamond Abrader: A New, Useful Adjunct for Dermabrasion. **J. Plast. Reconstr. Surg.,** 39:521-522, May 1967.

Meyerowitz, B. R.: Pneumatic Drill for Tissue Biopsy. **Amer. J. Surg.,** 109:536 to 538, April 1965.

Spira, M. et al.: Discussion of Methods of Management of Lower Extremity Soft Tissue Trauma in Arteriosclerotic Patients. **J. Trauma,** 9:874-886, 1968.

Introduction

The rapid growth in number and types of surgical procedures in the past few years has resulted in an increased need for products to implement these activities. Thus, the nursing profession and auxiliary personnel, especially in the operating room, face a new challenge in using and evaluating the many commercial products which come into the hospital.

Having been used successfully for several years, air instruments have meritoriously fulfilled the demands of the new surgical era. Indeed, they have benefited the patient to such an extent that a genuine breakthrough in surgical techniques has been a-chieved.

Instruments that formerly limited surgical versatility and effectiveness have now been implemented by air-powered equipment. Both patient and surgeon have bene-fited by the time saved and the improved cosmetic results.

What information does the skillful and alert O. R. nurse need to direct her "team" (surgical staff and hospital staff) intelligently in the use of air-driven instruments? First, she must understand the instructions thoroughly. Comprehension of mechanics is an asset. An understanding of the construction of these extremely useful tools and a pronounced regard for their maintenance are important. The advantages of nitrogen (the power source for the instruments) should be understood.

Explanation and demonstration are necessary before implementation. These are provided by Air Instrument Surgery – Volume 3. This book is not only a ready and dependable reference for the surgeon, but also for nursing personnel.

Mabel Crawford R.N.

LOS ANGELES, CALIFORNIA

Contents

Air Pressure Regulator

Regulator

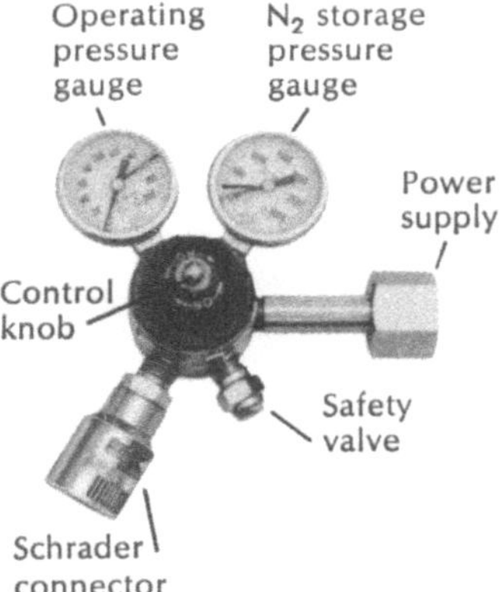

Twin Regulator

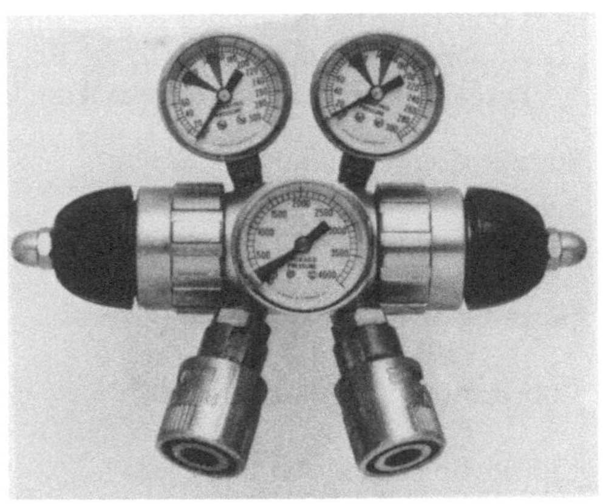

The regulator is manufactured specifically for use with H. I. air instruments. For safety, it is designed to limit pressures to a maximum of 220 psi and to transmit to the instruments any selected lower pressures.

This regulator is designed with twin outlets, necessary when two air instruments are required for the same procedure.

Connecting the Regulator to the Nitrogen Tank

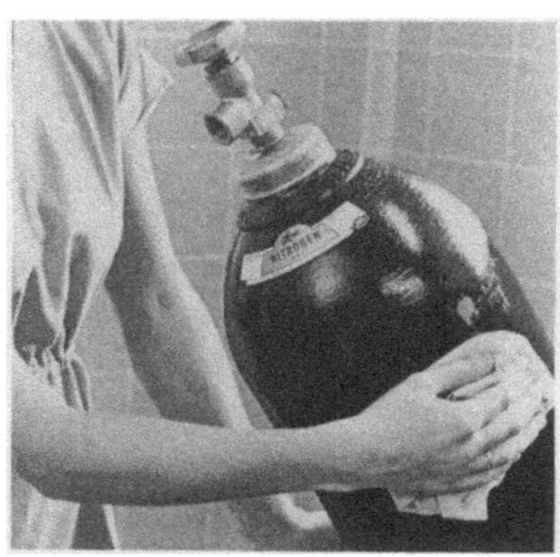

A. To attach regulator to nitrogen tank:

1. This should be done outside of operating room. Wipe off the outside of the cylinder and carrier. (These industrial cylinders are not normally used in clean areas such as operating rooms).

178

2. Open cylinder valve and blow off briefly to clear lines of debris (rust particles, etc.).

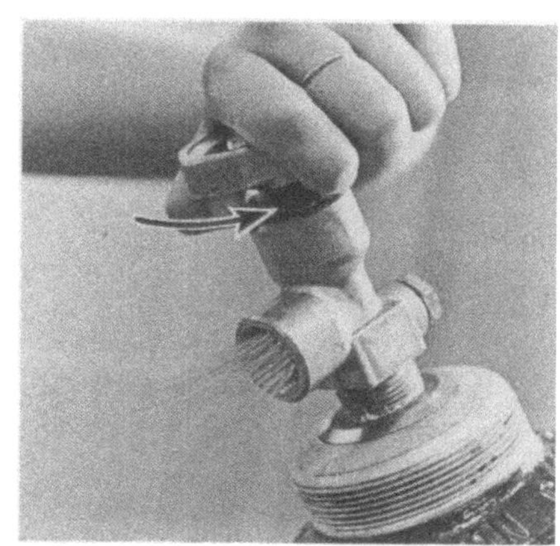

3. Attach regulator by hand.

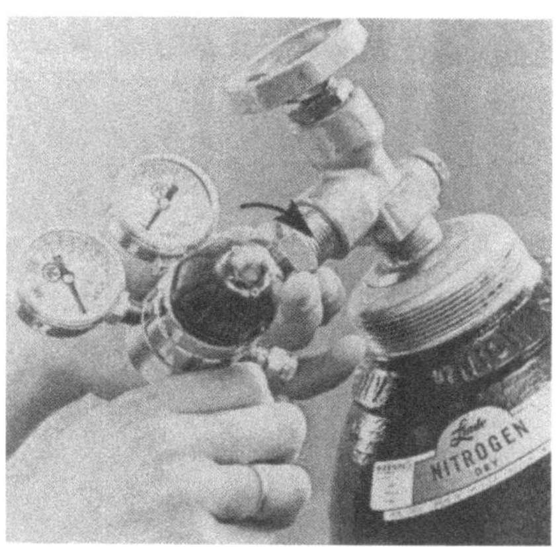

4. Secure with a 1 1/8 inch wrench.

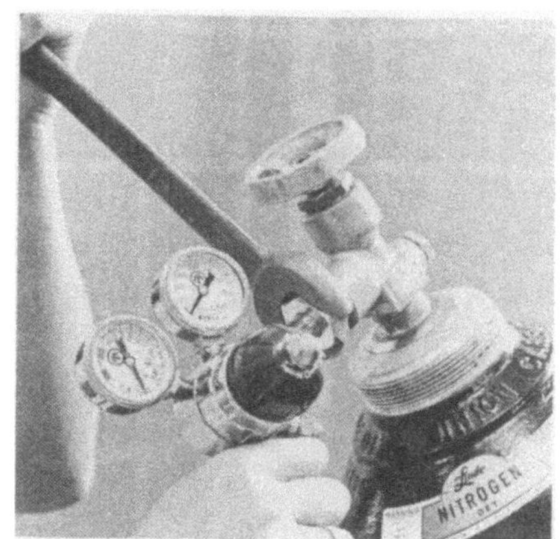

Regulator Assembly *(continued)*

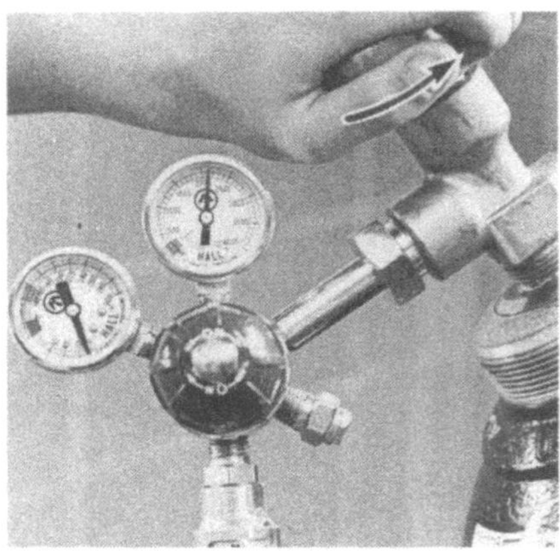

5. To check the connection for air leaks:

   a. Turn on the main tank by slowly turning knob counterclockwise.
   b. The pressure within the tank should register approximately 2,000–2,500 psi when full.
   c. Listen for air leaks.

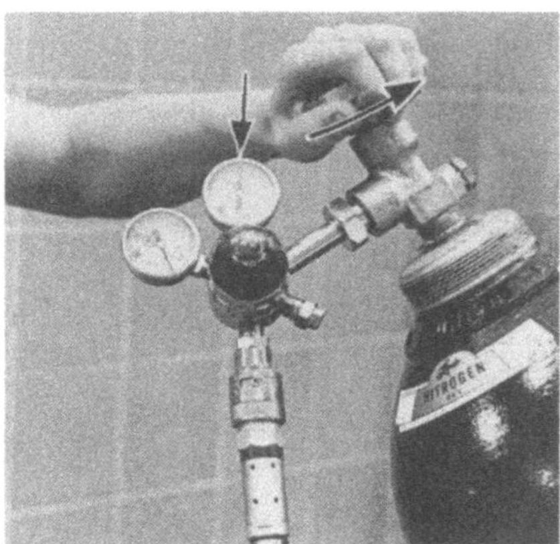

6. Replace the tank when the cylinder pressure gauge shows less than 500 psi or when the indicator is in the red zone. At 500 psi the pressure passing to the instrument is considerably lower than recorded by the regulator. Always have a spare tank available for emergency. Wheel the tank into the operating room and place on surgeon's side of the operating table.

Attaching Air Instruments to the Regulator

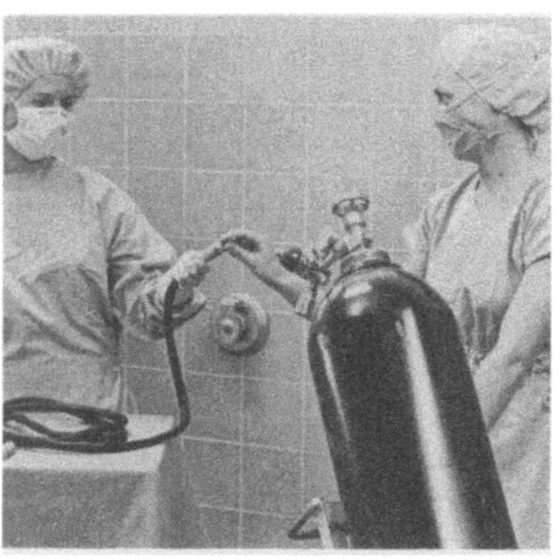

B. To connect instruments to regulator/tank:

1. The circulating nurse takes the connector end of the instrument from the scrub nurse.

2. The connector end of the instrument is thrust into the regulator outlet. Open the tank valve fully (counterclockwise) if this has not been done outside the operating room.

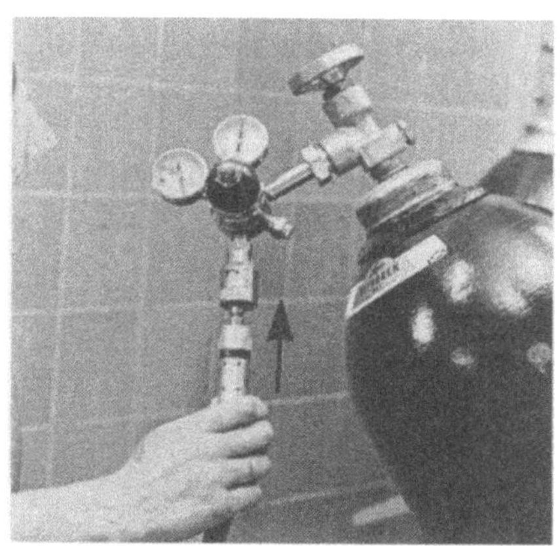

3. Turn the green knob on the regulator "ON" (as indicated by the arrow) according to the requirements of instrument and surgeon.

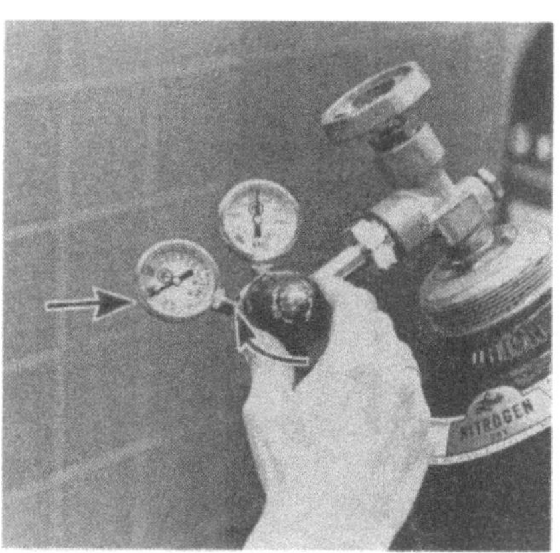

4. Actuate the throttle to set correct pressures at the regulator. Pressure settings must be made while the instrument is running.

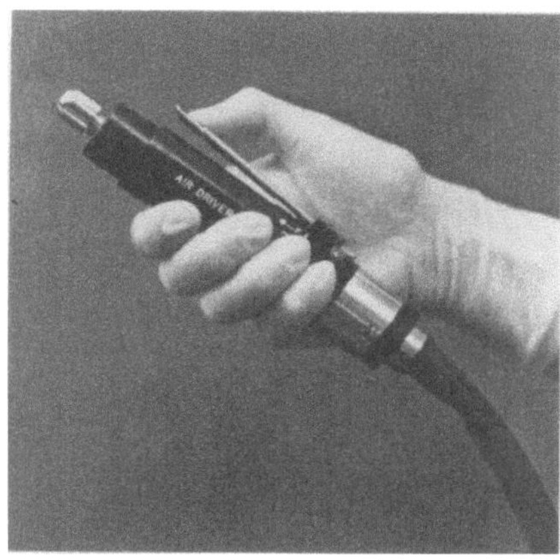

REGULATOR PRESSURE SETTINGS:

Instrument	*Speed*	*Pressure*
Air Drill 100	100,000 rpm max.	90–110 psi (7atm–8.5atm)
Air Driver II	20,000 rpm max.	90–110 psi (7atm–8.5atm)

NOTE: Pressure to the Air Drill 100 can be increased to 160 psi. The speed is increased to between 110,000–115,000 rpm. The change in pressure and speed also increases the torque.

The instrument torque of the Air Drill 100 can also be significantly increased if the exhaust hose is removed. The air is exhausted behind the drill. Drills are available with the single hose.

Disconnecting Air Instruments from the Regulator

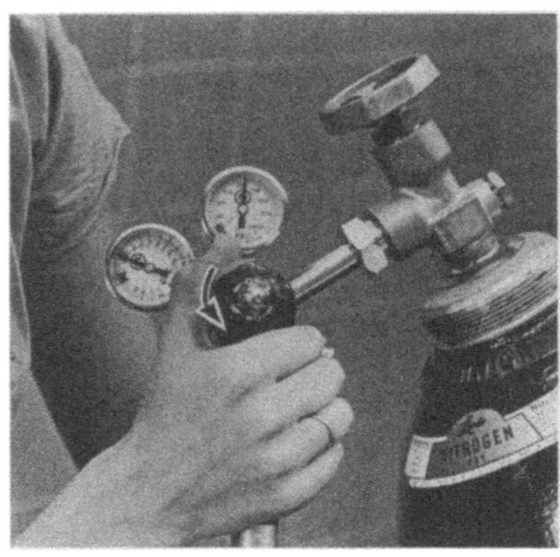

C. To disconnect instruments from regulator:

1. Turn off the green knob on the regulator (as indicated by arrow).

2. Activate control throttle to release ("bleed off") excess air from within the tubing. Regulator should read zero.

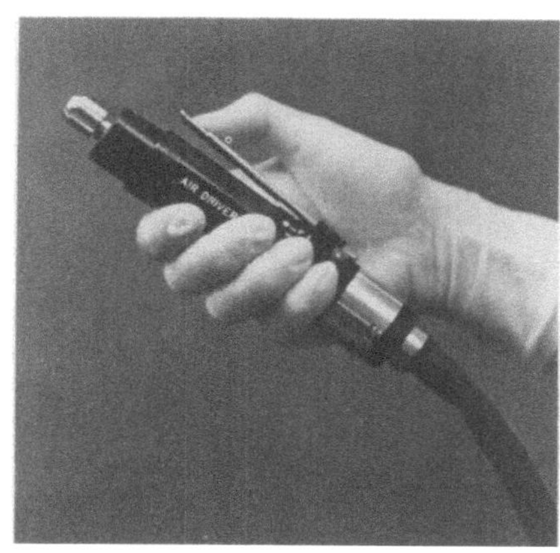

3. Turn connector end clockwise; it will "pop" out.

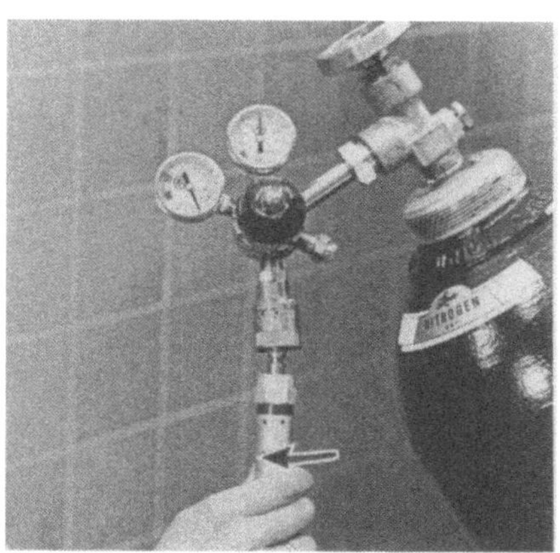

D. Return tank to storage area. Check the nitrogen volume; if the pressure is below 500 psi change the tank. If pressure is 500 psi or more, turn off the valve at the tank (clockwise).

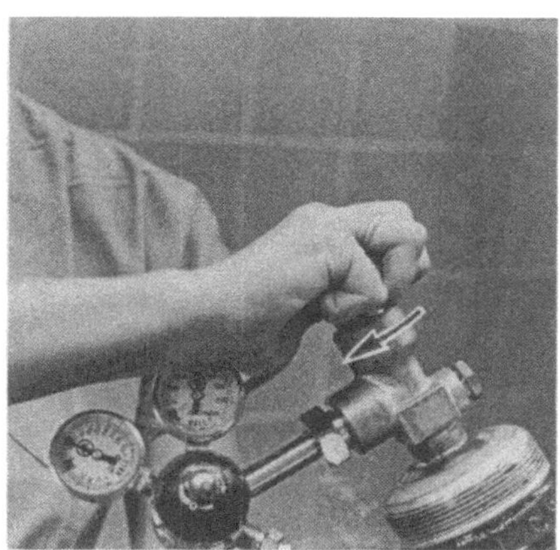

Sterilization of Equipment: Steam

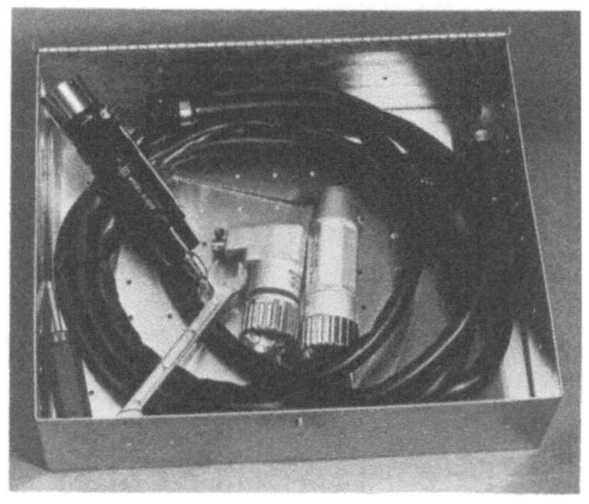

1. Dismantle all attachments from the main motor. Assemble all the equipment required, including an adequate number of burs, blades, etc., into the autoclave box.

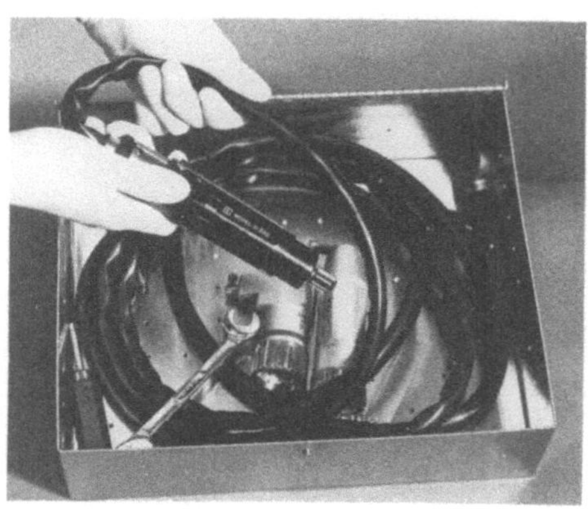

2. Do not kink hose at the instrument connection; (kinking will cause early hose deterioration).

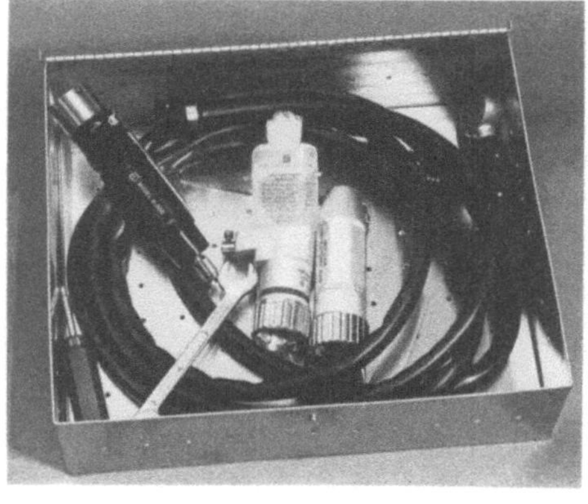

3. Do not include plastic bottle of oil, plastic protectors used to mail the equipment, or the regulator.

4. Steam-sterilize unwrapped instruments (in autoclave box):

   Steam under pressure at:–

   250 – 254 °F for 30 minutes
   (122 – 125 °C)
   270 – 275 °F for 20 minutes
   (132 – 135 °C)

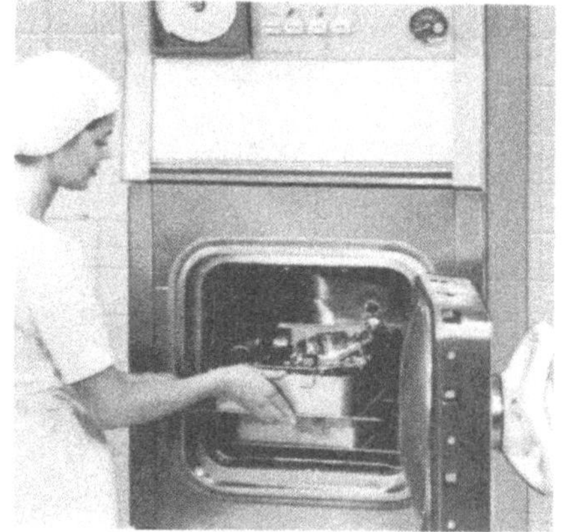

5. Instruments in autoclave box and box wrapped in double-thickness muslin:

   Steam under pressure at: –

   250 – 254 °F for 60 minutes
   (122 – 125 °C)
   270 – 275 °F for 40 minutes
   (132 – 135 °C)

   NOTE:
   Place absorbent muslin in the base of the autoclave box to absorb excess moisture and reduce risk of contaminating or staining the equipment.

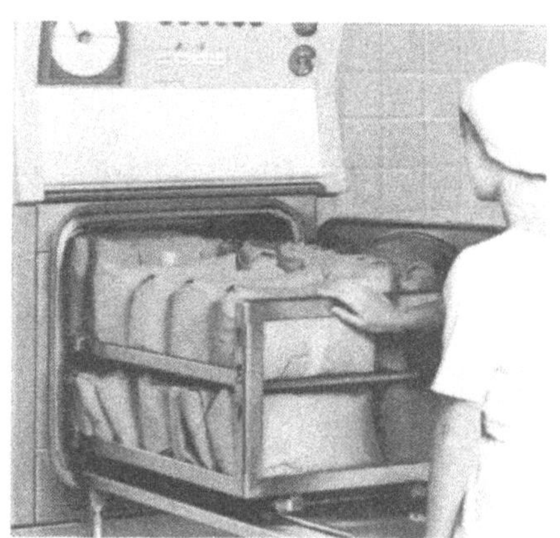

6. Do not use the equipment until cooled to room temperature. *Do not immerse* in cold liquid. Cool by exposure to room temperature or activate throttle and cool with nitrogen. If a warm instrument is plunged into cool liquid (especially saline) the air inside the instrument will contract and the solution will be drawn into the mechanism. The presence of this liquid would prevent the lubricant from lubricating the power system and the instrument would be permanently damaged.

Sterilization of Equipment: Gas

The four factors necessary to effect gas sterilization are temperature, gas concentration, humidity and exposure time.

1. Temperature

   Normally, ethylene oxide sterilization is conducted at temperatures of 120–140°F, (40–60° C), as this is the uppermost temperature range tolerable to many plastic materials.

2. Ethylene oxide concentrations and exposure

   There should be a minimum ethylene oxide concentration of 650–750 milligrams/liter of chamber space for most practical sterilization processes requiring exposure periods of up to 16 hours, dependent upon temperature. (Increased temperature reduces exposure time.)

3. Relative Humidity

   Moisture is an important factor for effective gas sterilization. Excessive drying or desiccation of materials to be gas sterilized should be avoided. The relative humidity or moisture content of the atmosphere in those areas where material packaging is conducted should be not less than 30% and preferably closer to 50% to avoid unintentional dehydration. Although moisture is the least critical factor in ethylene oxide sterilization, it does play a role in achieving sterilization.

4. Exposure Time

   Exposure times vary, and are influenced by:

   a. Level and degree of hydration.

   b. The microbial contamination on the material to be sterilized.

   c. The type of wrapping material to be used.

   In practice, relatively short exposure periods can be employed in gaseous sterilization with ethylene oxide at temperatures of 130–140°F (54.5–60°C) and concentrations of 700–1000 mg/l, provided all articles or materials are thoroughly cleaned and properly wrapped in approved wrapping materials prior to exposure.

NOTES: 1. Refer to manufacturer instructions for correct chamber pressures, ethylene oxide concentration, cycle and exposure times.

2. Gas sterilization of burs will eliminate rusting.

Cleaning of Air Instruments

1. Remove the equipment to the cleaning and processing area as soon as possible following surgery. Remove all attachments from the handpiece.

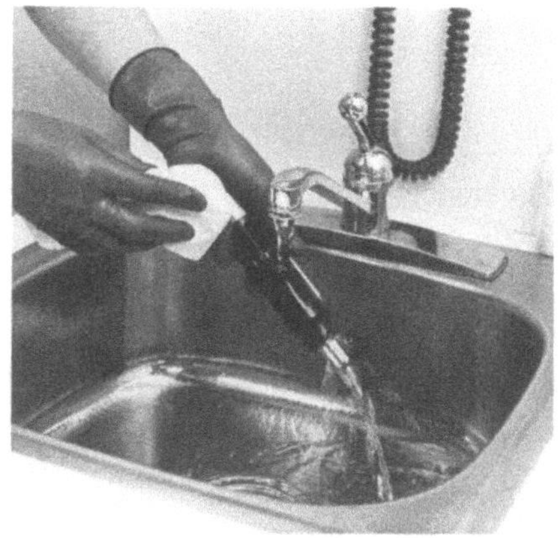

2. Thoroughly scrub the instruments with a soft brush and mild detergent. All traces of blood, coagulated material, etc. should be completely removed. During this scrubbing do not immerse the instruments in the soap solution or rinse water.

3. After the instrument has been thoroughly scrubbed, rinse all traces of soap off the instrument under a running faucet, not by immersing in pan or basin. Rinse the surface free of tap water with distilled water to prevent metal discoloration.

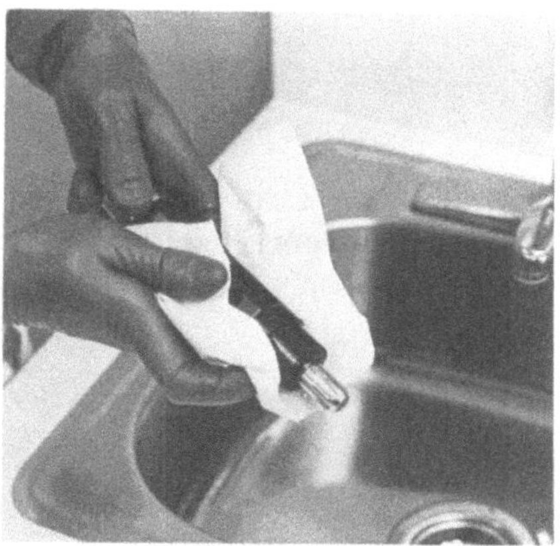

4. Shake the instrument free of water and wipe dry with a clean lint-free towel.

CAUTION:

1. Do not clean equipment in ultrasonic cleaners; this will dislodge oil from the bearings, causing irreversible damage.

2. Do not immerse this equipment in ANY liquid. Saline solution will cause corrosion of the metal and delicate moving parts.

3. See that no water enters the collet of the air drill and air driver.

4. Do not use any liquid chemical disinfectants.

Lubrication of the Air Drill 100

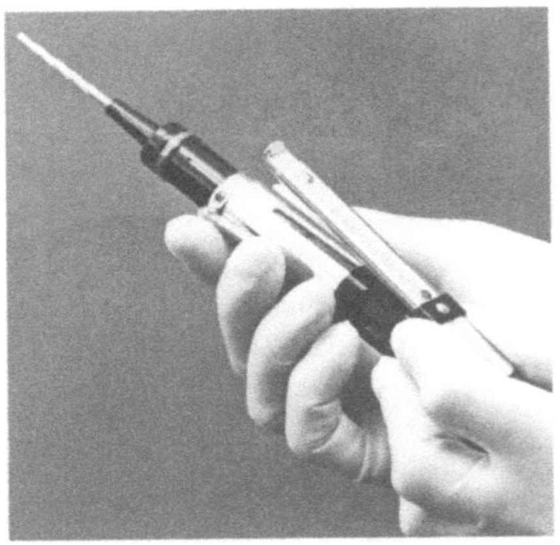

1. Thoroughly clean the drill. With the unit disconnected from the air hose, slide on safety lock.

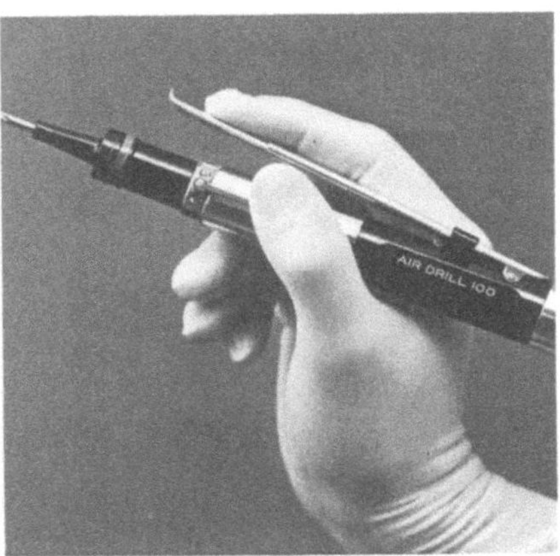

3. Connect the drill to the hose and air supply and run the motor at full speed (100 – 110 psi) for not less than one to three minutes. This allows an oil film to coat the moving parts.

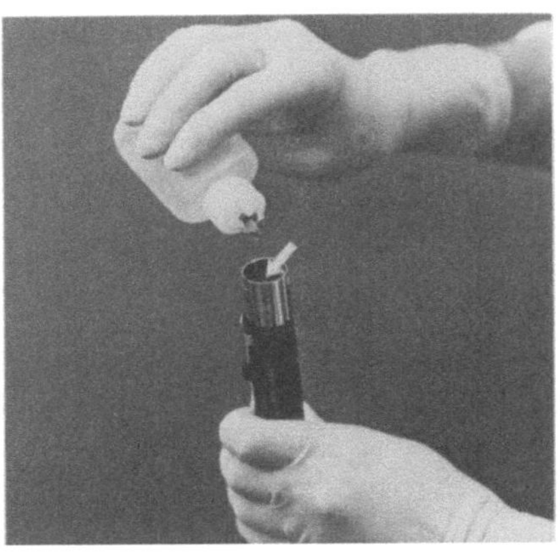

2. Depress throttle and place one or two drops of oil into the inlet stand-pipe at the connector end of the drill.

CAUTION: Do not immerse in any liquid. In the event that the unit is immersed by accident, shake off excess fluid, hook up air supply, hold spindle rigid and depress throttle until all moisture is blown from the unit. Lubricate the drill.

4. The air drill must be used for 30 minutes of running time before further lubrication is necessary. Too much or too little oil will damage the turbine. Indications of either of these conditions are:

    a. Slowing of the drill.
    b. Low torque.
    c. Low-pitched whine.
    d. Heat at the drill nose.
    e. Excess oil at the diffuser.

If one or more of these conditions occur, insert a medium bur into the drill and spray the drill nose with the blitz cleaner and run until the speed increases. The spray dilutes accumulation of oil and removes debris from the front nose bearing.

Lubrication of the Air Driver II

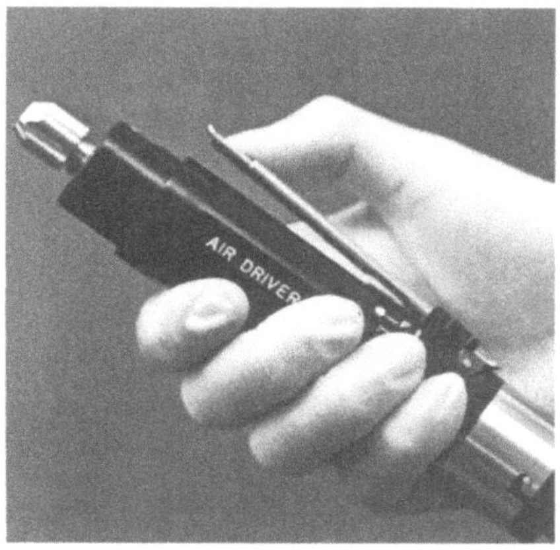

1. Thoroughly clean the drill. Depress throttle with safety lever forward.

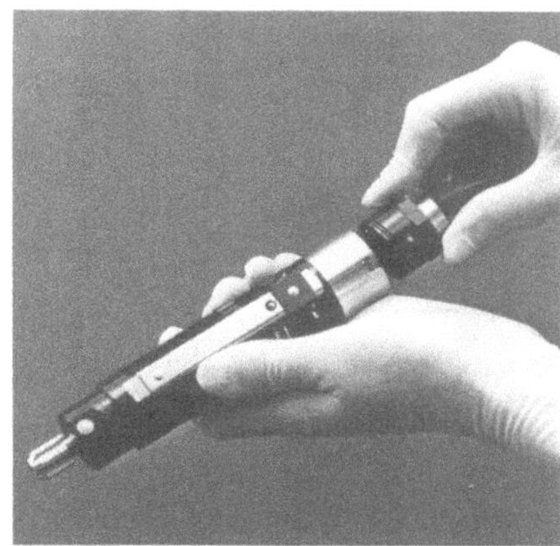

3. Attach motor to hose and regulator and run for several seconds.

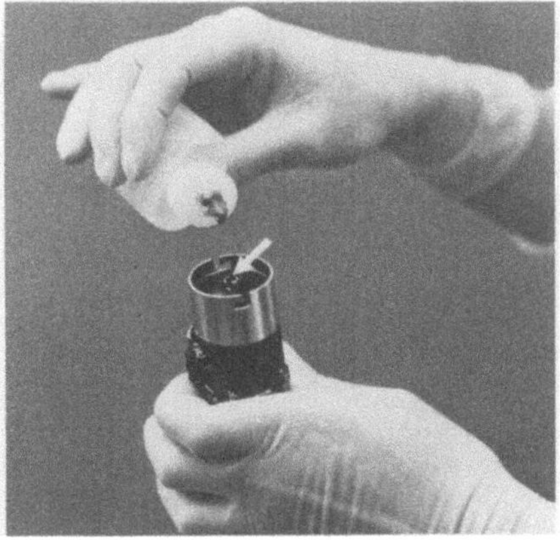

2. Place three drops of oil into the center standpipe.

CAUTION: Use oil supplied by manufacturer for these instruments.

HANDLING

Fine precision air instruments should be handled with same care as other surgical equipment. They should never be dropped, thrown or tumbled. They should not be banged against hard surfaces or other instruments. We recommend that as soon as the instruments have been cleaned and lubricated they should be returned to the autoclave box and stored until used again.

NOTE: The life of an air turbine or air motor is significantly increased if it is run for a few minutes each month.

Tips for Improving Care of Instruments

Probable Causes	*Corrections*
1. CORROSION	
Poor cleaning; residual soil.	Improve cleaning. Do not allow soil to dry on instruments.
Moisture.	Check sterilizer for drying efficiency. Store in a dry area.
Exposure to harsh chemicals: acids, iodine, sodium chloride, detergents, etc.	Do not expose instruments to these chemicals. If exposure occurs, rinse thoroughly as soon after contact as practicable.
Metallic deposition resulting from galvanic reaction with sterilizer components and other instrument metals.	Keep sterilizer chamber and trays clean. Use detergent recommended by manufacturer.
2. SPOTTING AND/OR STAINING	
Mineral deposits on instruments.	Wash with soft water and detergent with good wetting properties.
Laundry compound from instrument wrappers.	Check laundry procedures.
Residual detergent from cleaning solutions.	Rinse instruments thoroughly.
Mineral deposits from tap water rinse.	Use distilled water for final rinse.
3. STIFF HINGES OR JOINTS	
Corrosion or soil in joint.	Clean joint with a warm, weak (10%) solution of nitric acid or a lapping compound (Grit 180-Clover Mfg. Co., Norwalk, Conn.). Rinse instruments thoroughly.

Bibliography

1. Tips for Improving Sterilizing Techniques. Education and Research Departments of AMSCO (American Sterilizer Co.) Erie, Pa.

2. Sterilization Aids. Education and Research Departments of AMSCO (American Sterilizer Co.) Erie, Pa.

3. Perkins, John J.: Principles and Methods of Sterilization in Health Sciences. 2nd Edition, 1969. Charles C Thomas, Publisher, Springfield, Illinois.

SPECIFICATIONS

Length:
6½ inches (165 mm)
Diameter:
¾ inch (19 mm)
Weight:
6 ozs (170 gm)
Speed:
100,000 rpm at 100 psi (7 atm)
Throttle:
Built-in extension
Safety lock
Operating Pressure:
90-110 psi (7-8.5 atm)
Nitrogen Consumption:
6.0 cfm max. (170 liters min.)
Collet:
Mechanically activated collet by means of automatic bur release.
Exhaust:
Rearward (diffused)
10 ft. from surgical field.
Hose:
Antistatic dual hose at least 10.5 ft. long, swivels 360°.
Braking Time:
3 seconds max.

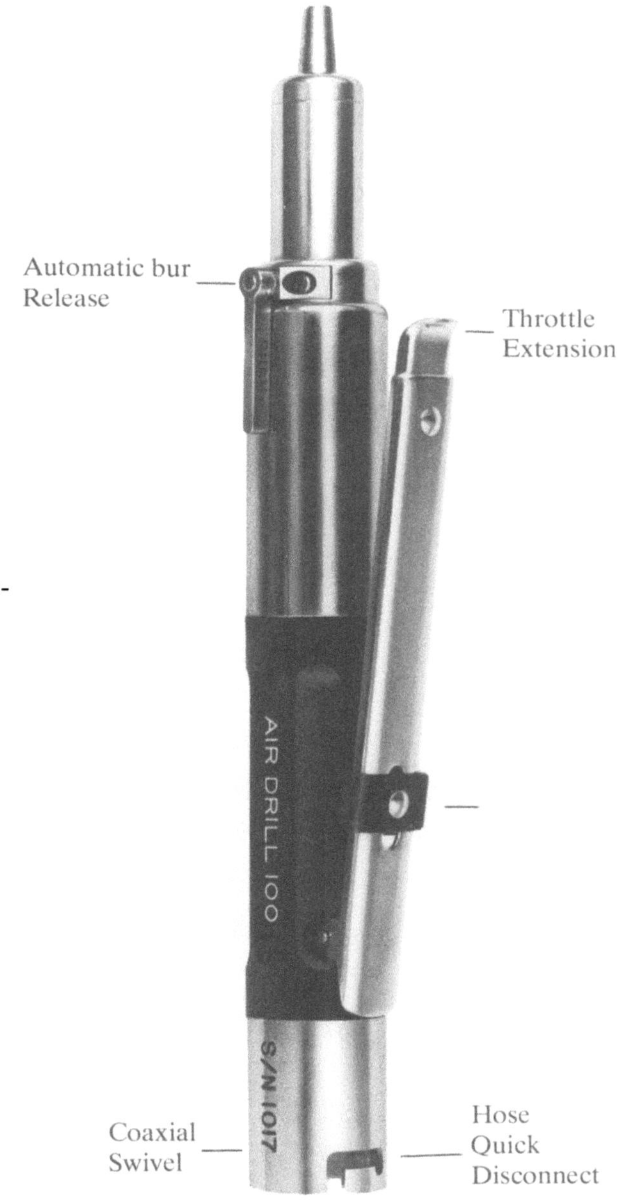

NOTE: Burs and attachments are interchangeable with all previous air drills.

Air Drill 100 Attachments

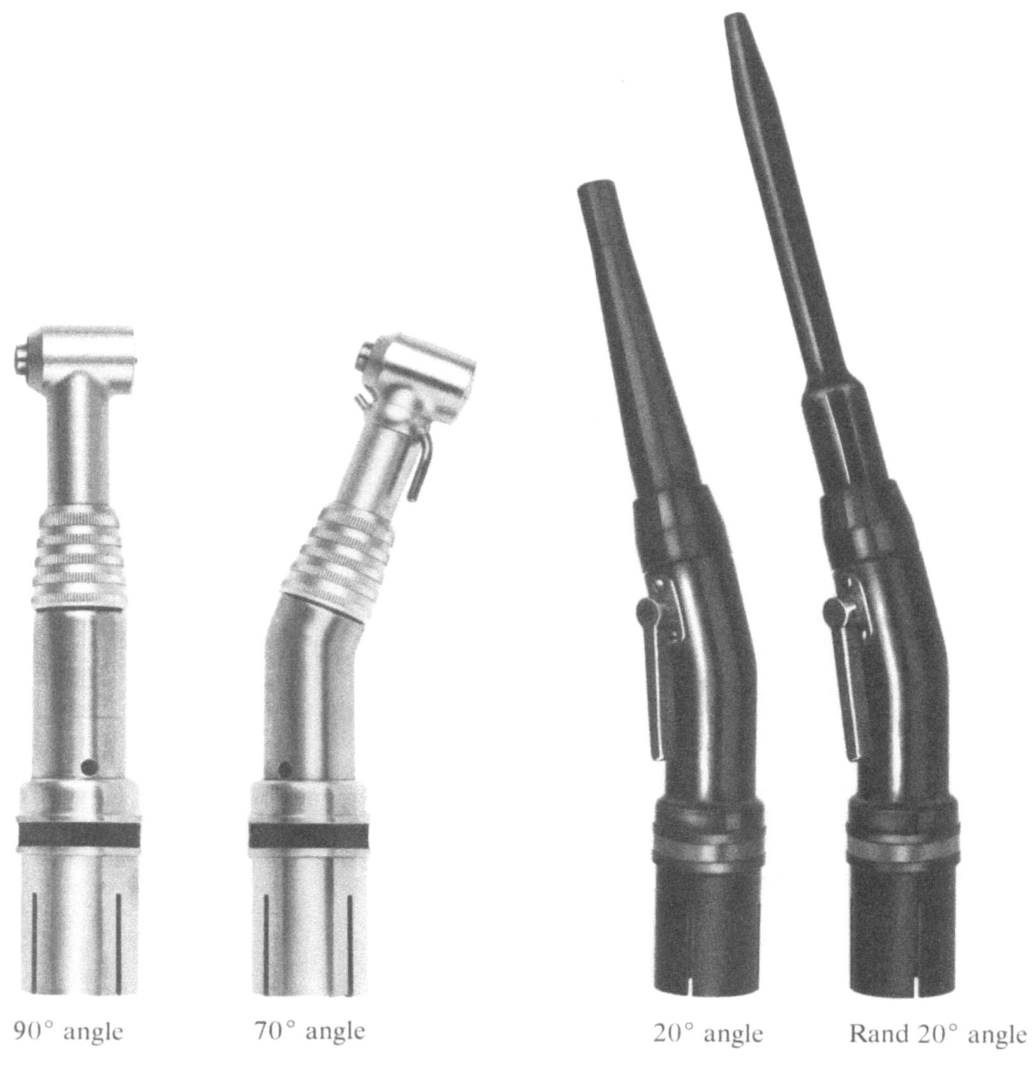

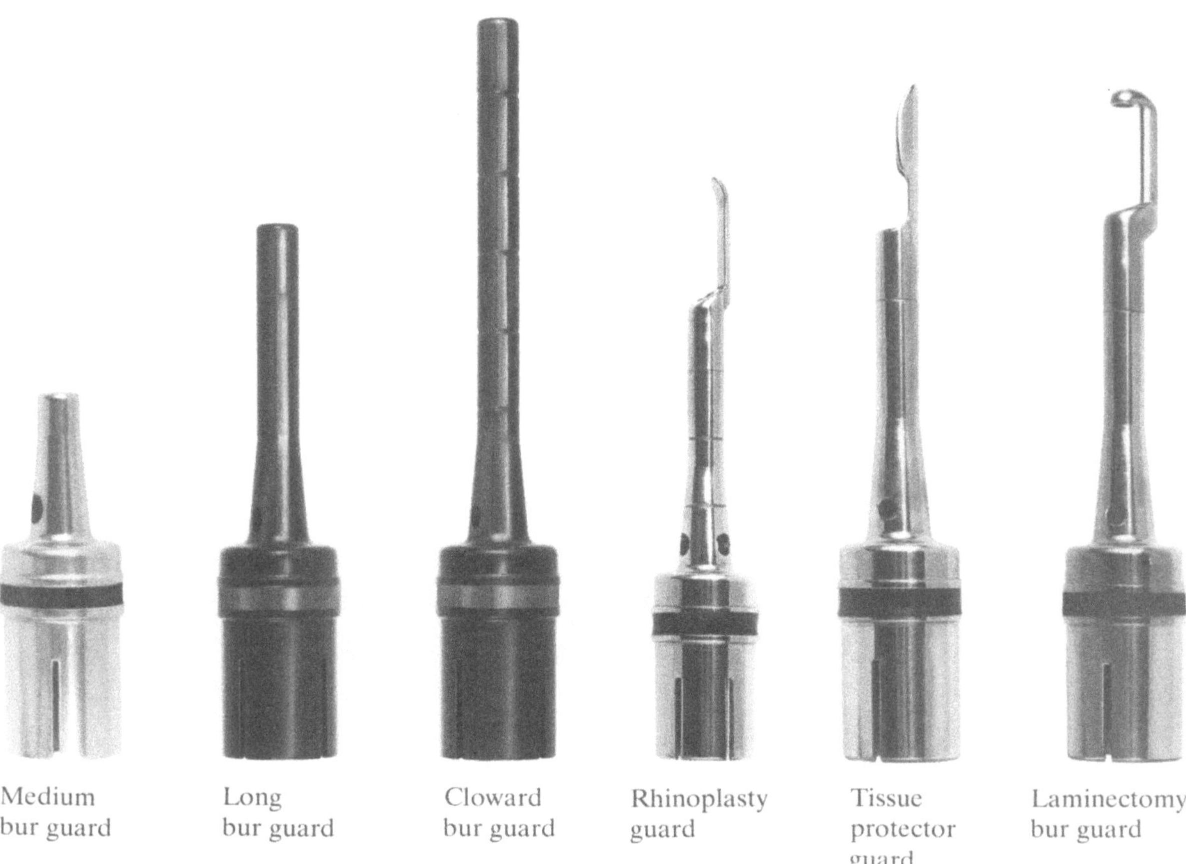

Medium bur guard

Long bur guard

Cloward bur guard

Rhinoplasty guard

Tissue protector guard

Laminectomy bur guard

Air Drill 100 Accessories

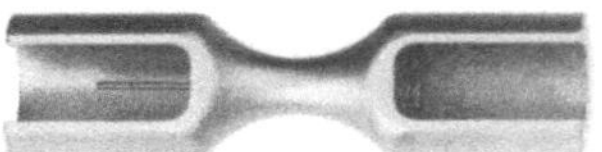

Bur changer

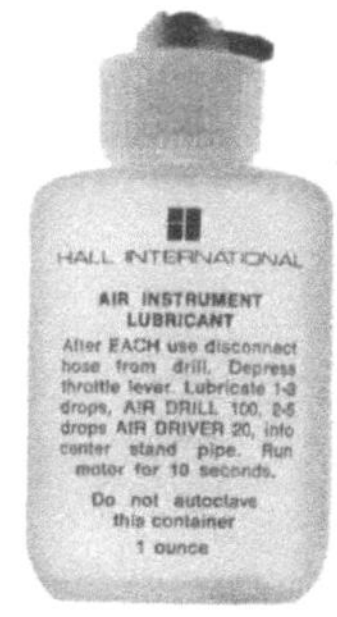

Lubricant

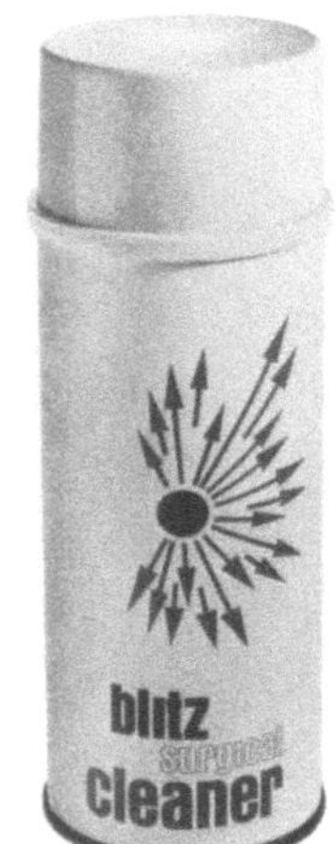

Blitz cleaner

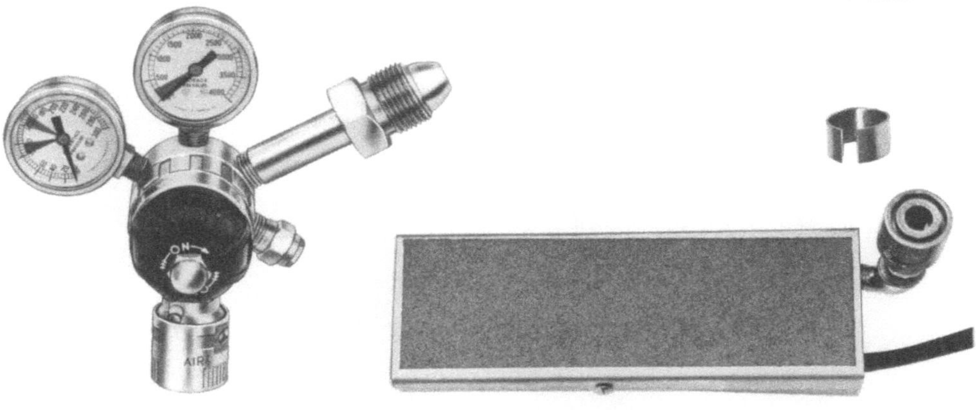

Nitrogen regulator   Foot control and throttle retainer

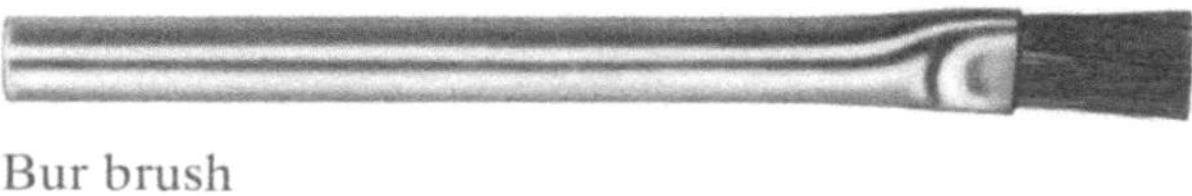

Bur brush

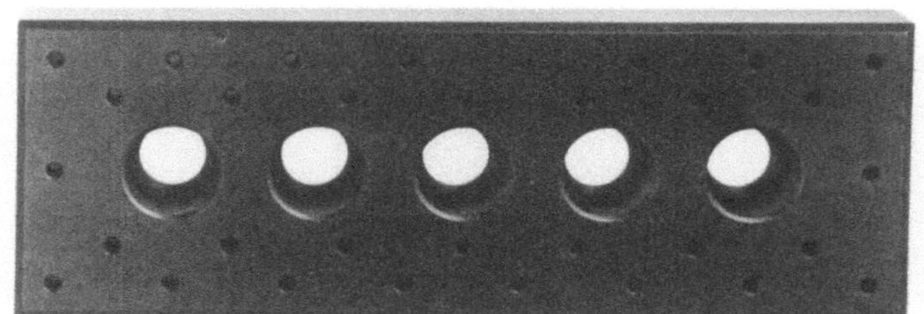

Bur and attachment rack

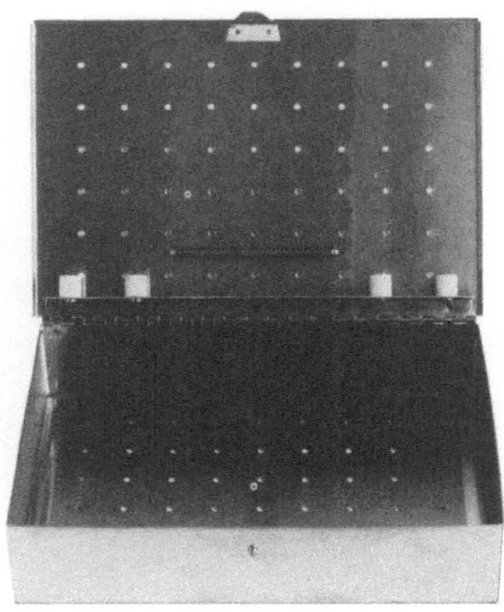

Autoclave case

Assembly of the Air Drill 100

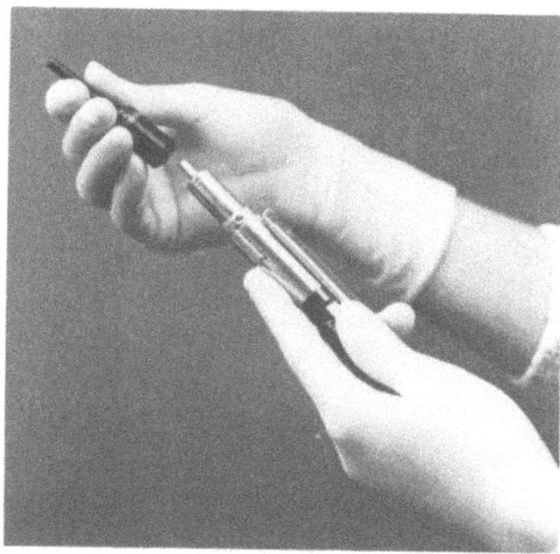

1. INSTRUMENT SAFETY
   SLIDE

   Pull safety lock back to release throttle; motor will not run. Assemble appropriate attachment or bur guard and bur.

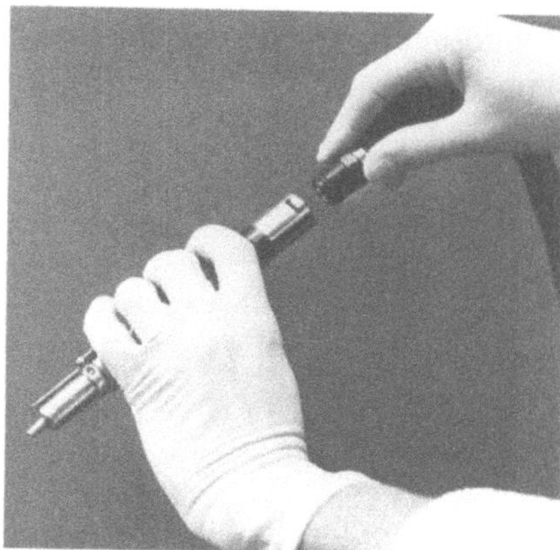

1. INSTRUMENT-HOSE
   DISCONNECT

   Pull safety lock back to release throttle, align pin and hole.

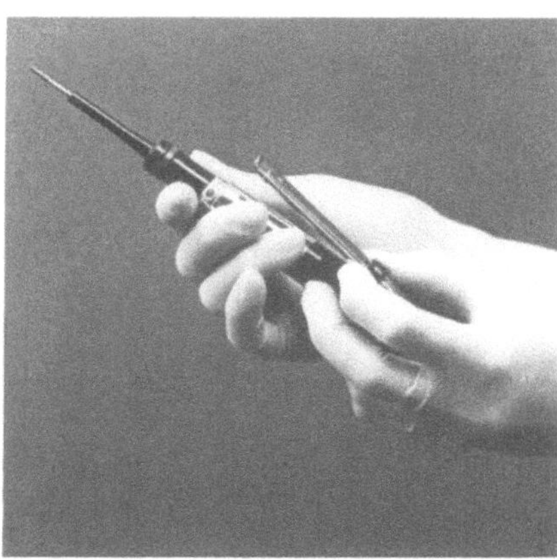

2. Lift throttle and push safety lock up. Press throttle; motor will run.

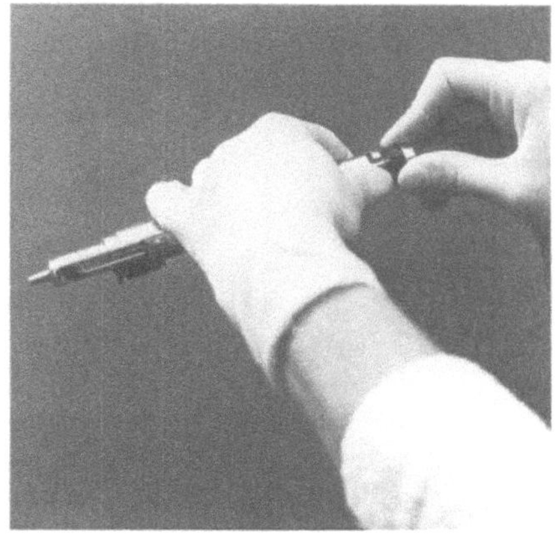

2. Press together. Grasp the end of the instrument to steady the swivel. Twist clockwise to lock.

THE INSTRUMENT-HOSE DISCONNECT ALLOWS:

A. Independent sterilization of hose and instrument.
B. Attachments can be assembled with the hose disconnected.
C. With an additional sterile hose, sterilization time between operative procedures can be significantly reduced.
D. Hose repairs can be made independently of the handpiece.

NOTE: The air drill and attachments are interchangeable with all previous air drills.

Burs*

There are many different types of burs varying in size, shape and cutting edge. The round and oval burs are for bone sculpting. The straight side-cutting burs are for bone resection.

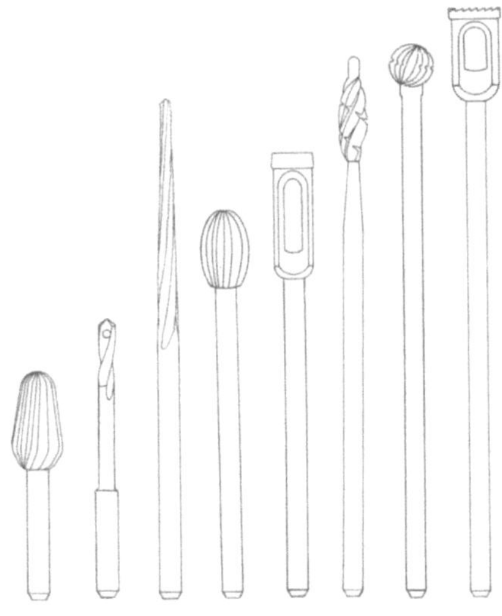

HIGH-SPEED STEEL BURS

The high-speed steel burs have sharp cutting edges, however, after one or two operations and autoclavings they become blunt. Autoclaving will not rust the burs and the only way to ensure sharpness is to use a new bur every time. High-speed steel burs are excellent for gross bone removal and bone sculpting. Use them in widely exposed areas as all soft tissue must be retracted to prevent entanglement with the burs.

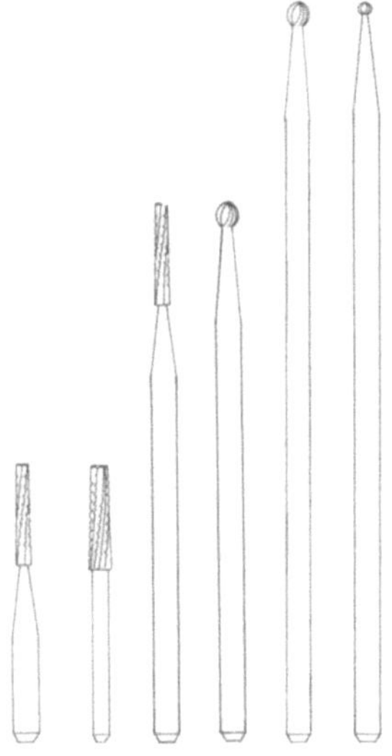

CARBIDE-TIP BURS

A completely different combination of metals makes up a carbide bur. Carbide is sharp and maintains its cutting edge for a longer time than a high-speed steel bur. Two disadvantages of carbide burs are brittleness of the metal and rusting due to autoclaving. Carbide burs sold by Hall International have stainless steel shanks and carbide tips. The shank minimizes breakage and rusting, while the carbide tip maintains the sharp cutting edge. The sharp edge is good for cutting tooth enamel and dense cortical bone. The (01-10) burs are less likely to lacerate soft tissue when working on dense cortical bone in confined areas.

---

* All burs are numbered according to the Hall International catalog.

DIAMOND BURS

Diamond burs are manufactured with a high-speed steel shank and a bur tip dipped in industrial diamond. These burs are not good for sculpting dense cortical bone, but because of their abrasive quality, they can be used next to vital nerves and blood vessels without danger of tissue laceration. The burs clog easily and must be cleaned periodically throughout the procedure to obtain maximum cutting performance. A diamond bur is an abrasive rather than a cutting bur.

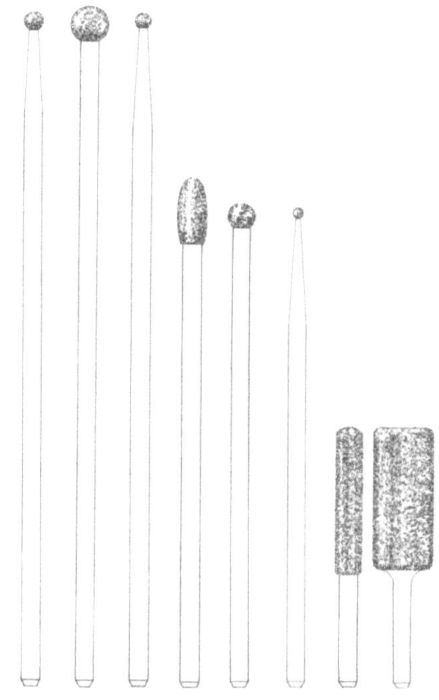

MAINTENANCE

All burs should be inspected carefully for shaft straightness and sharp cutting edge before autoclaving. A bent bur will whip and may snap during surgery.

It is possible to have bent bur shanks that are barely perceptible. All burs should be checked by placing each bur in the drill without a guard and spinning it manually.

Use the appropriate bur guard with the bur. A long bur with a medium bur guard may snap off during the procedure. Do not use the air drill without a bur guard.

A dull bur will create the impression of a loss of torque in the air drill.

Clean the burs during surgery with the autoclavable bur brush.

No bur should be used for more than three operations. Ideally the surgeon should have a new bur for each procedure.

Bur Guard and Bur Assembly

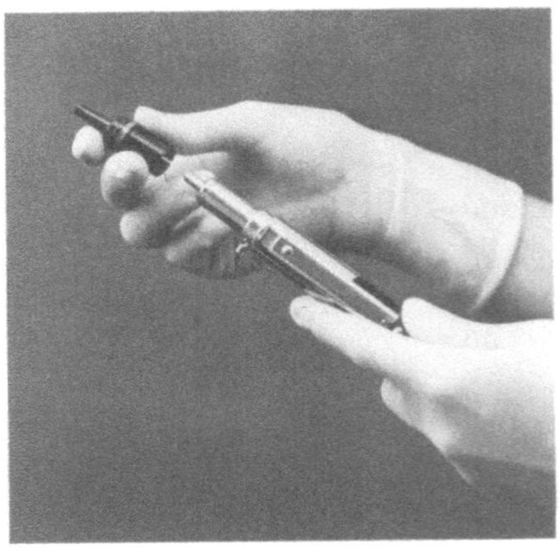

1. Place the bur guard over the drill shoulder. Completely seat.

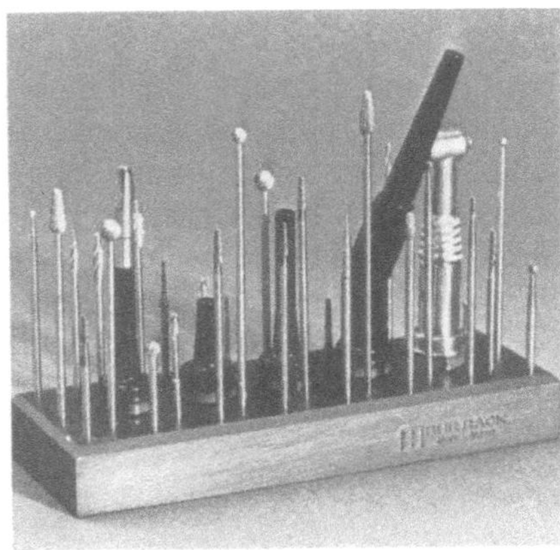

4. Keep burs and guards in the bur and attachment rack during surgery.

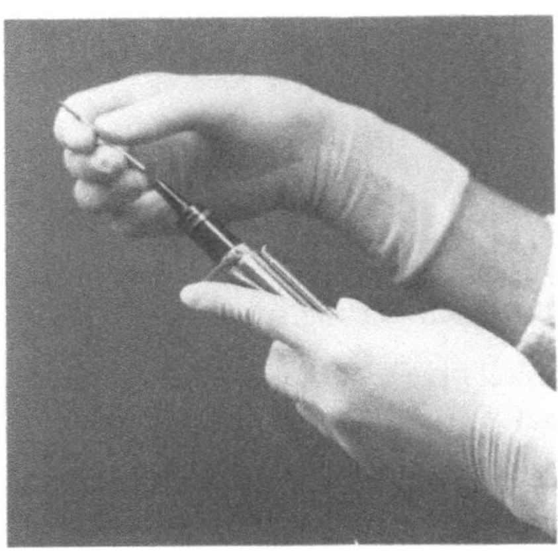

2. Push the release lever forward 90° and insert bur into the collet.

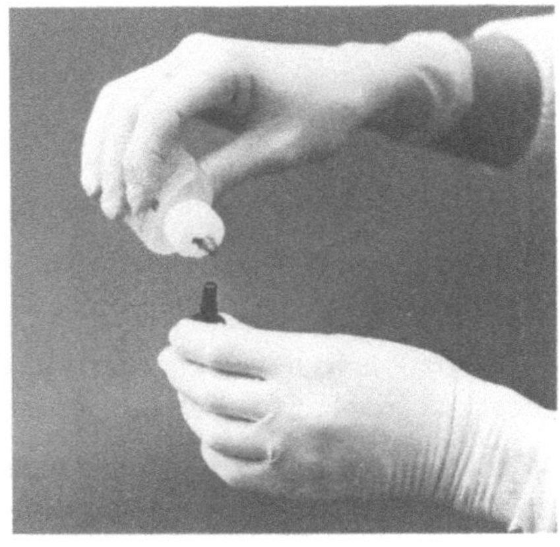

MAINTENANCE: Lubricate the bearing in the tip of all bur guards with one drop of lubricant.

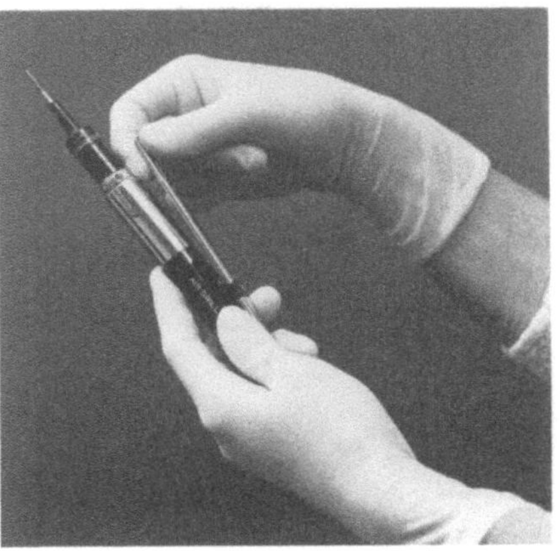

3. Lock the bur securely by returning lever flush against the drill. Reverse these steps to release burs.

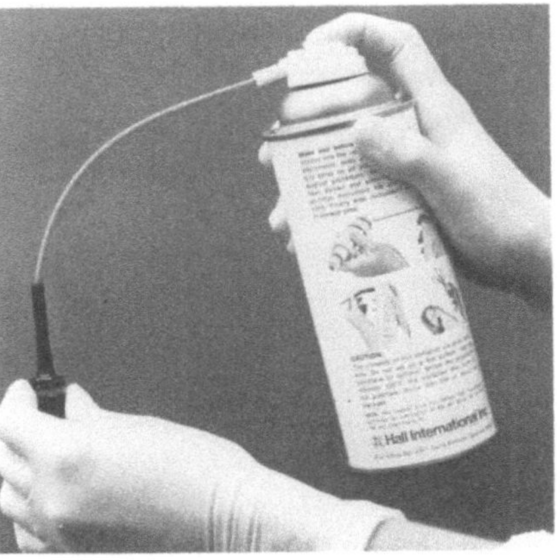

Flush the guard with blitz spray after cleaning to remove debris and to lubricate internal parts.

Specific Bur Guards and Bur Assembly

The laminectomy and tissue protector guard must be assembled in the following manner:

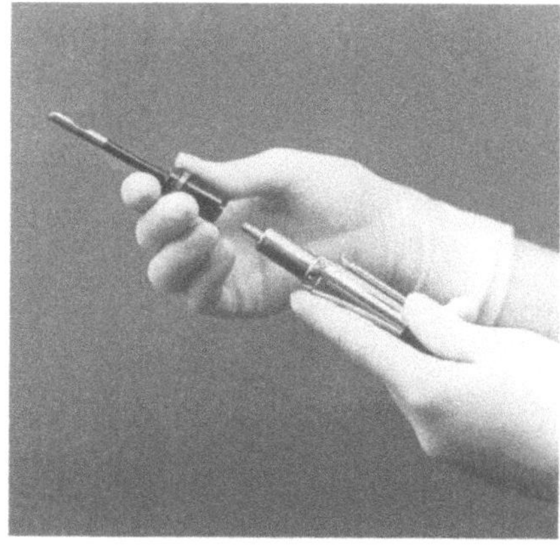

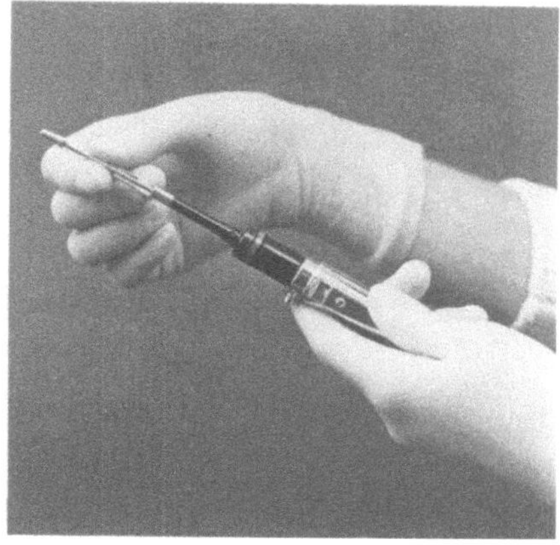

1. With safety lock off, place guard over drill and seat bur firmly.

2. Push bur release lever forward 90° and insert bur deep into collet. Return lever flush against drill.

TISSUE PROTECTOR BUR GUARD: The protective shield over the 19 long steel bur is ideal for surgical techniques where cortical bone must be removed while overlying soft tissue is preserved. Lubricate the tip of the bur guard after use.

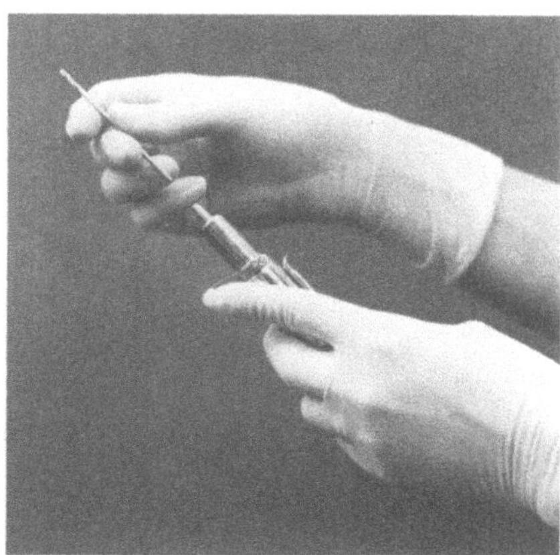

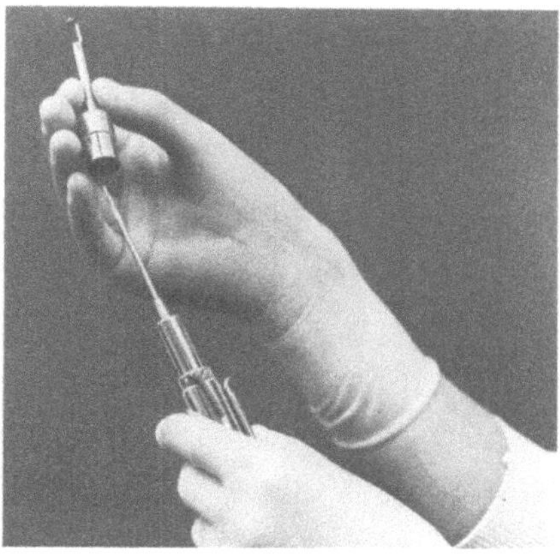

1. Insert the 03 long steel bur into the collet while the bur release lever is at 90°.

2. Slip attachment over bur and drill shoulder. Seat the bur into the tip of the attachment.

LAMINECTOMY BUR GUARD: The laminectomy bur guard will only accept the 03 long steel bur. The side-cutting bur rests in the tip of the protective foot. During excising of laminae, the foot protects the dura from the rotating bur.

Attachment and Bur Assembly

20° Angle Attachment (Long burs only) and Rand 20° Angle Attachment (Extra long burs only)

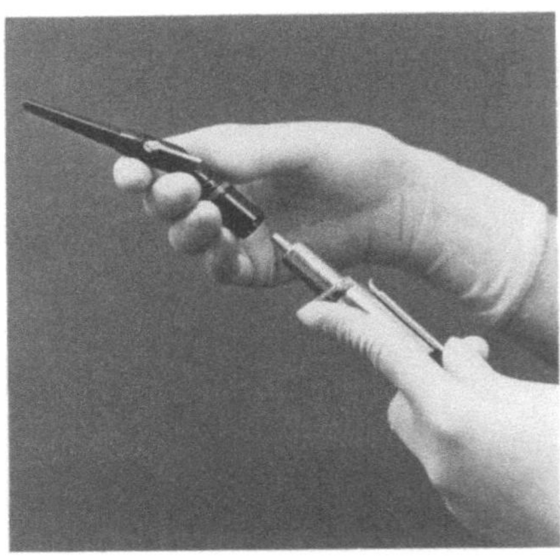

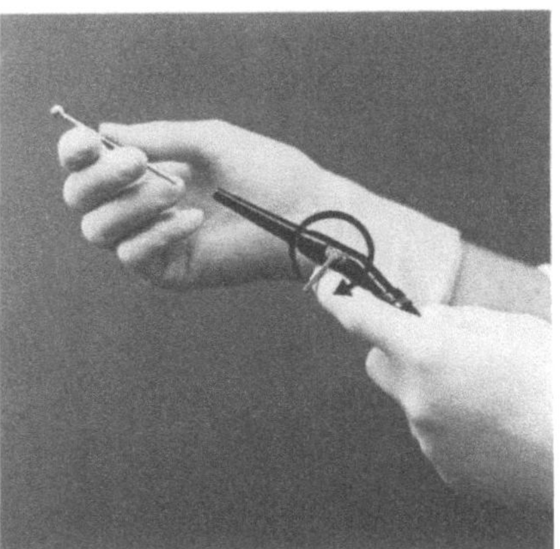

ASSEMBLY:

1. Pull back throttle safety lock. Press release lever forward 90° and hold. Seat attachment over drill shoulder.

3. Using a long bur only for 20° angle, or an extra long bur for the Rand 20° angle, press release lever on attachment 90° to insert or remove bur. If the bur release is pressed further than 90°, or while returning lever strong resistance is encountered, do not continue. Push lever forward and round 180° to lock bur.

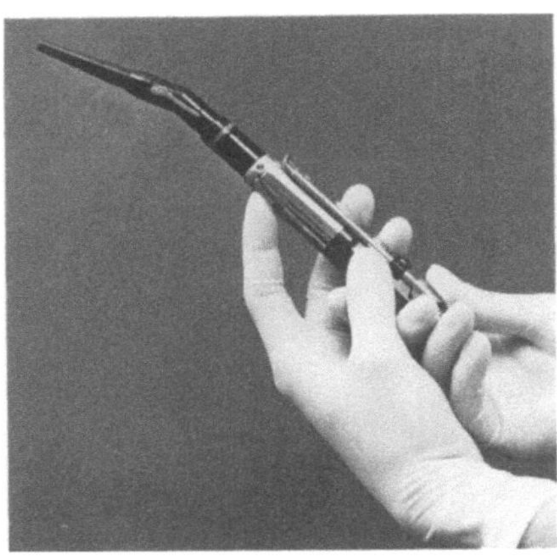

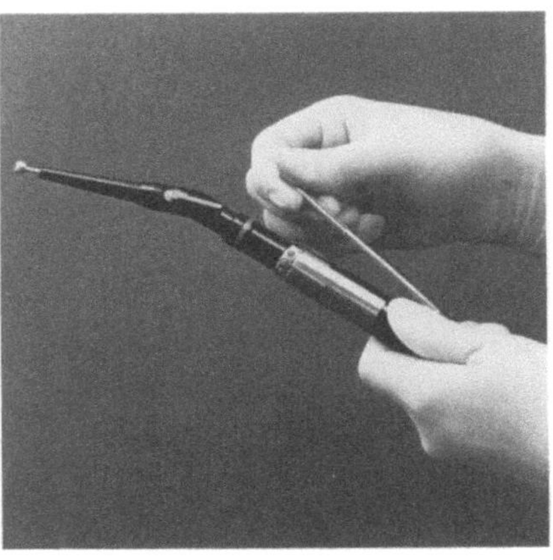

2. Return lever flush against drill to lock attachment.

4. Pull out throttle extension lever for added convenience and control.

MAINTENANCE:

1. Disassemble attachment and bur. Scrub with soft brush and mild detergent. Rinse under running faucet. Wipe dry.

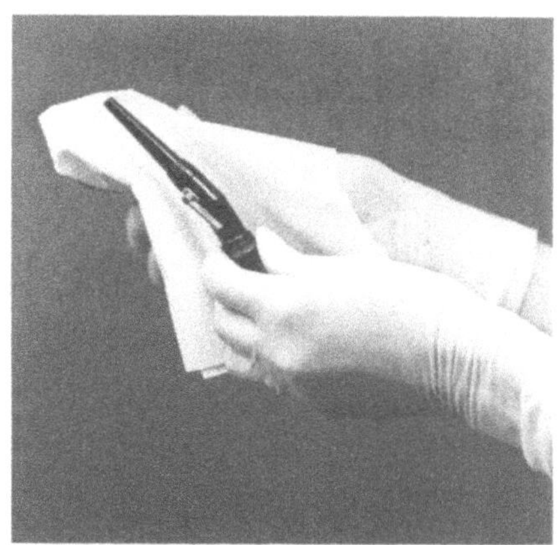

2. Flush internal parts with blitz cleaner. Shake off excess cleaner and wipe dry with a lint-free cloth.

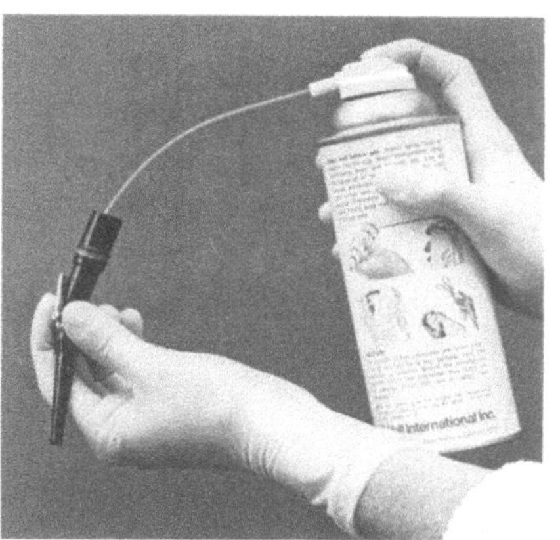

3. Lubricate the bearing at the end of the attachments with one drop of oil.

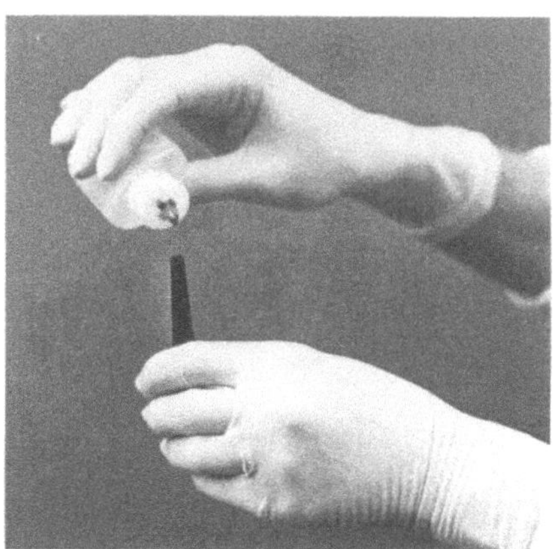

90° Angle Attachment (short burs only)

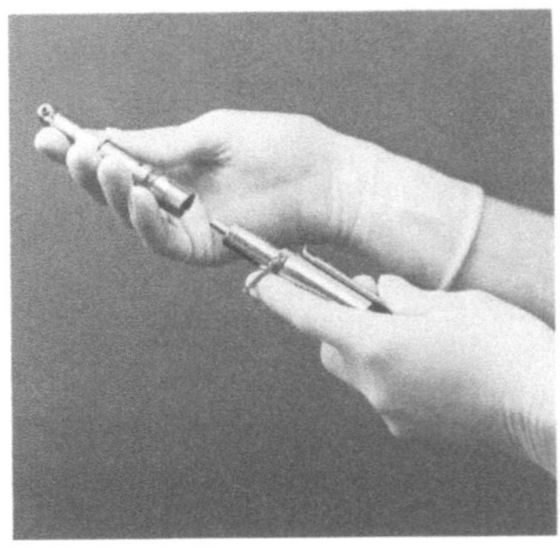

ASSEMBLY:

1. Push bur release lever forward 90°
   to assemble attachment. Completely seat.

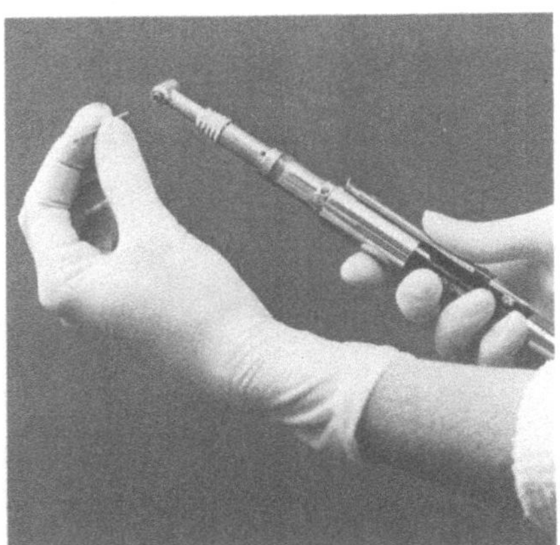

3. Place bur into collet.

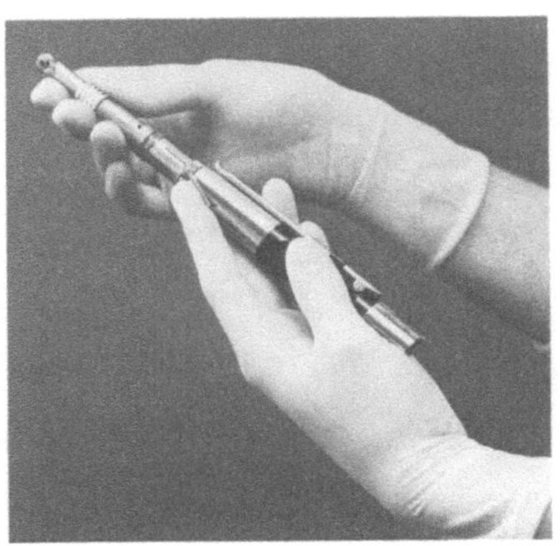

2. Return lever flush against drill to
   lock attachment.

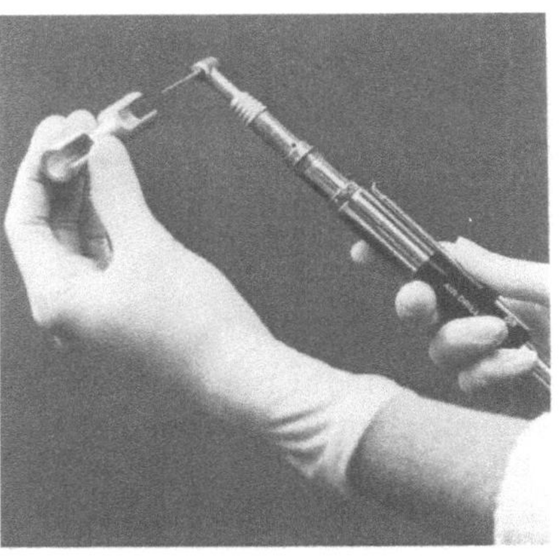

4. Slide hollow side of bur changer
   over bur. Press the bur firmly into
   place.

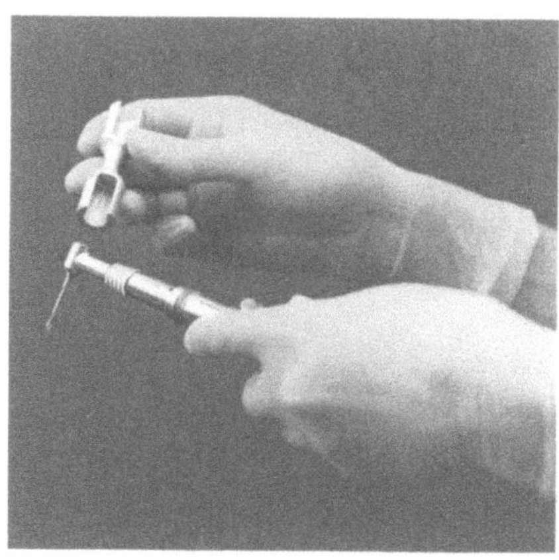

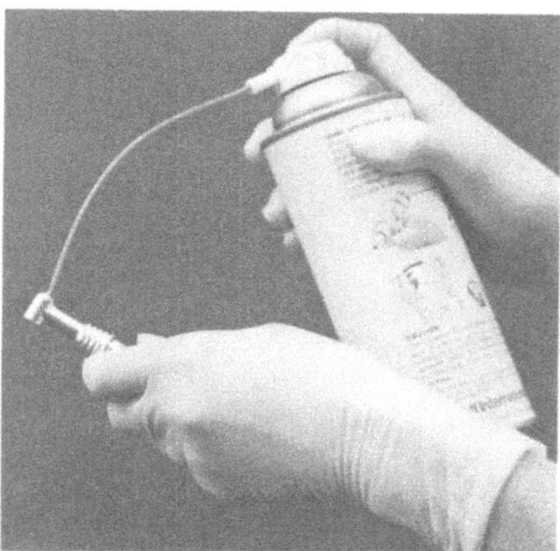

DISASSEMBLY:

1. To remove bur, insert pin of bur changer into hole in attachment head.

MAINTENANCE:

1. After cleaning flush bur hole and head housing with blitz spray.

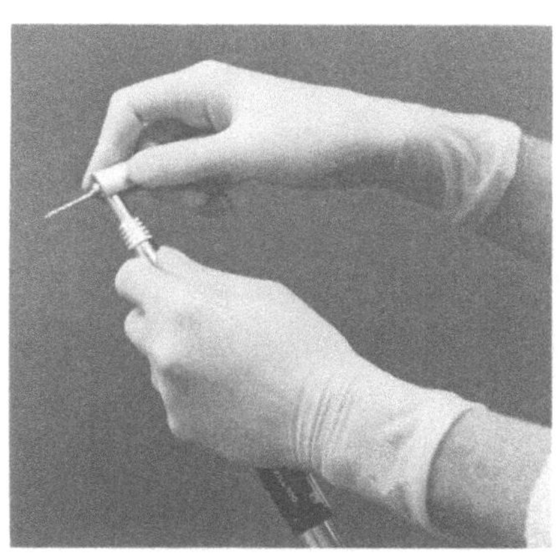

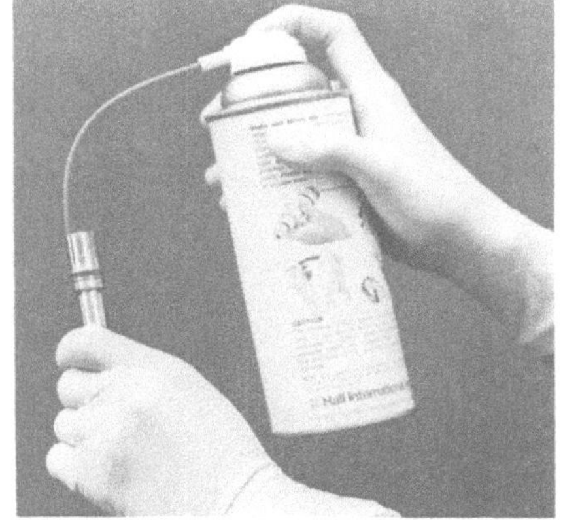

2. Press firmly to release bur.

2. Flush attachment end with the same spray. Wipe dry.

NOTE: If blitz spray is not available, use the regular lubricant used for the motor to lubricate the attachment.

3. Push release lever forward to remove attachment.

Contra 70° Angle Attachment (Friction grip [F. G.] dental burs only)

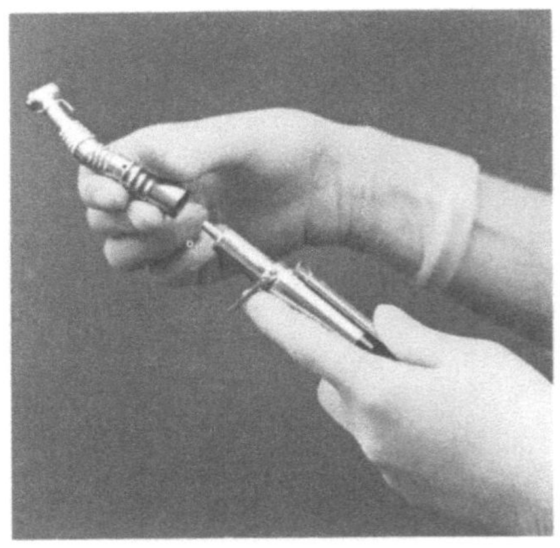

ASSEMBLY:

1. Push bur release lever forward 90° to assemble attachment. Completely seat.

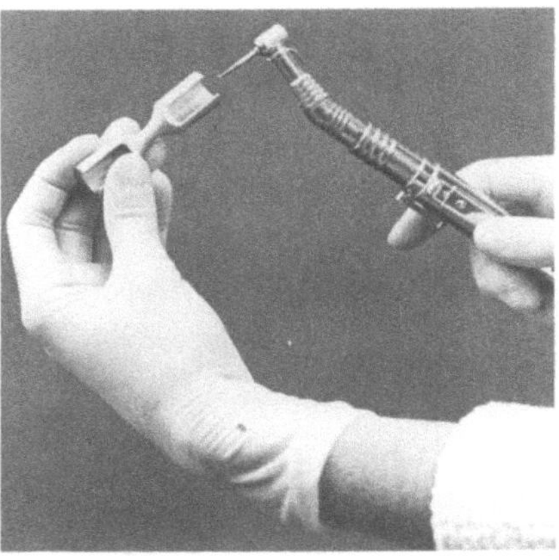

3. Place bur into collet. Slide hollow side of bur changer over bur.

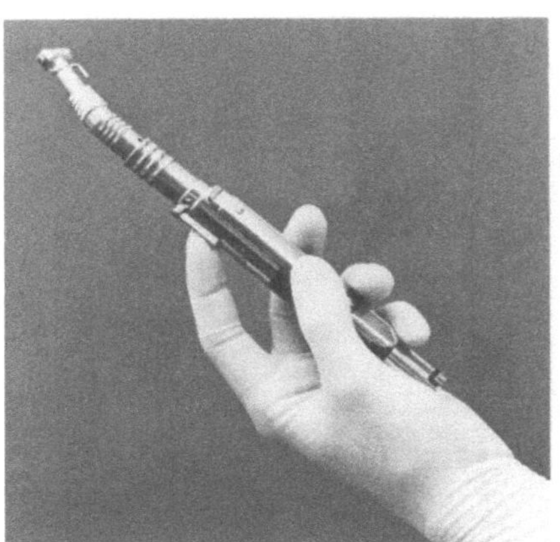

2. Return lever flush against drill to lock attachment.

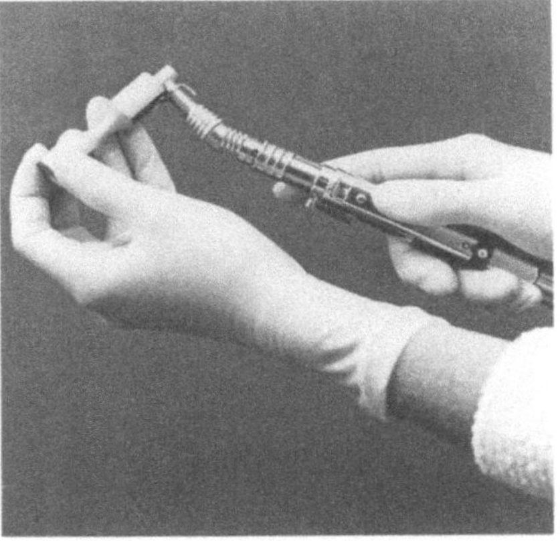

4. Press the bur firmly into place.

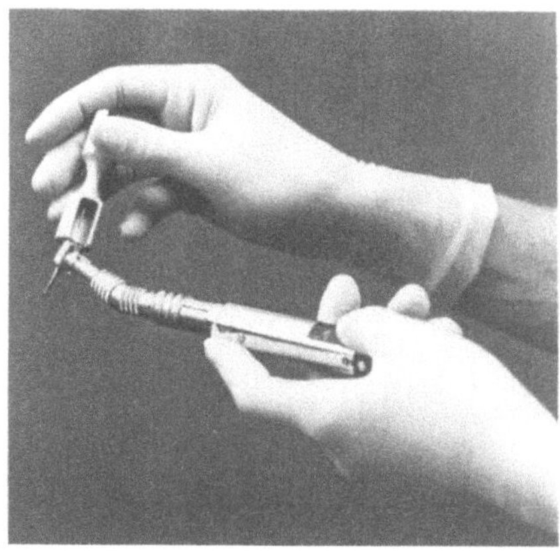

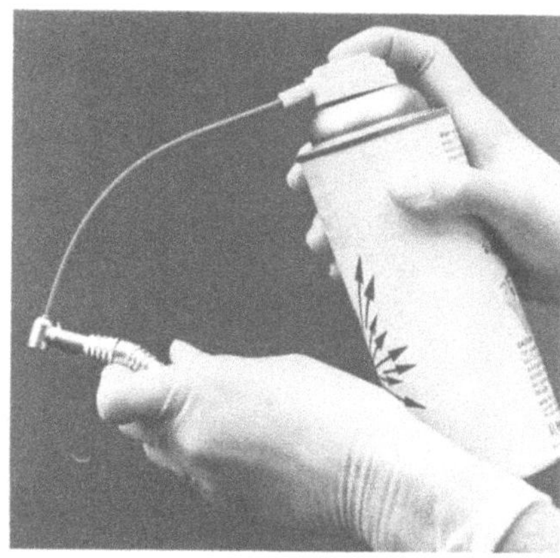

DISASSEMBLY:

1. To remove bur insert pin of bur changer into hole in attachment head.

MAINTENANCE:

1. After cleaning, flush bur hole and head housing with blitz spray.

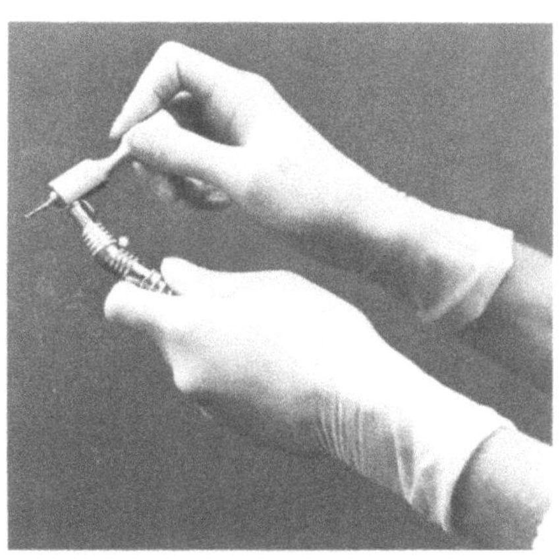

2. Press firmly to release bur.

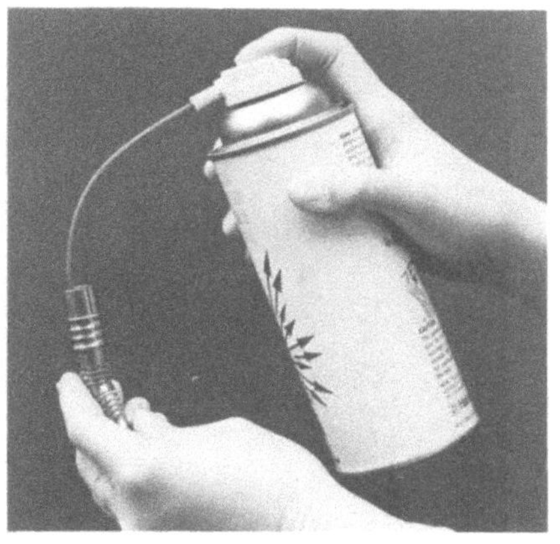

2. Flush attachment end with the same spray. Wipe dry.

NOTE: If blitz spray is not available use the regular lubricant used for the motor to lubricate the attachment.

3. Push release lever forward to remove attachment.

Air Driver II Accessories

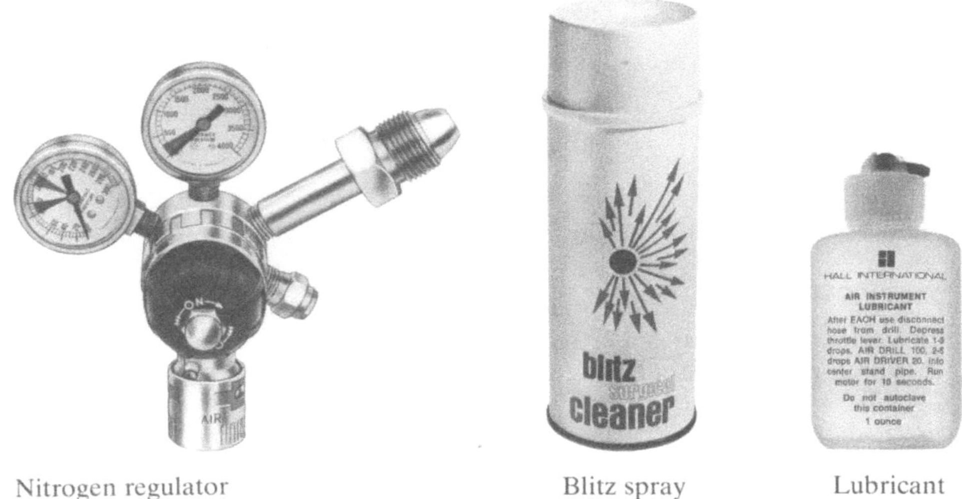

Nitrogen regulator   Blitz spray   Lubricant

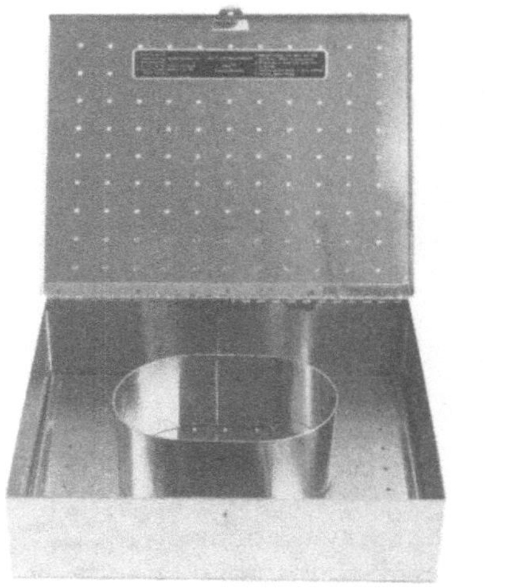

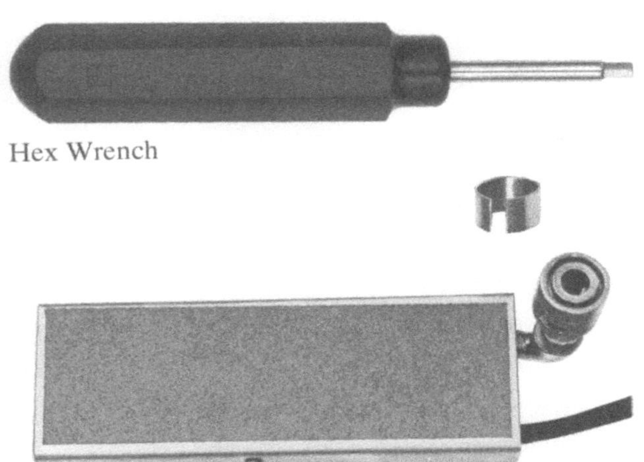

Hex Wrench

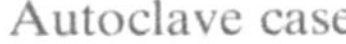

Autoclave case   Foot control and throttle retainer

SPECIFICATIONS

Length:
6 inches (152 mm)
Diameter:
$1\frac{1}{8}$ inches (27 mm)
Weight:
11 ozs (312 gm)
Speed:
20,000 rpm at 100 psi (7 atm)
Throttle:
Built-in extension, safety lock and variable control.
Operating Pressure:
90-110 psi (7 atm-8.5 atm)
Nitrogen Consumption:
10 cfm (280 liters min.)
Exhaust:
Rearward (diffused) 10 ft from surgical field.
Hose:
Antistatic dual disconnect hose. At least 10 ft long, swivels 360°.
Braking Time:
1 second max.

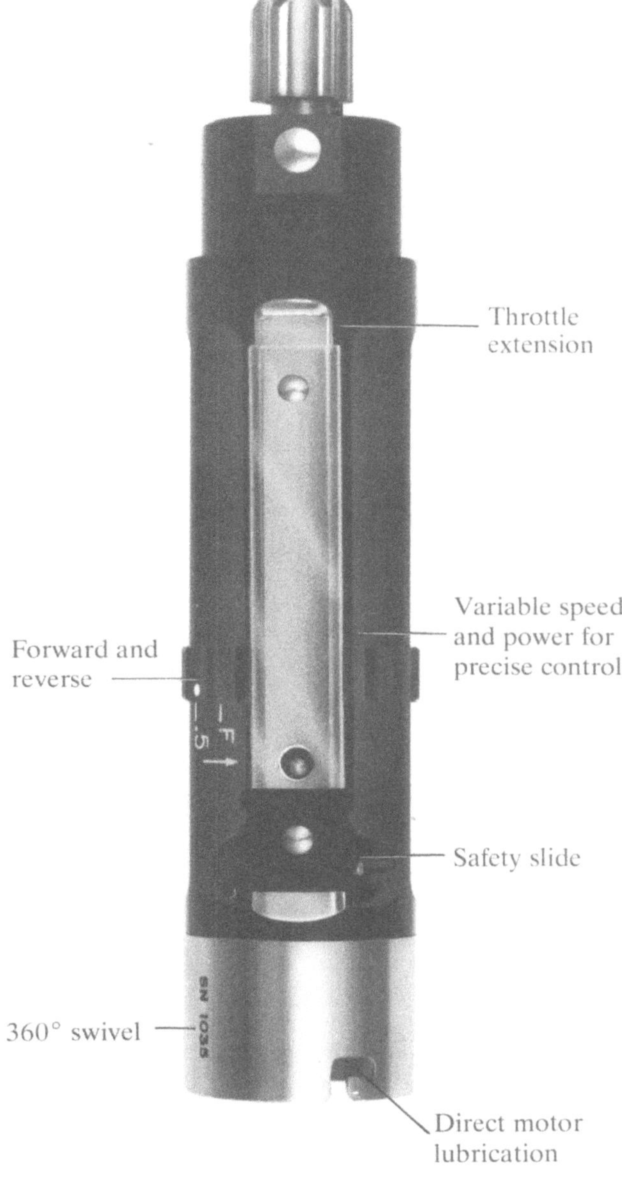

NOTE: This motor drives any attachments designed for previous Hall air motors with the hex drive-shaft.

RECIPROCATING SAW ATTACHMENT
shown actual size

This saw operates at 20,000 reciprocations per minute at full-speed. The unit is completely sealed and requires no lubrication. A set-screw secures the saws, hooks, extractors and impactor. The right-angled head gives an unobstructed view.

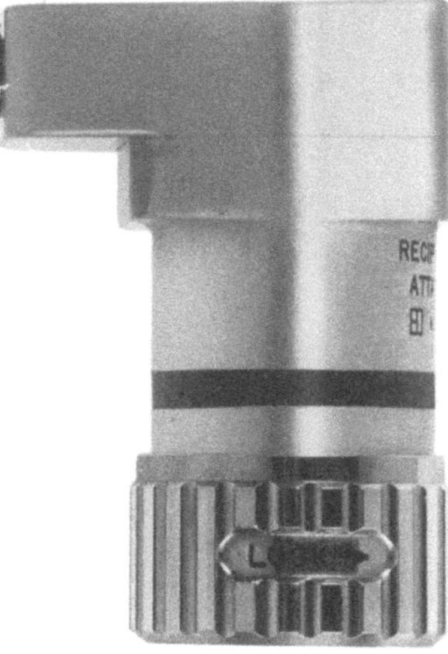

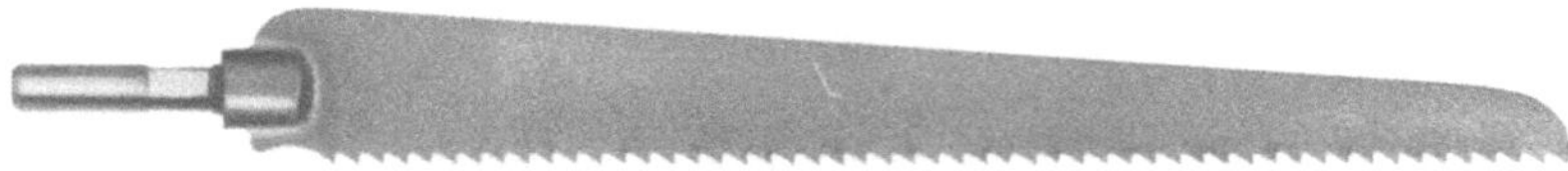

Regular saw blade

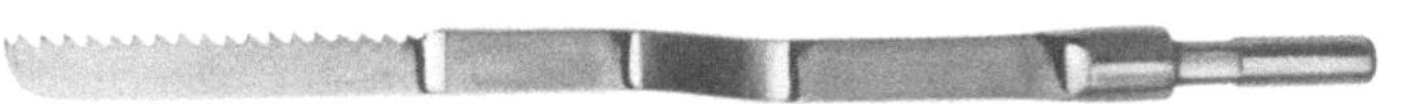

Heavy duty saw blade

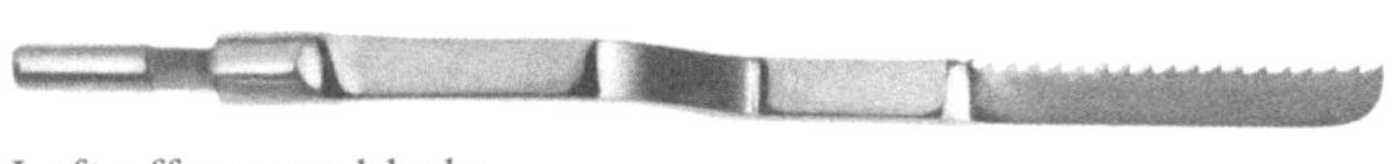

Right offset saw blade

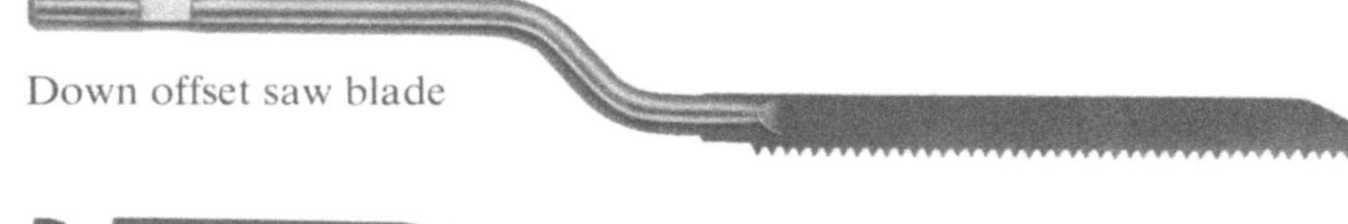

Left offset saw blade

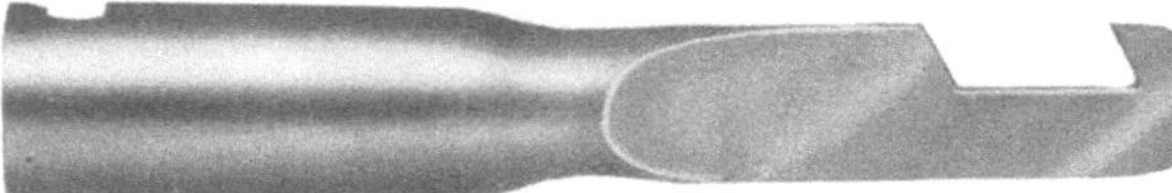

Down offset saw blade

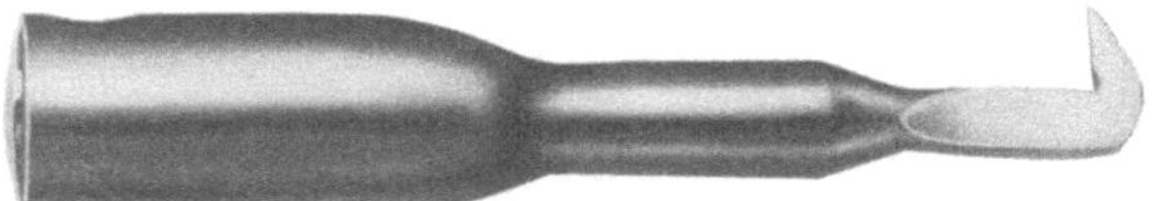

Küntscher nail extractor, large

Küntscher nail extractor, small

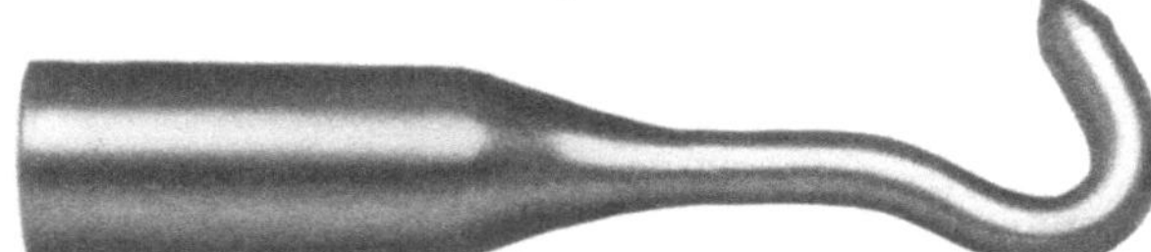

Moore prosthesis extractor

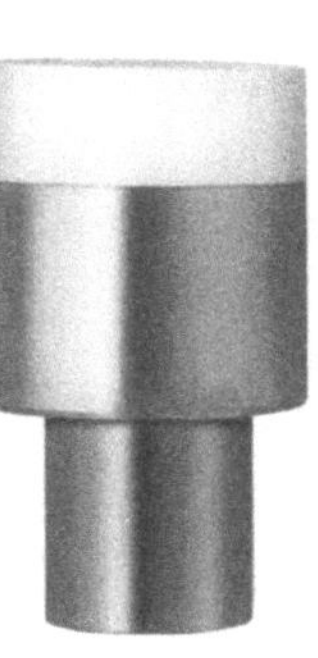

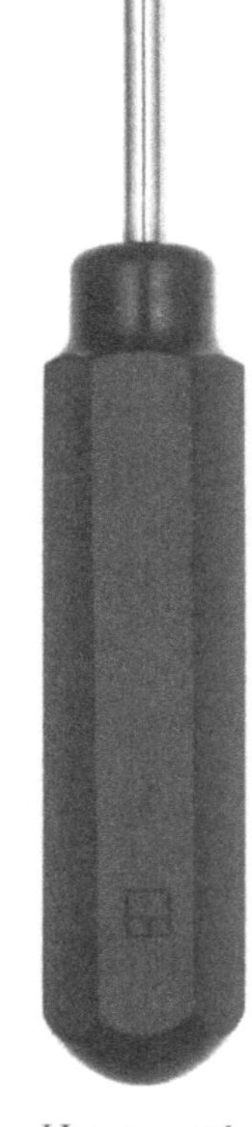

Head impactor   Hex wrench

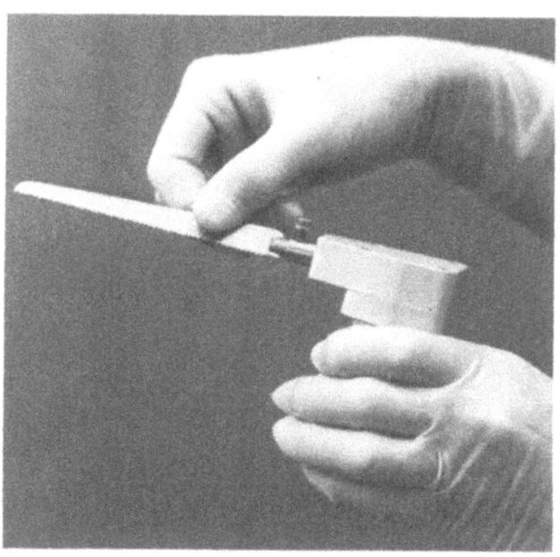

BLADE ASSEMBLY:
1. Loosen hex nut and insert blade with cutting edge at the correct angle.

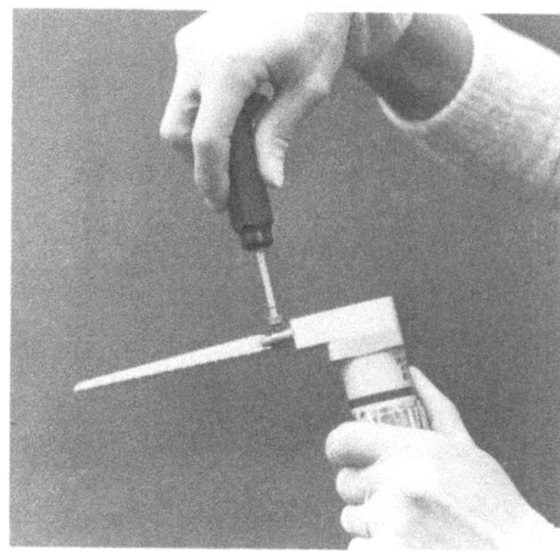

2. Tighten blade securely with hex wrench.

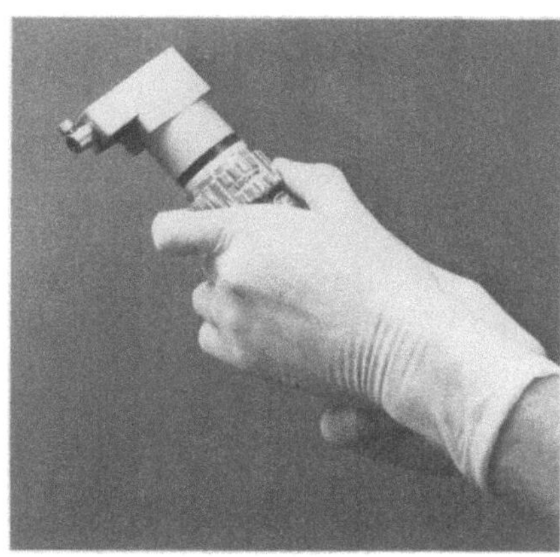

ATTACHMENT ASSEMBLY:
1. Seat attachment over air driver, engage hex drive-shaft. Turn lock-ring to secure.

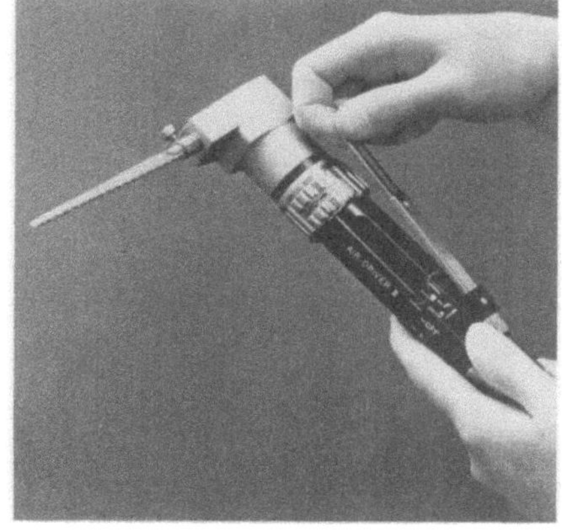

2. Use extension handle and run at full speed for maximum cutting efficiency.

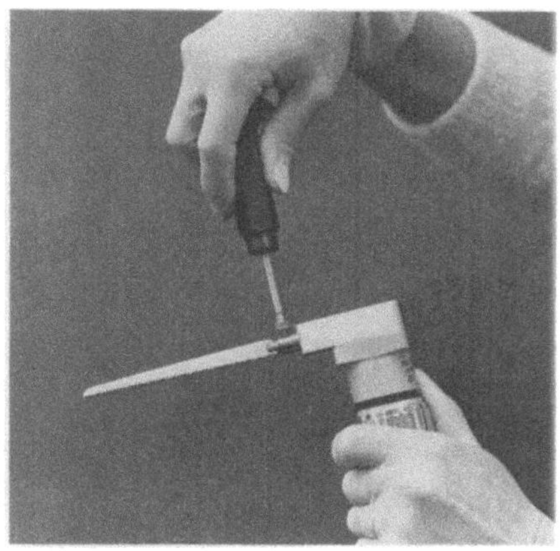

MAINTENANCE:
1. Disassemble blades before cleaning and sterilization. Do not remove set-screw completely.

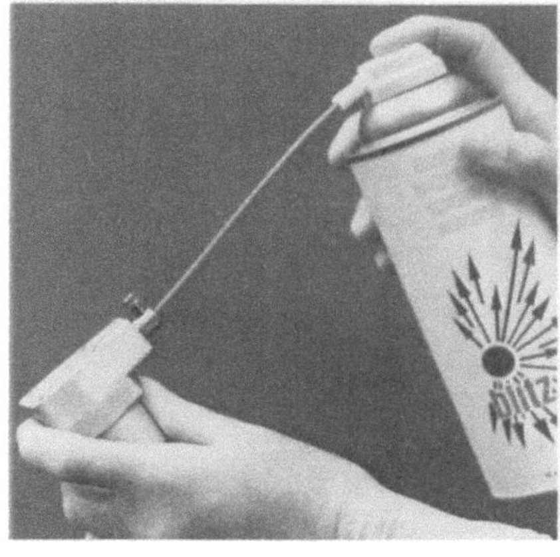

2. Clean attachment end thoroughly. This unit requires no lubrication.

OSCILLATING SAW ATTACHMENT
shown actual size

At full speed the saw moves at 20,000 oscillations per minute within a quarter-inch arc. This unit is completely sealed and requires no lubrication. The self-retaining set-screw is for securing the blades and gouges.

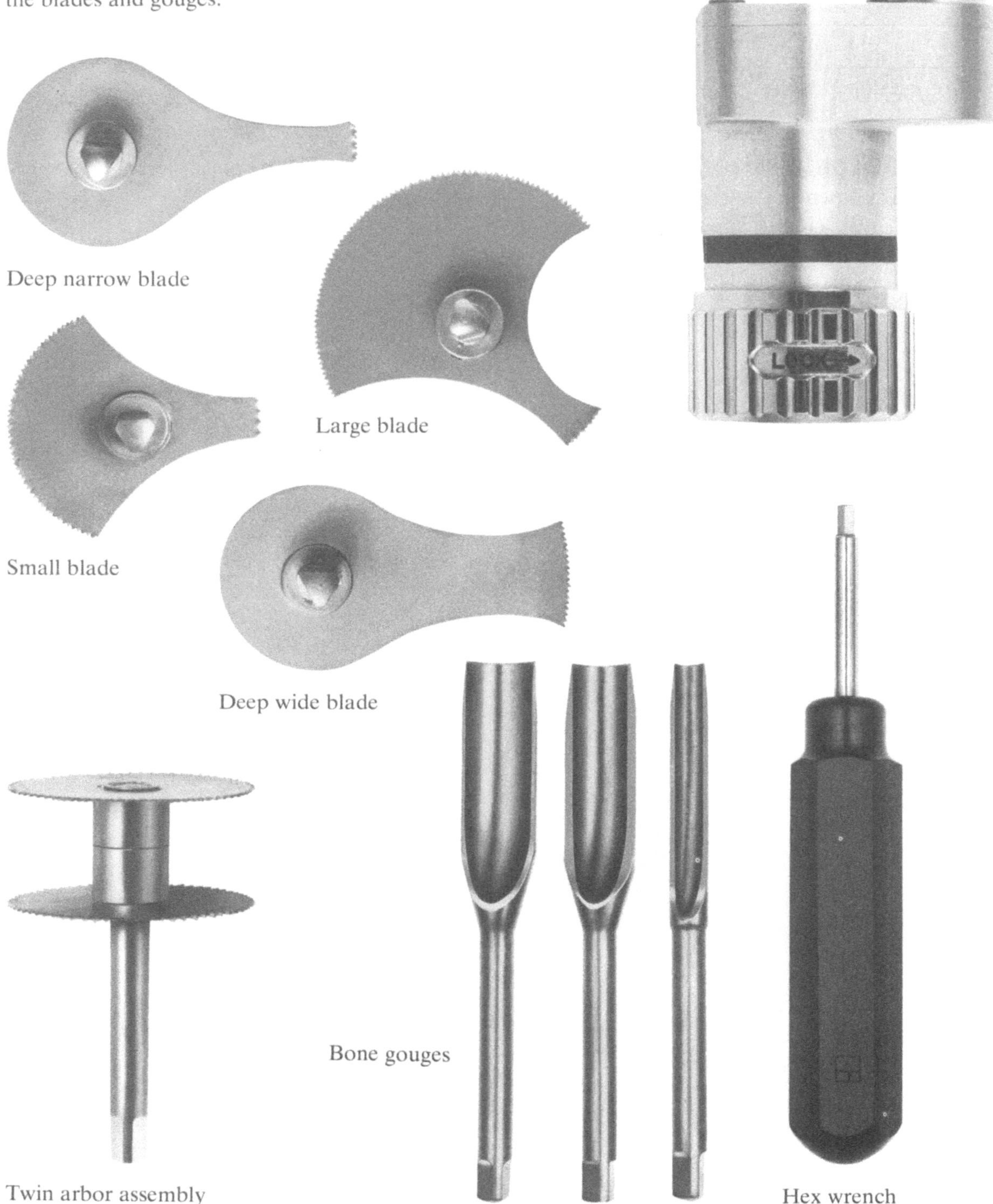

Deep narrow blade

Large blade

Small blade

Deep wide blade

Twin arbor assembly

Bone gouges

Hex wrench

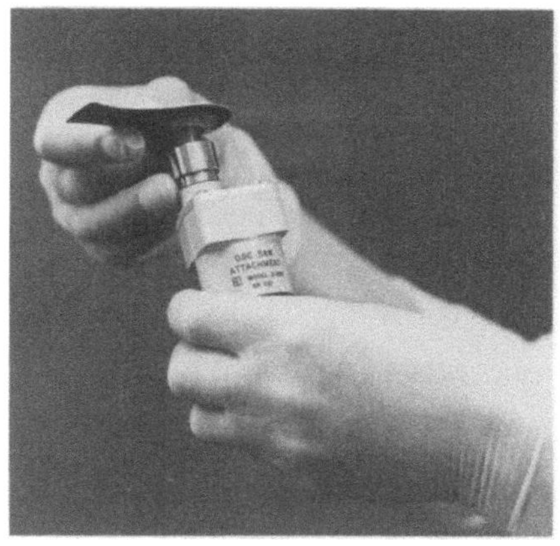

BLADE ASSEMBLY:
1. Loosen set-screw to insert triangular arbor. Set blade at the required angle.

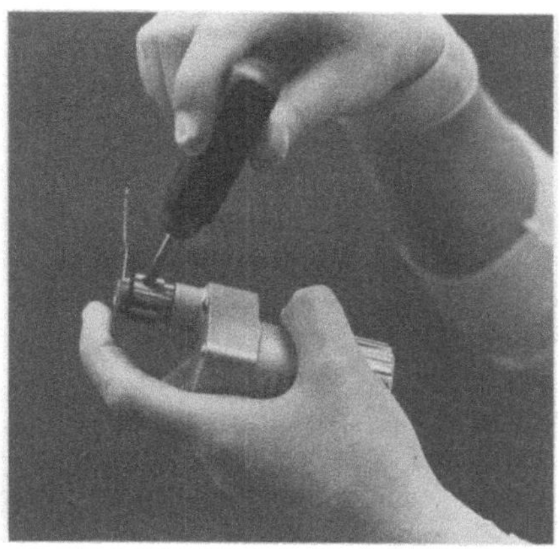

2. Tighten blade securely with the hex-wrench.

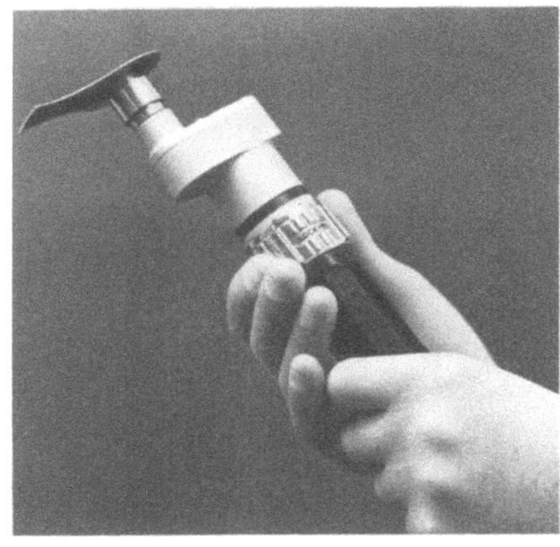

ATTACHMENT ASSEMBLY:
1. Seat attachment over air driver, engage hex drive-shaft. Turn lock-ring to secure.

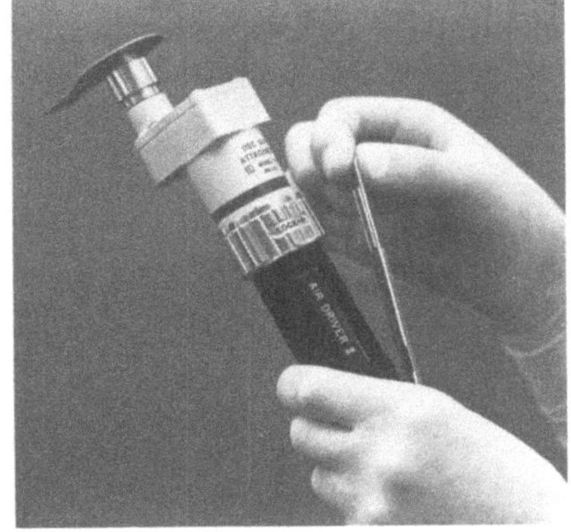

2. Use the extension lever if necessary. Run at full speed for maximum cutting efficiency.

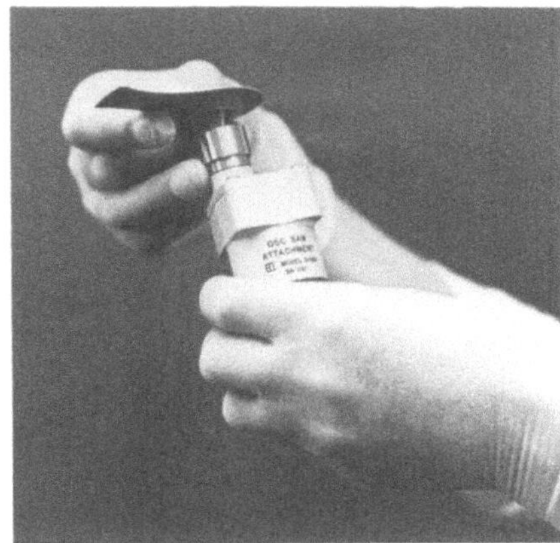

MAINTENANCE:
1. Disassemble blades prior to cleaning.

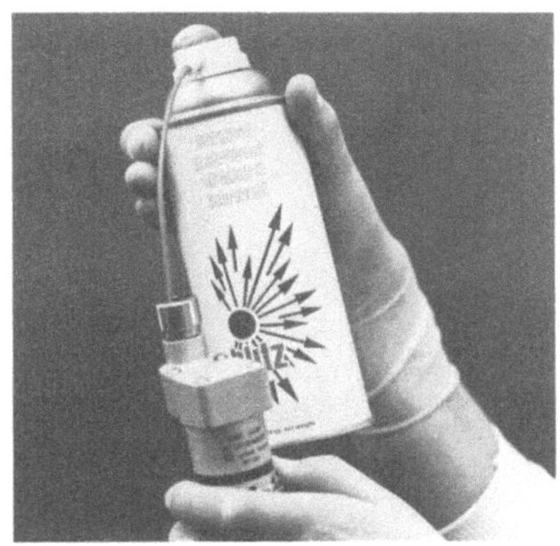

2. Clean attachment end thoroughly. This attachment requires no lubrication.

WIRE AND PIN DRIVER
shown actual size

The wire and pin driver has a full 5/32″ cannulation. The gear reduction in this unit reduces the speed from 20,000 rpm to 10,000 rpm. At .5 on the speed selector ring the instrument can be reduced to a variable of 0–5,000 rpm. The unit is completely sealed and requires no lubrication.

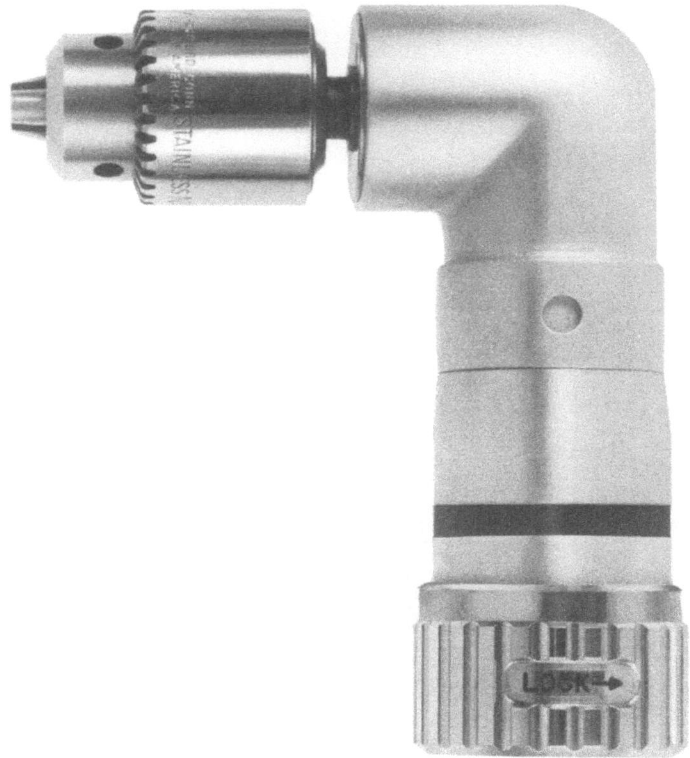

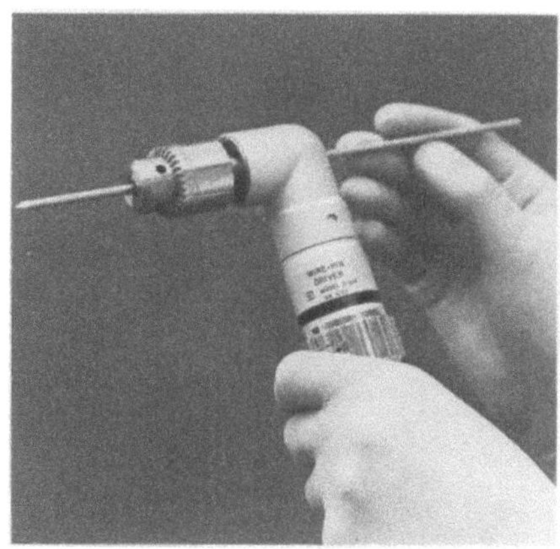

PIN ASSEMBLY:
1. Open Jacobs chuck to receive pin or wire.

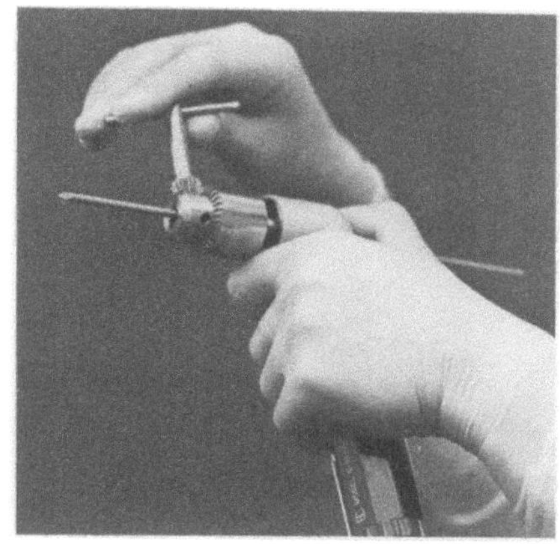

2. Place pin through cannulated angle. Tighten chuck and pin with key.

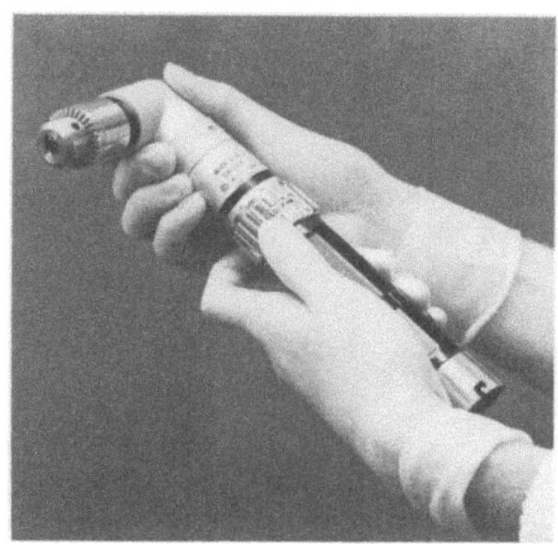

ATTACHMENT ASSEMBLY:
1. Seat attachment firmly over air driver shoulder. Turn ring to lock.

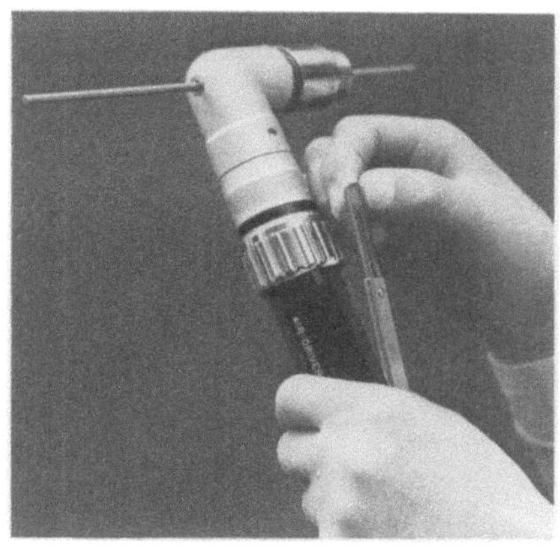

2. Use extension handle for additional throttle control.

MAINTENANCE:
1. Keep chuck clean and lubricate.

2. Clean attachment end thoroughly. This attachment requires no lubrication.

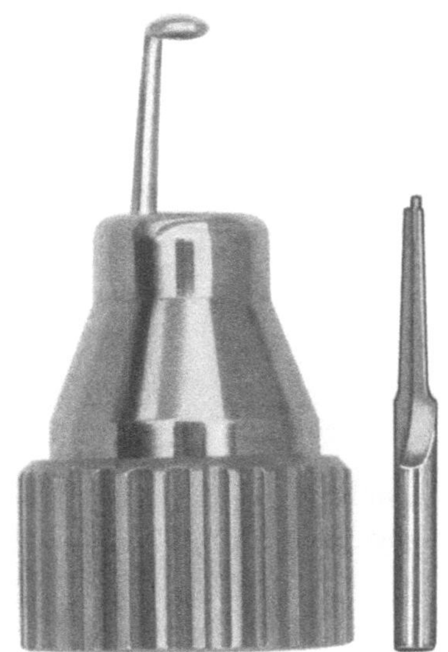

STERNUM GUARD AND BLADE
shown actual size

The sternum guard has a long reinforced stem designed to accommodate the heavier bone of the sternum. The tip of the bur is accurately aligned into the foot of the guard to protect the pleura from the fast-rotating blade.

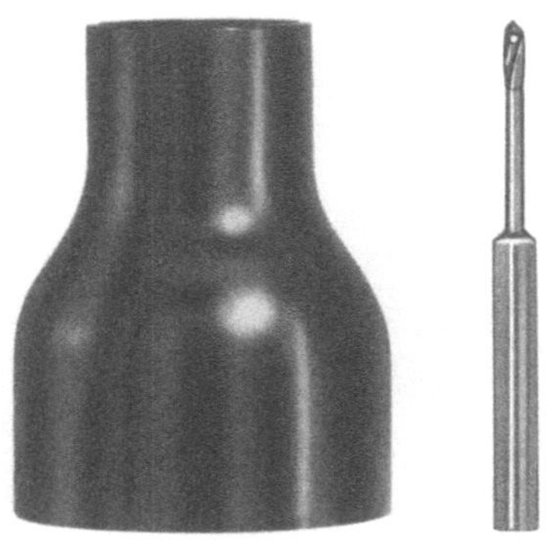

WIRE-PASS GUARD AND WIRE-PASS BUR
shown actual size

For closure of the sternum, pass the wires through the hole in the tip of the wire-pass bur. The guard protects the operator from the rotating hex-nut.

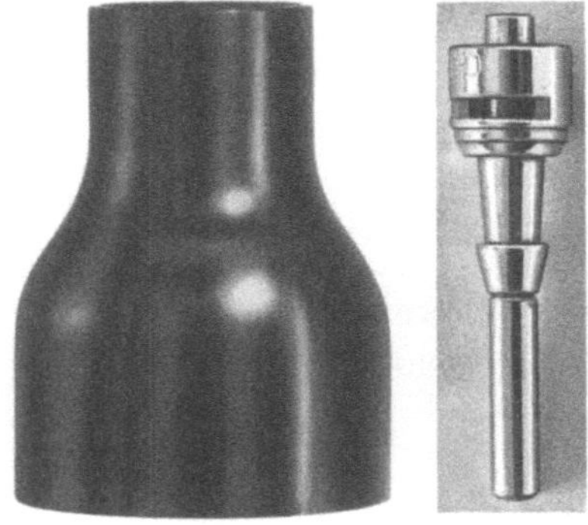

WIRE-PASS GUARD AND BIOPSY-NEEDLE ADAPTER shown actual size

The attachment is designed for the assembly of a liver or lung biopsy needle for removal of a biopsy specimen.

NOTE: These attachments can only be used on the Air Driver II and neurosurgical handpieces.

Biopsy-Needle Adapter and Biopsy-Needle Assembly:

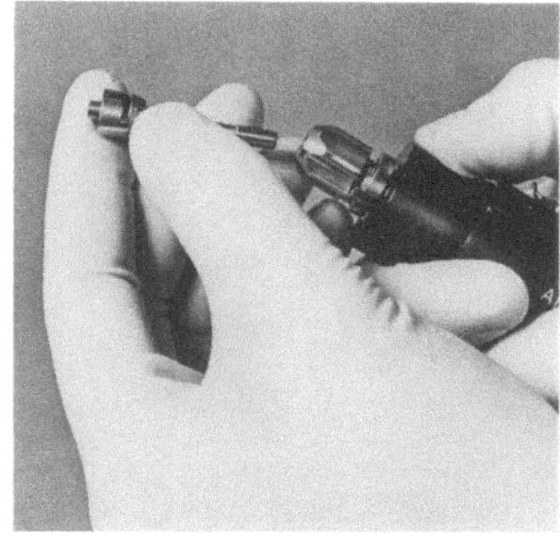

1. Hold thumb over collet release button and insert needle biopsy adapter.

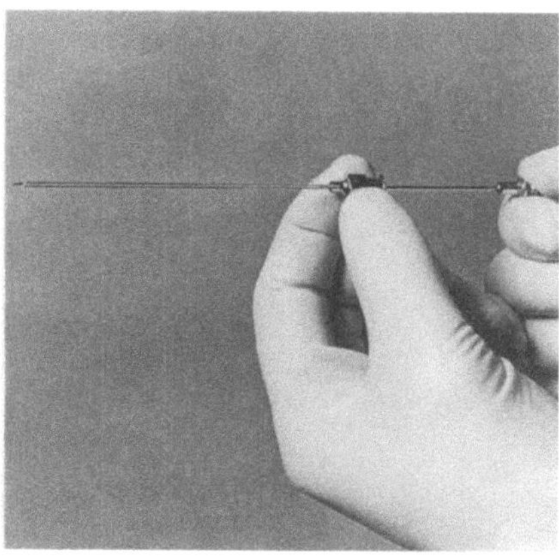

4. Remove trocar point from cannulated biopsy needle.

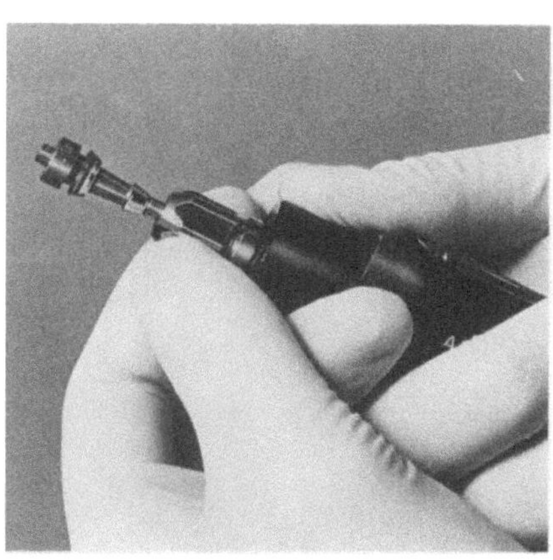

2. Maintain hold on button and turn collet to secure adapter.

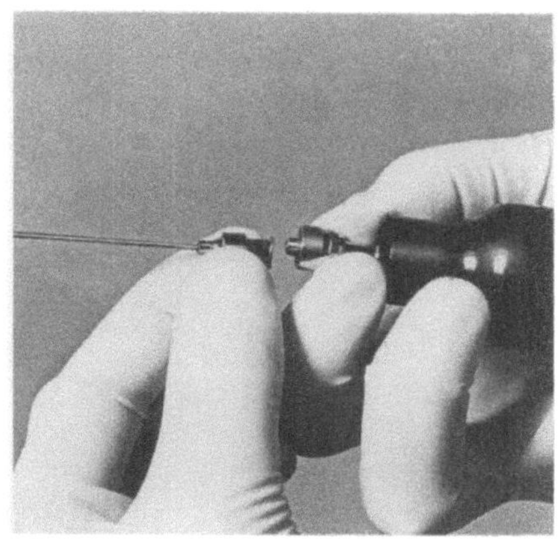

5. Place the needle into the biopsy-needle adapter.

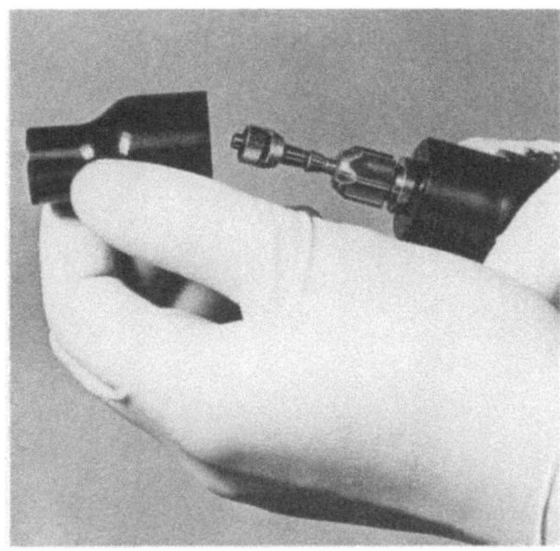

3. Place wire-pass guard over adapter and air-driver shoulder. Seat firmly.

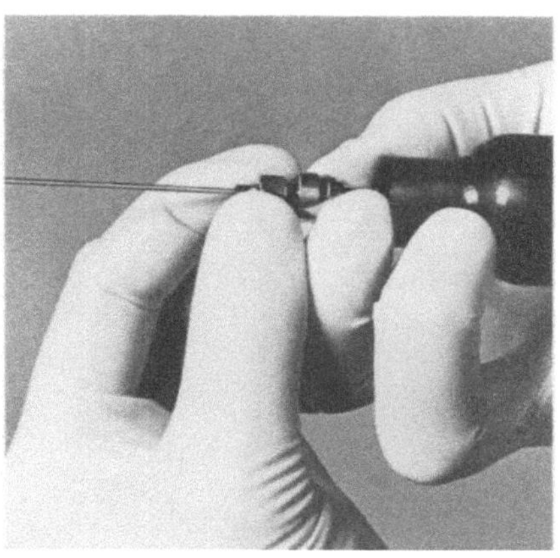

6. Turn the needle within the biopsy-needle adapter to secure needle.

Assembly of Air Driver II

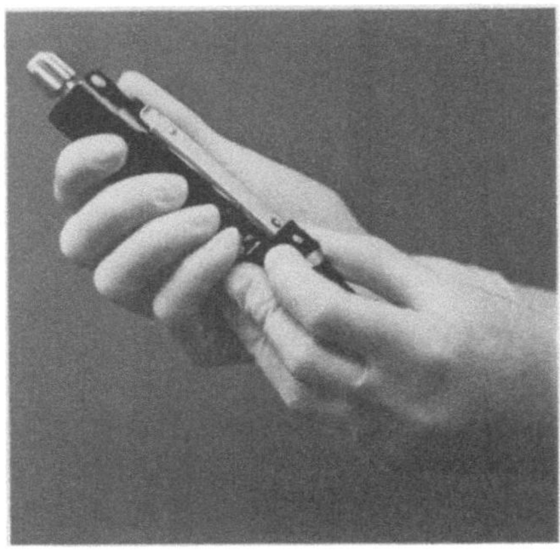

INSTRUMENT SAFETY:
1. Pull safety lock back to release throttle; motor will not run.

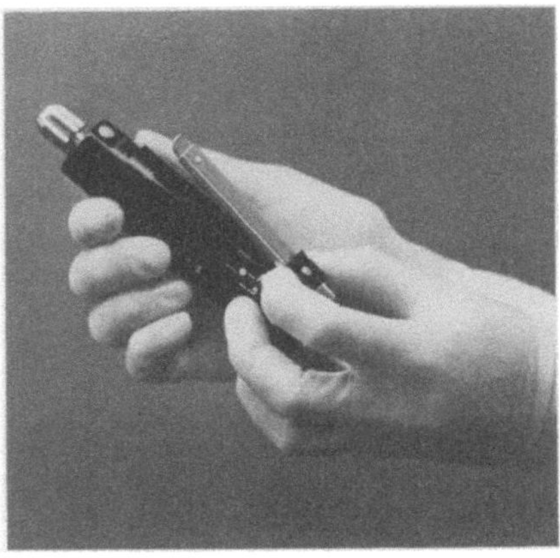

2. Lift throttle and push safety lock up. Press throttle; motor will run.

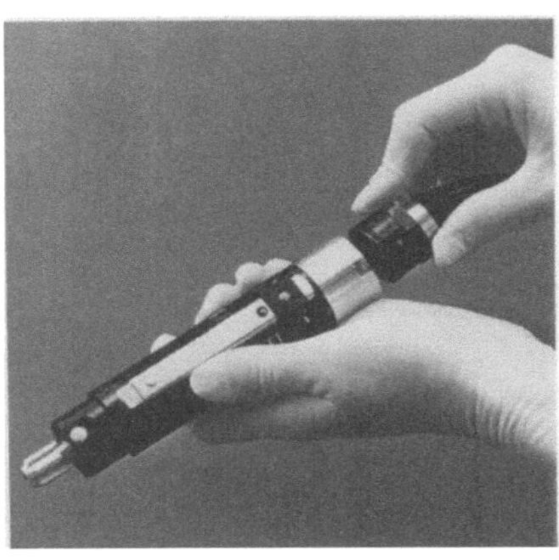

INSTRUMENT-HOSE DISCONNECT:
1. Pull safety lock back to release throttle. Align pin and hole.

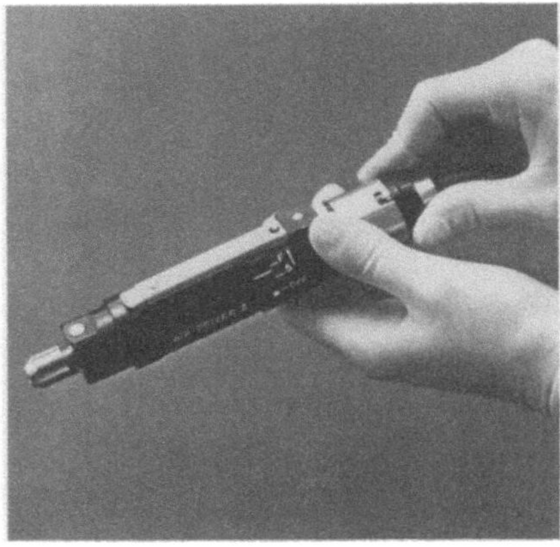

2. Press together. Grasp the end of the instrument to steady the swivel. Twist clockwise to lock.

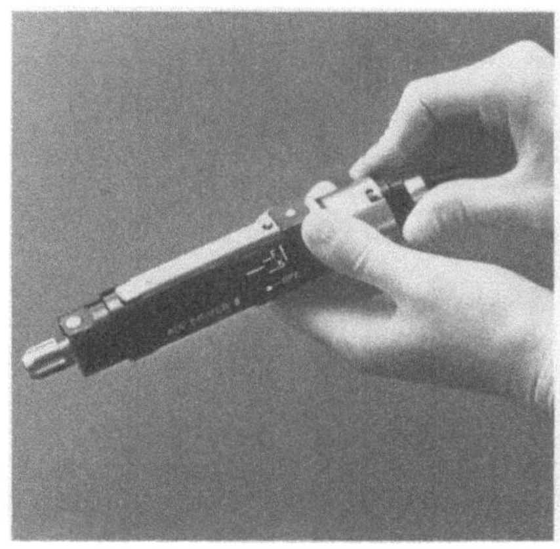 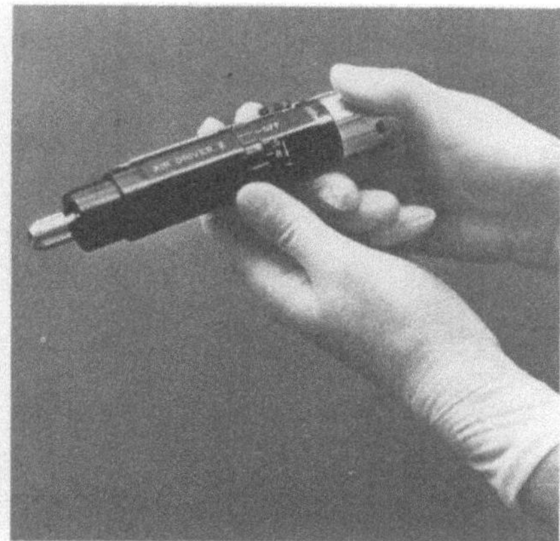

SPEED-SELECTOR RING:

1. The off position of the selector ring (the dot aligned with OFF) deactivates the air driver and can be used as an additional safety device.

3. Turn the ring to half speed (.5) for speed reduction in both forward and reverse. Move the ring until a detent is felt at the (.5) position.

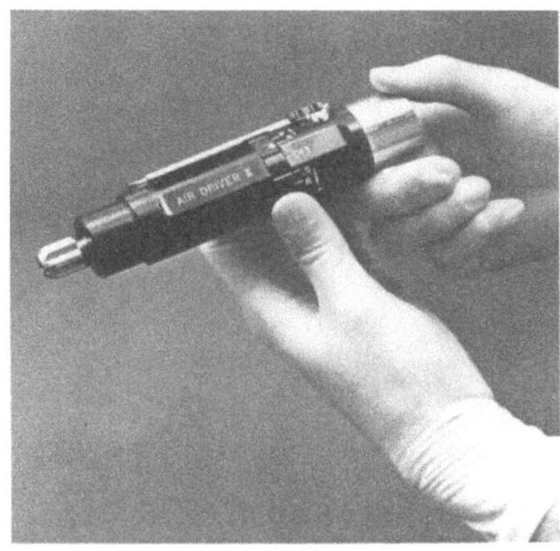 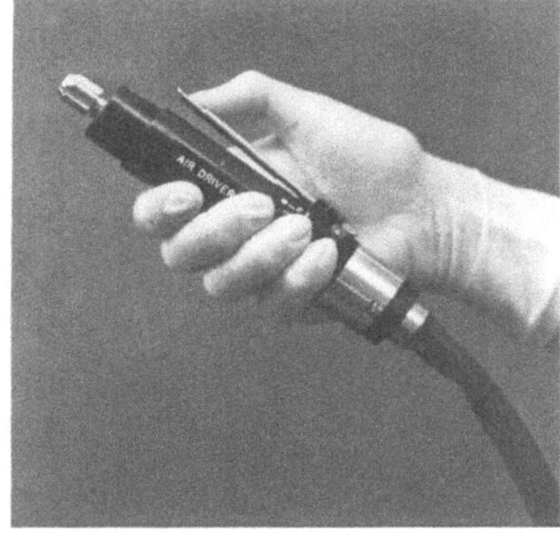

2. Turn the ring fully to forward (F) or reverse (R) for full speed.

4. For additional speed control use the throttle.

Repair and Maintenance Guide

Instrument	Symptoms	Probable cause	Cure
Air Drill 100	Air leaks from hose; loss of power and torque.	Worn or damaged hose.	Do not kink hose when storing or sterilizing instrument. Remove hose from instrument. Return for repair.
	Collet will not hold burs.	Sterilized with burs in place. Hall International burs are not being used.	Use Hall International burs. If malfunction persists return for repair.
	Burs locked in collet.	Other manufacturer's burs used.	Use only Hall International burs. Return for service.
	Excessive heat and noise. Do not use. *Bearing will disintegrate and cause serious damage.*	Worn bearings.	Return for repair immediately.
	Loss of speed and torque.	Accumulation of debris and oil at the front nose bearing.	Flush the front nose bearing with blitz spray.
Attachments			
Bur Guards Long Medium Extra Long	Burs whipping.	Burs are bent, incorrect guard is being used with bur. Bur is not fully seated.	Replace burs. Always use guard with companion bur. Always insert until fully seated into collet.
	Bur does not attain high speed.	Worn bearing at tip of guard.	Lubricate with one drop of oil at narrow end of guard. If malfunction persists, return for repair.
Laminectomy Guard and Bur	Bur does not cut.	Wrong bur is used. Bur is very dull.	Use only 03 long bur. Always use new bur.
	Bur does not rotate.	Worn bearing in tip of guard.	Lube at narrow end with one drop of oil. Return for service.
	Bur is not seated into foot of guard.	Foot of guard is full of bone dust. Guard is bent.	Clean with H. I. cleaner. Return for service.
Tissue Protector Guard and Bur	Bur does not cut.	Wrong bur is used. Bur is dull.	Use only 19 long bur. Always use a new bur.
	Bur does not rotate.	Wrong bur is used. Worn bearing in tip of guard.	Lubricate at narrow end with one drop of oil. Return for service.

Instrument	Symptoms	Probable cause	Cure
Rhinoplasty Guard and Bur	Bur does not fit.	Wrong bur is used.	Use only 40 long diamond bur.
	Bur does not rotate.	Worn bearing at tip of guard.	Lubricate bearing with one drop of oil. Return for service.
Rand 20° Attachment 20° Attachment 90° Attachment 70° Attachment	Difficulty in inserting burs.	Dry blood may accumulate at head of 90° or 70° attachment.	Clean with Hall International blitz spray cleaner. Flush thoroughly through bur hole with water or blood solvent before lubrication.
	Bur does not rotate.	Lack of lubrication. Worn bearing in guard tip.	Clean properly and lubricate tip.
Steel, Carbide-Tip and Diamond Burs	Bur whipping.	Bur may be bent. Guards are not being used.	Use new burs. Seat all burs.
	Dull burs.	Bur re-used.	Use new burs.
	Worn exhaust hose.	Kinking of hose in storage or autoclaving.	Store with hose disconnected.
		Locking attachments with handpiece connected.	Assemble attachments with hose disconnected.

All burs should be removed from attachments and cleaned with the autoclavable bur brush before sterilization.

Air Driver II	Motor loses speed.	Lack of proper lubrication.	Lubricate after use with 3-5 drops of H. I. lubricant in the stand pipe at the disconnect end of drill. Run motor.
	Excessive noise and heat.	Worn bearings.	Return for service.
Attachments			
Sternum Guard	Guard is bent.	Rough handling.	Keep guard protector over guard when not in use. Return bent guard for repair.
	Blade does not seat correctly into foot of guard.	Poorly cleaned. Guard tip is packed with bone dust.	Clean tip of guard with H. I. spray cleaner.
Sternum Blade	Blade cuts slowly.	Blades are dull.	Replace blades after one use.
	Blades break.	Poor technique.	Check blade alignment in tip of guard.

Instrument	Symptoms	Probable cause	Cure
	Excessive heat at guard tip.	Bent guard, lack of irrigating fluid, or guard foot clogged with bone dust.	Clean foot with H. I. spray cleaner. Return guard for inspection.
Oscillating Saw	Attachment does not run.	Dirty.	Clean thoroughly. Return for repair.
Reciprocating Saw	Loss of set-screw.		Replace at factory.
Wire and Pin Driver 10,000 rpm	Jacobs chuck is stiff.	Lack of lubrication and cleaning.	Clean with H. I. cleaner.

Power Systems for Air-Driven Surgical Instruments*

Many new hospitals and those undergoing remodeling are attempting to provide the necessary high-pressure gas service required to drive the air-driven surgical instruments. The purpose of this chapter is to assist the hospital in making decisions as to the type of power source to be used, and how to provide that service to the surgical area.

Pressurized Gas Power Sources

The increasing acceptance of using air-driven surgical instruments in the operating room has generated its own unusual set of problems. The greatest single obstacle to their implementation as an "everyday" surgical tool has been the slow evolution of a completely satisfactory pressure system for powering the turbine handpiece. Generally speaking, three types of compressed gas systems have been considered: air; carbon dioxide (CO_2); and nitrogen (N_2). All of these are capable of being supplied from cylinders, through a regulator and supply hose to the instrument. These three gases can also be manifolded** from cylinders onto a pipeline system, and piped to the required area of the hospital (compressed air would most likely be supplied from a motor-driven compressor, rather than from cylinders).

Selecting a Compressed Gas Power Source

1. Compressed Air

Based on cost alone, the cheapest and most abundant power source is air. The raw material is free for the taking, and is in the gaseous state over a wide range of temperatures and pressures. However, the application of compressed air to the task of driving the surgical air-instrument demands that certain exacting prerequisites be met: air must be compressed under precisely controlled conditions, which include producing "oil free" compressed air, with provision for proper drying and filtering. The tiny turbine motors, some of which operate at 100,000 rpm, are precision instruments and will not tolerate impurities in the pressurized gas source. Regardless of the brand of air instrument employed, impurities such as dirt, oil and moisture must be eliminated from the pressurized gas source prior to delivery to the handpiece. Purchasing, installing and maintaining an air compressor system of sufficient quality and capacity for this specific application, is usually a rather costly undertaking.

Assuming that an air compressor system of sufficient quality was to be utilized, it is then necessary to examine the pressure and flow requirements of that system. It is not inconceivable that in a large hospital, three "light" drills and three "heavy" drills might be in service simultaneously. With the "light" drills requiring up to 6 cubic feet per minute (cfm) each, and the "heavy" drills up to 15 cfm each, peak flow requirements would total 63 cfm. While this potential maximum demand would seldom occur, the compressed air system would have to be capable of delivering this flow, while maintaining a line pressure of 200 pounds per square inch (psi).

---

* For additional information on "Pressurized Gas Powered Systems for Turbine-Driven Surgical Tools" request Form No. 2549, Ohio Medical Products, Madison, Wisconsin.

** Jackson, F. E.: Shipboard Installation of High Pressure Air System for Actuation of Turbine Craniotomes. **Military Med.** Vol. 133, No. 2, Feb. 1968.

These characteristics necessitate a two-stage compressor system, which should be of the duplex type, providing for occasional shutdown of one unit for maintenance and repair. Either unit of the duplex compressor system should be capable of supplying 75% of the peak flow and pressure requirements. The system must also be equipped with electrical controls that will automatically allow both compressors to operate simultaneously during peak flow and pressure demands. As previously stated, these compressors must be of the "oil free" type, with provision for cooling, drying and filtering the air before delivery to the pipeline system.

In summary, the primary objections to compressed air as a source of power are the very high initial cost of purchasing the system, coupled with the above average routine maintenance required to assure a constant supply of clean, dry air at the proper flow and pressure.

2. Carbon Dioxide (CO_2)

Carbon dioxide is also readily available, but at a cost that is approximately 25% greater per hundred cubic feet than nitrogen. This gas is easily obtained in a purified form which exceeds U.S.P.* requirements. On the surface, at least, it appears that CO_2 should be considered as a source of power for turbine-driven surgical tools.

The greatest obstacle to utilizing CO_2 in this manner is that it is a liquid when stored in a cylinder at 70° F (839 psi cylinder pressure). In order to vaporize a sufficient amount of the liquid CO_2 to meet high flow requirements, special equipment must be employed to add heat to the gas, which will increase normal vaporization rates. Since vaporization of a liquified gas is a cooling process, and the fact that manifolds are frequently placed outdoors in geographic areas subject to extremely cold temperatures, additional problems of reduced vaporization seriously compound an already difficult situation. It is generally uneconomical and unsound, practically speaking, to attempt to maintain a satisfactory power source in this manner.

3. Nitrogen (N_2)

Research and experience have shown that "dry, water-pumped" N_2 is the ideal power source for air-driven instruments. It possesses the necessary favorable characteristics to provide a source of power that is satisfactory in every respect. The gas is 99.995% pure, dry and relatively inert (will not support combustion or corrosion). Nitrogen, throughout the normal range of temperatures and pressures, is in the gaseous state and instantly available at the desired pressure. Flow rates are limited only by the type of regulating device utilized. Unlike an air compressor, the capacity of a nitrogen supply system can easily and inexpensively be enlarged to meet increasing demands, simply by adding additional cylinders.

---

* United States Pharmacopeia.

Advantages of Nitrogen as a power source are:

1. Nitrogen is non-inflammable and self-cooling, The elimination of an ignition source for flammable anaesthetics reduces the danger of fire or explosion.

2. Because nitrogen is the sole source of power, the instruments do not require sizable motors or additional attachments, and consequently, can be made small, light weight and self-contained. This also eliminates the number of cords, motors, stands, flexible cables and "foot pedals" from the floor.

3. Nitrogen is independent of any other power source, therefore, maximum output is sustained throughout surgery.

4. The power source is portable and can be carried into military situations.

Types of water-pumped dry nitrogen grades recommended are:

1. Dry High Purity Nitrogen – 99.995 % vapor free
      – 73° F dewpoint at maximum moisture content
2. Ultra Dry High Purity   – 99.998 % vapor free
      – 84° F dewpoint at maximum moisture content

CAUTION: Neither oil-pumped nor commercial grades of nitrogen should be used because of the high-moisture content.

Delivery Systems

The preceding discussion is based on the assumption that one of these pressurized gases would be delivered to the operating room through a pipeline system, from either a compressor or a cylinder manifold.

Advantages of a piped system are:

1. The nitrogen pipeline system eliminates the necessity of introducing a nonsterile cylinder into the operating room environment.

2. It eliminates unnecessary and potentially hazardous traffic in the hospital's halls and elevators, resulting in damaged walls, doorways and elevator interiors.

3. Valuable labor is saved as hauling cylinders and making repairs is eliminated.

4. A piped nitrogen system completely solves another problem associated with the use of cylinders; that is, the single surgical procedure utilizing a turbine-driven tool which frequently consumes more than one-half the contents of an "H" cylinder of nitrogen. Should a second procedure be initiated using the remaining contents of the cylinder, a mid-procedure cylinder exchange might well be required. This is undesirable for a number of reasons, not the least of which is patient safety. If a full cylinder is utilized for each procedure, the remaining contents of each partially exhausted cylinder will probably be wasted.

5. A piped nitrogen system supplies an uninterrupted flow of gas at optimum pressure. Manifolded cylinders are economically scavenged to the minimum residual level (approximately 250 psi).

Alternative to a piped-in system:

A common method of furnishing the power source in the operating room is with the H, K or T cylinder supported by a cylinder carrier.

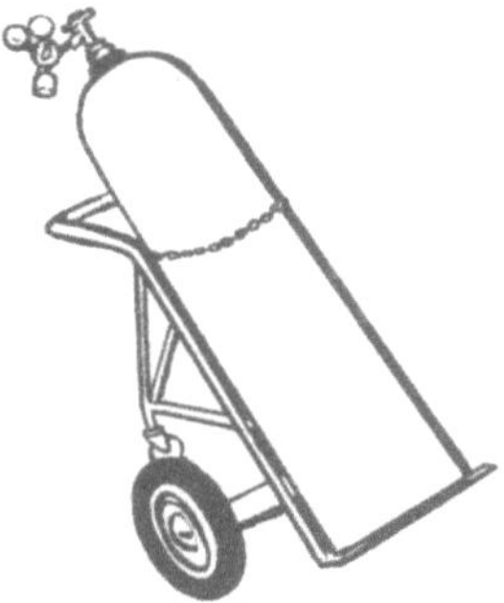

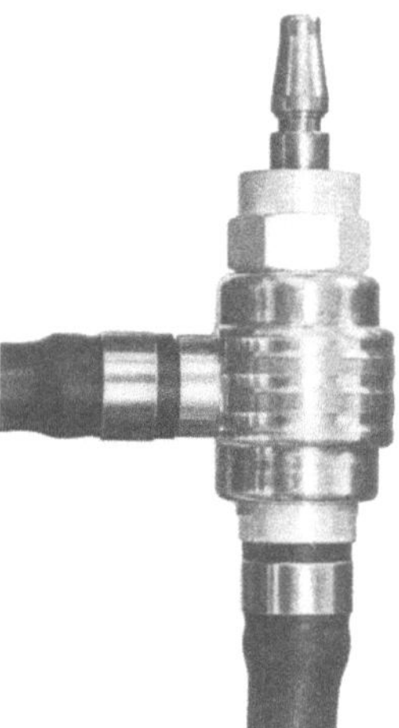

Exhaust hose extender

A piped-in system may require additional hose length to reach the operating table. An exhaust hose extender (above) enables additional lengths of hose to be run from the cylinder to outside the operating room. Any instrument can be made with extra hose length when desired.

Codes and Regulations

There are presently no nationally recognized codes or recommendations specifically covering the piping of nitrogen, as now exists for oxygen and nitrous oxide (NFPA* Pamphlet # 565). Until such codes are established, it is recommended that NFPA Pamphlet # 565 be followed in the design and installation of piped nitrogen systems, except for obvious deviations which must be applied. These deviations would occur primarily in the sections dealing with line pressure levels and types of outlet connections. A safe, functional system can thereby be assured.

---

* National Fire Protective Association.

Components of a Nitrogen Pipeline System

The following nitrogen pipeline system equipment components are consistent with the intent of the recommendations set forth in the NFPA Pamphlet # 565.

Supply System

A duplex manifold (two banks of cylinders) is considered to be the best means by which cylinders may be utilized to provide nitrogen to the pipeline. When the "in use" cylinder bank is depleted from a full 2,200 psi to approximately 250 psi, the manifold controls automatically begin supplying the pipeline from the "reserve" bank of cylinders. Manifolds are customarily located in an area convenient to the hospital's loading dock, to facilitate cylinder exchange. Both the unimatic and economy models are available in a range of capacities which will handle the requirements of any nitrogen pipeline system.

Manifolds

Air-powered surgical instruments are basically of two general types: the "light" turbine drills, which require maximum flows of 6 cfm and a supply pressure variable up to 110 psi; and the "heavy" orthopedic and neurosurgical air motors, requiring an adjustable supply pressure up to 160 psi, and maximum flow rate of 15 cfm. Assuming we are dealing with a typical situation anticipating average use of the air-driven surgical instruments, the following chart can be used to select a suitable nitrogen manifold to handle various size installations.

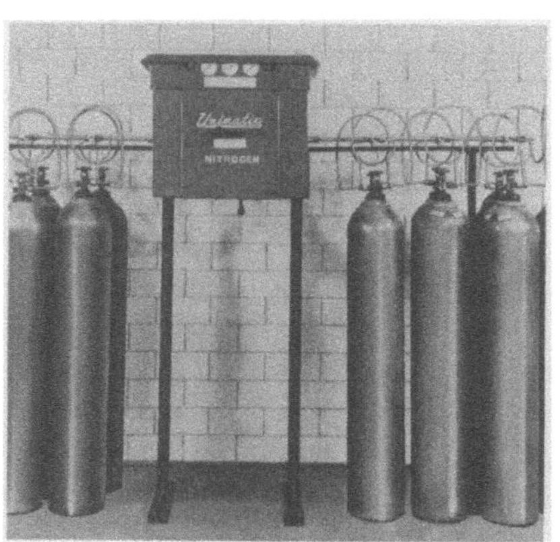

A stand-mounted nitrogen manifold with "in use" and reserve cylinder banks.

Number of Operating Rooms Piped with Nitrogen	Recommended Sizes of Cylinder Manifold
1	2 cylinders (1 each side)
2 to 4	4 cylinders (2 each side)
5 to 8	6 cylinders (3 each side)
9 to 12	8 cylinders (4 each side)
13 to 16	10 cylinders (5 each side)
17 to 20	12 cylinders (6 each side)
21 to 24	14 cylinders (7 each side)
25 to 28	16 cylinders (8 each side)

Valves

One of the most important aspects of any piping system is the valving which is employed. Valves must be properly sized so that flow is not restricted. They must be positioned in the line so that either partial or total shut-off of the system may easily be accomplished, should maintenance or an emergency so require. The typical pipeline system will employ valves in a number of places, which include: main line shut-off; a shut-off at each riser base; and a shut-off valve for each operating room. Valves accessible to other than authorized hospital personnel must be installed in properly labeled valve boxes with frangible windows.

The ball-type main line shut-off valve is located near the nitrogen manifold. A quarter turn of this valve will completely shut off the flow of nitrogen to the entire pipeline system.

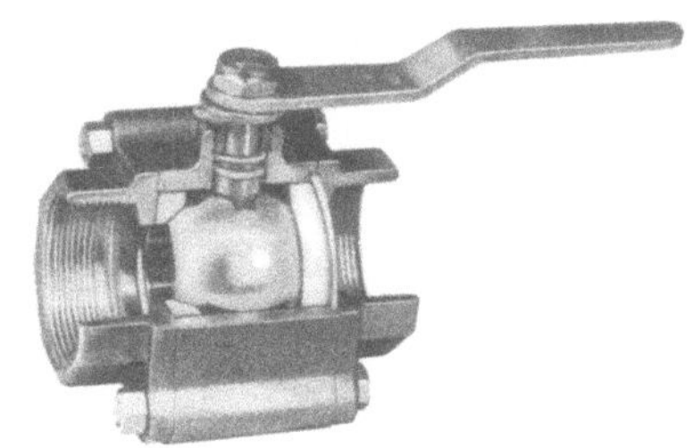

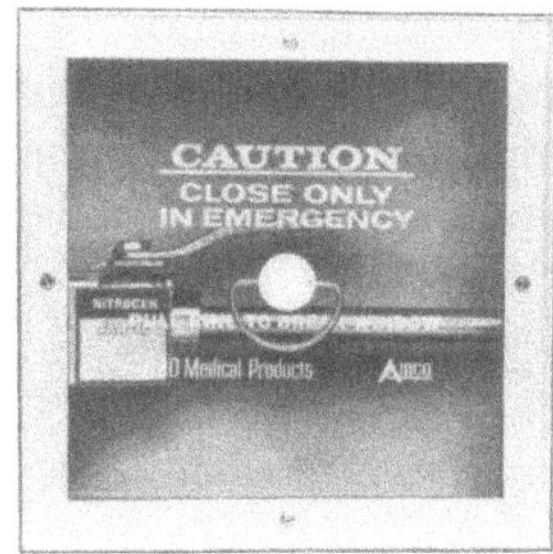

Recessed valve box with single nitrogen valve.

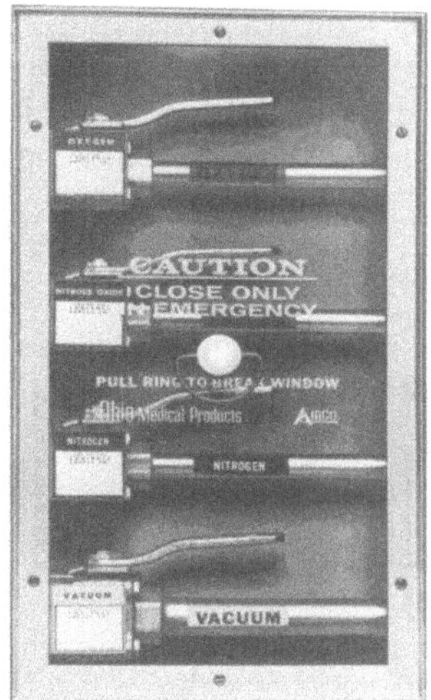

Recessed valve box with four valves.

Pressure Control Cabinet

The operational characteristics of available air instruments are such that it is necessary to have a means of adjusting line pressure in the operating room, to match the various air-instrument pressure requirements. The required pressure adjustments range up to 160 psi at full rated turbine flow. Pressure regulation is accomplished by means of an adjustable regulator, located either up or downstream of the nitrogen service outlet, to which the turbine supply hose is connected.

While the use of a downstream pressure-reducing regulator is slightly less costly, it is the least desirable method of pressure regulation from the standpoint of convenience, utility and appearance. This is particularly true in the typical situation where two or more nitrogen service outlets are installed in an operating room. This situation requires either a separate regulator for each outlet or removal and re-attachment of a single regulator each time a different outlet is selected for use. The external downstream regulator is generally bulky, subject to physical damage, and is a potential hazard to operating room personnel who may bumb into it, particularly when it is connected to various types of ceiling-mounted service outlets.

It is recommended by Ohio Medical Products that an upstream pressure regulator be used, and they have available a nitrogen pressure control cabinet for this purpose. This control cabinet, in addition to the upstream regulator, contains the room shut-off valve, line and wall outlets, pressure gauges, and a D.I.S.S.* service outlet

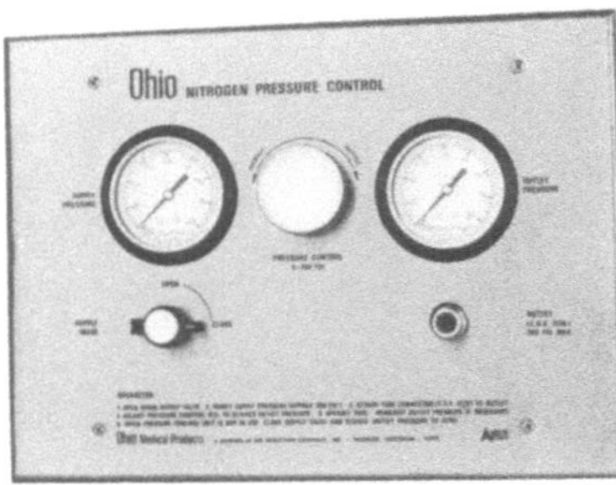

Nitrogen pressure control cabinet.

All of these components are housed in a single box, designed for recessed mounting in the wall of the operating room. An important feature of the nitrogen pressure control cabinet is the incorporation of a connection for piping regulated, pressurized gas to remote nitrogen service outlets. Operating room personnel are then able to regulate pressure at all nitrogen outlets in the surgery, from a single point.

Alarm Systems

A properly designed nitrogen pipeline system should include the following audio-visual alarm signals:

1. Switch-over warning signal

Indicates that the "in use" bank of cylinders on the manifold has been depleted and the pipeline is being supplied from the "reserve" bank: This operating signal allows adequate time to replenish the empty bank with full cylinders insuring that the supply of nitrogen gas will never be completely exhausted.

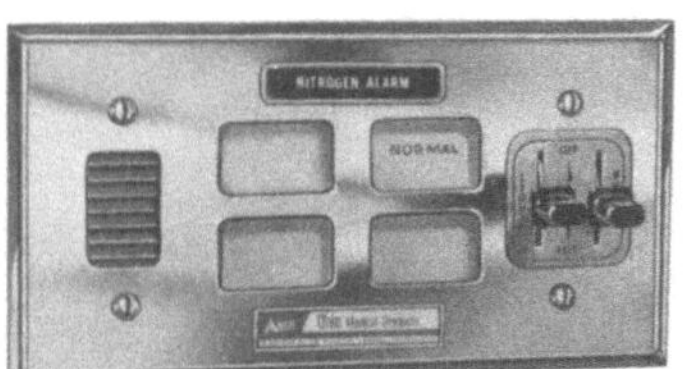

Four-light audio-visual alarm panel combines switch-over Warning Signal (1) and High and Low Main Line Pressure Warning Signals (2a) into a single unit.

2. High and low main line pressure warning signals

   a. Since the system is designed to operate at a constant 200 psi, it is important to have an audio-visual warning of any significant fluctuation in main nitrogen supply line pressure. Pressure switches, connected to the main near the mani-

---

* Diameter Index Safety System.

fold, together with a relay control box, are employed to activate high and low line pressure warning signals. These are commonly adjusted to energize the alarm systems should line pressure drop to 175 psi or increase to 225 psi.

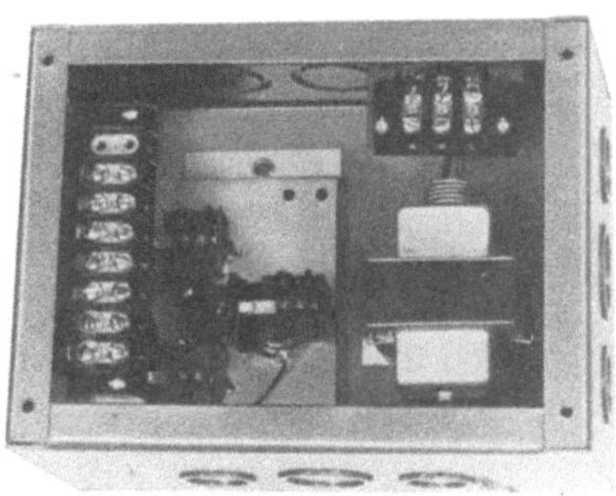

Relay control box which connects high and low main line pressure switches to audio-visual alarm panel.

b. The nitrogen manifold and the surgical suite are generally located on different floors of the hospital, separated by a considerable distance. There are one or more valves in the pipeline interspaced between the two areas. These valves could inadvertently be closed. It is strongly recommended that separate audio-visual warning signals monitoring high and low line pressure be installed in the surgical suite.

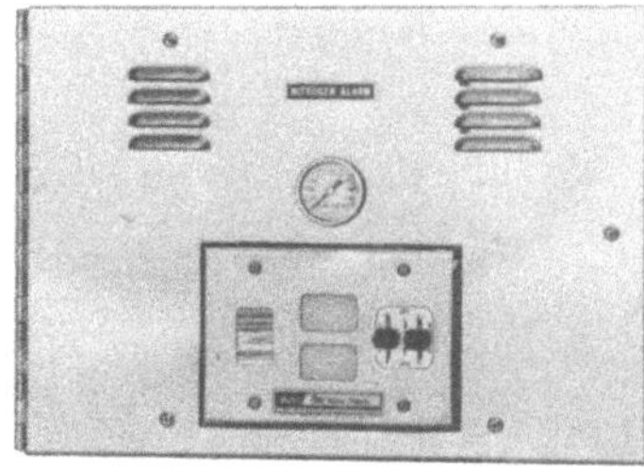

This is a completely self-contained alarm panel monitoring the nitrogen system in the surgical suite for abnormal line pressures.

To assure optimal utilization of the nitrogen pipeline system, experience has shown that a few basic rules regarding alarm system design and location should be observed. First, the switch-over alarm warning signal and the high-low main line pressure warning signals should be combined into a single multi-signal alarm panel, and be located within the hospital so as to assure 24-hour surveillance. To accomplish this objective, one set of signals is usually installed at the telephone switchboard. A duplicate set is usually installed in the engineer's office, or master control station. Second, normal/abnormal main line pressure warning signals, for location in the surgical suite, should be incorporated into a complete self-contained line pressure alarm panel, with a pressure gauge, to facilitate installation in the corridor wall approximately five feet above floor level, for easy observation and accessibility. Third, all alarm panels, in addition to having a horn or buzzer and signal lights, should include a buzzer-silencing switch and a means of quickly testing all lights and audible alarms for functional integrity.

Piping

The piping of nitrogen, like all medical gases, is accomplished through the use of pre-cleaned Type "K" seamless copper tubing. All joints are silverbrazed, while threaded connections utilize a suitable sealing compound. Prior to being placed in service, the pipeline system should be blown clean of moisture and foreign matter, through the use of "oil free" compressed air or "dry, water-pumped" cylinder nitrogen. This procedure is recommended even though the tubing is delivered pre-cleaned and capped by the manufacturer. Suitable testing procedures should be performed, including a 24-hour standing pressure test, to determine if leaks are present in the system.

NOTE: If this method is used, a Regulator is not required. To connect Hall instruments to the wall, a D.I.S.S. Nitrogen Adapter is necessary.

CAUTION: Do not connect the D.I.S.S. Nitrogen Adapter to a wall or ceiling outlet without verifying correct Hall operating nitrogen pressures.

The use of the upstream pressure control cabinet also includes the important safety feature of allowing equipment connections to be made at zero pressure, rather than at 200 psi. (Without a nitrogen pressure control cabinet, the downstream regulator would require attachment and removal from an outlet at full line pressure).

Service Outlets

Because a nitrogen pipeline system deals with line pressures up to four times greater than those found in medical gas pipeline systems, more attention must be given to the potential safety hazards that may exist, particularly for uninformed and/or untrained personnel. Safety has been a primary consideration in the design of all components for nitrogen pipeline systems, and in the hands of trained personnel, represents a minimal hazard to the user. What hazard does exist is that which is associated with the connection and removal of the turbine supply hose adapter, at elevated pressures.

To provide complete non-interchangeability of gas services and maximum personnel safety, Ohio recommends the exclusive use of the D.I.S.S. threaded connection (Compressed Gas Association = 1120) for all nitrogen service outlets. For 200 psi nitrogen pipeline applications, the D.I.S.S. connections have the desirable feature of providing several threads of engagement between the nut and male thread, before the supply valve opens. The adapter is thereby prevented from blowing off, as is possible with quick-disconnect fittings not properly engaged. Existing surgical instruments equipped with a Schrader compressed air quick-disconnect-type connector can readily be converted to a threaded-type D.I.S.S. nitrogen adapter.

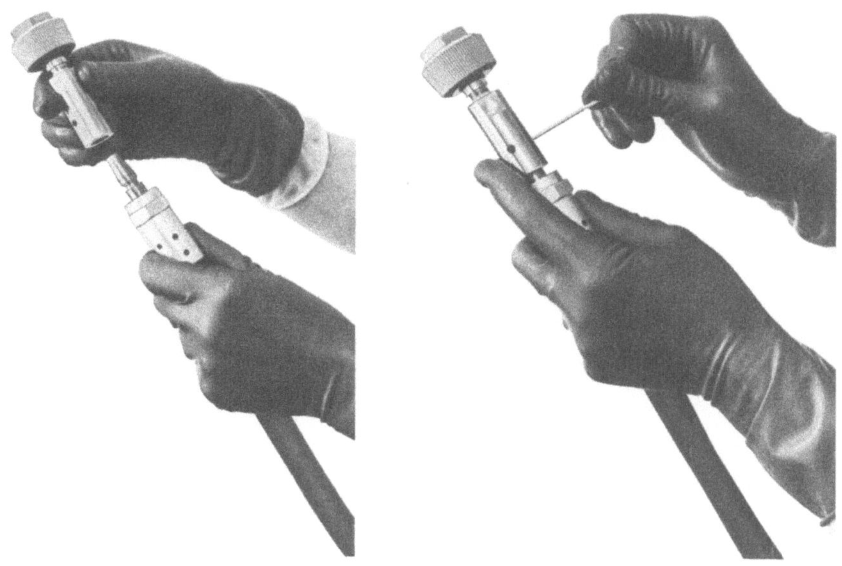

Attach the Schrader fitting to the D.I.S.S. adapter. Secure the adapter with a hex wrench.

The D.I.S.S. nitrogen adapter permits safe, sure connection to the nitrogen pressure supply without altering the Schrader compressed air connector.

Service outlets for nitrogen, in addition to being wall-mounted, can be included in ceiling-mounted equipment, such as ceiling columns and straight gas tracks, together with the medical gas and vacuum outlets.

All of the foregoing information and data has been presented to aid those who are contemplating the use of air-driven instruments for surgery. We believe that this information will provide them with some idea of the problems and considerations to be examined when attempting to utilize these instruments in the hospital. The information is by no means complete; however, it does represent a basic picture of how provision can be made for air-driven surgical instruments, considering th
design and economic aspects of the situation.

Engineering and Air Instrument Glossary

atn: Atmosphere; an European unit measuring the air pressure in storage or when operating the instruments.

Braking Time: Elapsed time (measured in seconds) between release of throttle and end of bur rotation.

Bur Safe Line: A line delineated by H. I. Inc. for every Bur; when Bur is placed in the instrument properly, the Safe Line will not be visible.

Bur Release: The tip of the Bur Release is inserted on the side of the H. I. 20°; this opens the Collet for insertion of Burs.

cfm: Cubic feet per minute.

cfh: Cubic feet per hour.

Carbide-Tip Bur: A Bur with a steel shank and carbide tip; the steel reduces chance of bur breakage; the carbide provides long-lasting sharpness.

Coaxial Hose: A pair of hoses, one running within the other.

Dry Nitrogen (High Purity): 99.995 % pure; 5 grains of water vapor/1000 cubic feet; approximate dewpoint at maximum moisture content: $-73°$ F and $-58°$ C.

Diffuser: A device to disperse a force (such as exhaust nitrogen) nondirectionally.

Exhaust: An arrangement for withdrawing gases (such as nitrogen).

H (or K) Nitrogen Cylinder: Colored black; 244 cubic feet; 2200 psi at 70° F; 9″ outside diameter; 56″ high; 149 pounds (full); 133 pounds (empty); CGA 580 thread. H and K cylinders are being replaced by T cylinders.

Lever Slot: The aperture into which the Bur Changer for the H. I. 20° is placed to release the Collet for inserting or extracting Burs.

Lubricate: To make smooth or slippery with a suitable lubricant.

Nitrogen: A colorless, tasteless, odorless gaseous element that constitutes 78 % of the atmosphere by volume.

Nitrogen Consumption: Amount of nitrogen consumed by an air instrument over a specified period of time.

psi: Pounds per square inch; unit measuring the pressure of air in storage or when operating the instrument.

Pull-Out Force: Amount of force (measured in pounds) required to manually pull a Bur from the Collet.

Quick Connector: A push-lock, ⅛-turn release device to couple H. I. tools to H. I. Regulator.

rpm: Revolutions per minute; unit measuring the speed of the instrument.

Runaway rpm: The natural rpm that a machine will seek at full speed.

Self-Lubrication: Internal lubrication of a unit by the manufacturer. There is no need for any further internal lubrication.

Strength: Quality or state of being strong; capacity for exertion or endurance; power to resist force.

Engineering and Air Instrument Glossary *(continued)*

Swivel: A device joining two parts so that one or both can pivot freely.

T Nitrogen Cylinder: Colored black; 300 cubic feet; 2640 psi at 70° F; 9 1/4 " outside diameter; 60" high; 165 pounds (full); 143 pounds (empty); CGA 580 thread.

Torque: Moment of force; the tendency of the force to rotate the shaft about an axis; commonly expressed in foot-pounds or inch-pounds. Torque is the measure of the capability of an instrument to do work.

Turbine: A rotor (assembly of axial vanes which form peripheral open-ended chambers) which causes a resistance to a directed pneumatic stream and creates a high-speed rotary motion.

Torque-Increasing Device: A patented device designed by H. I. Inc. to automatically increase the torque, or work capability, of the Air Drill 100 as the unit is being used.

Variable Speed: Controlled speed change through a H. I.-patented valve mechanism.

Vane Motor: A pneumatic displacement motor utilizing moveable phenolic strips, or vanes, as chambers. High-pressure nitrogen expands in the chambers, creating rotary movement.

Vulcanized Rubber: Crude or synthetic rubber treated chemically to give it useful properties (as elasticity, strength, and stability).

Index

AIR INSTRUMENT SURGERY

Volume 1*
Cranial Surgery
Intracranial Surgery
Temporal Bone
Surgery
Vertebral Surgery

Compiled and edited by **R. M. Hall**
Over 200 illustrations by T. Bloodhart
291 figures. VIII, 262 pages. 1970
With an Addendum:
Cranio-Spinal Surgery with the Ronjair ®
32 illustrations by T. Bloodhart, 37 pages. 1973
Vol. 1 and Addendum: Cloth DM 108,–; US $40.00

Advances in medical science have resulted in a need
for new types of surgery. Consequently, operative
procedures have increased in number, and the
surgical team has been challenged to maintain a
demanding pace. Fortunately, airpowered instruments
help meet that challenge. Now the surgeon has the
fast, dependable instrumentation he needs for many
procedures he formerly had to perform laboriously
and often with a disturbing lack of confidence in the
only instruments available.
Air instrumentation has been effective in establishing
a sensible relationship among specialists. Former
"boundaries" of operative areas have been expanded
so that now a single type of air instrument can be

readily adapted to serve for many surgical procedures.
The procedures, techniques and statements are not
intended as necessarily applicable in any particular
situation, only as a guide to the understanding
and use of air instruments in surgery.

Volume 2*
Orthopedics

Compiled and edited by **R. M. Hall**
356 illustrations by T. Bloodhart
XIV, 509 pages. 1972
Cloth DM 140,–; US $ 51.80

This volume is the first thorough compilation of
surgical orthopedics with special emphasis on the
application of air-driven surgical instruments. Its
illustrations carefully detail the assembly and
maintenance of the various instruments. Surgical
techniques are depicted and all sections include
important safety and engineering information.
Surgeons already familiar with air instruments will
find this book a useful manual; for those to whom
these instruments are new, it will serve as a valuable
detailed reference source for their use.

* Distribution rights for Japan: Nankodo Co. Ltd.,
Tokyo

Prices are subject to change without notice

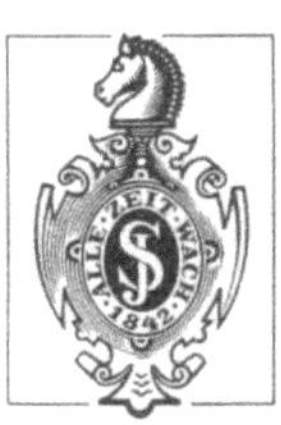

Springer-Verlag
Berlin · Heidelberg · New York

München · London · Paris · Sydney · Tokyo · Wien

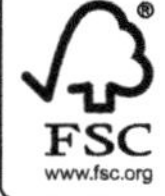